BUDDHIST FASTING PRACTICE

Buddhist Fasting Practice

The Nyungne Method of Thousand-Armed Chenrezig

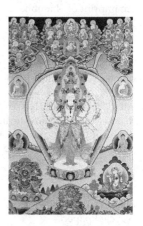

Wangchen Rinpoche

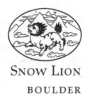

SNOW LION

BOULDER

DEDICATION

May the virtue of writing this book be the cause for all the
enlightened gurus to live long and for the buddhadharma to
flourish, and in particular, may it be the cause for the practicing
tradition of Nyungne to be cherished by all.

Snow Lion
An imprint of Shambhala Publications, Inc.
2129 13th Street
Boulder, Colorado 80302
www.shambhala.com

Printed in the United States of America

Shambhala Publications makes every effort to print on acid-free,
recycled paper.

Snow Lion is distributed worldwide by Penguin Random House,
Inc., and its subsidiaries.

Designed and typeset by Gopa and Ted2, Inc.

Library of Congress Cataloging-in-Publication Data
Wangchen, 1963–
Buddhist fasting practice: the Nyungne method of thousand-armed
Chenrezig / Wangchen Rinpoche.
p. cm.
ISBN 978-1-55939-317-1 (alk. paper)
1. Fasting—Religious aspects—Buddhism. I. Title.
BQ7805.W37 2009
294.3′4447—dc22
2008055819

Contents

SECTION SIX

Prayers

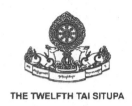

Foreword
The Twelfth Tai Situpa

LORD BUDDHA'S TEACHING manifested as various practices in order to benefit all sentient beings, to liberate them from the suffering of samsara, and to achieve the realization of ultimate Buddhahood. Of these numerous practices, fasting (Nyungne) is among the most important and transformative, as it involves all levels of discipline at once. It includes physical discipline, oral discipline, mental discipline, and the most essential applications of bodhichitta and transformation.

At this time there are many books about Nyungne available in a multitude of languages. This one, written by the Venerable Wangchen Rinpoche, provides a very precise explanation that is simple, clear, and to the point. Those wishing to learn and practice Nyungne will find this book of tremendous benefit.

The material covered stems not only from the Venerable Wangchen Rinpoche's own academic knowledge on this subject but also from his application and practice of this pure lineage throughout the course of his own life. With his genuine dedication to the buddhadharma, Rinpoche has transmitted this practice and acted as a guide to many students practicing Nyungne, helping them build this immeasurably beneficial connection to the Buddha of Compassion (Avalokiteshvara).

I sincerely pray that this book will benefit many individuals and provide them with genuine knowledge and wisdom through the blessing of the Buddha of Compassion.

March 18, 2010

Foreword
H.H. the Dalai Lama

THE FASTING PRACTICE known as Nyungne, which involves eating only one meal on the first day and fasting completely on the second, is often done in conjunction with taking the eight Mahayana precepts. Following the tradition established by the fully ordained nun Bhikshuni Lakshmi, who we Tibetans remember as Gelongma Palmo, people pay special attention to the practice of Avalokiteshvara, the Bodhisattva of Compassion, and recite the six-syllable mantra, Om mani padme hung. This is an excellent practice that, because it is simple to do, anyone can perform, yet at the same time can be a source of great merit and spiritual benefit.

It gives me great pleasure, therefore, to know that in this book Wangchen Rinpoche has given clear and comprehensive instruction on how to undertake the Nyungne practice. Not only that, but by including stories of the great past masters who have undertaken the practice, accounts of the benefits it has brought, as well as auxiliary practices and recitations, he offers a wealth of background information that will serve as a rich source of knowledge and inspiration. Nyungne is an authentic and effective Buddhist practice employing the actions of our body, speech, and mind that has been enthusiastically followed in India, Tibet, and the surrounding regions for many centuries past, and which those who are interested can easily undertake wherever they are today.

With prayers that all who try to put what they read here into practice shall be blessed with success.

December 19, 2007

Introduction

Definition of Nyungne Practice

The fasting practice of Nyungne is a well known, very popular, and profound purification practice that is widely performed in Tibet. One set of Nyungne consists of two days of practice. The first day is the preliminary day, and the second day is the actual fasting day. One takes what is called the Tekchen Sojong vow, the mahayana vow of Restoring and Purifying Ordination, with a total of eight precepts, and on the preliminary day one eats only one meal with drinks for the entire day. The meal is completely and purely vegetarian, which means it is free from any meat substance as well as onions, garlic, eggs, etc. The next day is a complete fast with no meals or drinks, and one must also be silent.

This important and well cherished fasting practice can be done by anyone. The only requirement is that if you are not a Buddhist, you must take the vow of refuge as well as the bodhisattva vow, and you must receive the empowerment for Thousand-Armed Chenrezig. As long as one is willing to receive these teachings, one is welcome to participate in the practice.

Source of the Practice

The source of this practice is a revered historical Buddhist figure known as Gelongma Palmo. She was actually an Afghani princess during a time when Afghanistan was a great Buddhist nation. Padmasambhava, who is considered second only to Lord Buddha, is also known to have come from that area. In Buddhist history books this place is known as Oddiyana, in what is now northwest India. Gelongma Palmo was a very learned, fully ordained Buddhist nun who overcame the dreaded disease of leprosy through her practice of Nyungne by means of a vision of Chenrezig. From her the lineage of this extraordinary Nyungne practice tradition began.

LEVEL OF PRACTICE
(WHERE NYUNGNE BELONGS)

Buddhadharma is generally classified into three vehicles (Skt. *yanas*). The three vehicles are shravakayana (hearers), pratyekabuddhayana (solitary realizers), and mahayana (Great Vehicle.) The path of mahayana is further divided into two paths, sutrayana and tantrayana. In tantrayana there are many levels, but generally we speak of four different tantras: kriya tantra or action tantra; charya tantra or performance tantra; yoga tantra; and anuttara yoga tantra, which is known as the highest yoga tantra. Within all these levels of tantric teachings, the practice of Nyungne belongs to the action and performance classes of tantra, kriya tantra and charya tantra.

Actually there is some debate with regards to the level of practice to which Nyungne belongs. Because Nyungne includes self-visualization, some historic masters consider it to be in the highest yoga tantra tradition practiced as action tantra. But enlightened masters, such as the Eighth Tai Situpa and Jamgon Kongtrul the Great, believe Nyungne is action tantra practiced as performance tantra. The main issue here is that there is no self-deity visualization according to action tantra doctrine, whereas in performance tantra there is. If the Nyungne practice of self-visualization were associated with highest yoga tantra, then strict physical practices would not be important. But in the historical tradition of Nyungne, physical discipline is an essential part of the practice, therefore the understanding and belief that this practice belongs to action and performance tantra makes perfect sense.

Action tantra here means that as practitioners we try to develop insight mainly through physical actions such as fasting, washing ourselves, and many other things that need to be done if the doctrine is to be followed strictly and precisely. Since Tibetan buddhadharma focuses primarily on highest yoga tantra, Tibetans pay less attention to action tantra and therefore some of the details of the physical practices are missing, such as bathing and changing one's clothes every day, etc. I have seen some of these traditional action tantra practices performed by Indians in India, but most Tibetans have no knowledge of them.

General Benefits of the Practice

Those who wish to make their human life meaningful must do one Nyungne practice at the very least. One practice is just two days, but those two days go a long way as far as your unending future is concerned. Because of the enormous benefits of the practice, we organize two Eight Nyungne sessions every year, one in the United States and one in Taiwan. We have been doing this for many years. In addition to this, we also have Nyungne practice one weekend every month. I am very happy that many of my students make every effort to participate in both sets of Nyungne every year, and I'm so glad the number of students who do Nyungne is growing.

A student once expressed a wonderful attitude, which I thought everyone should adopt. Since he was a new student, I asked him what made him come to do Nyungne. He told me that upon hearing about all the beneficial results of practice, he decided to participate in a complete set of Eight Nyungne. He said he realized that sixteen days out of a lifetime was nothing considering the benefits. He correctly recognized the benefits of the practice, and saw that the sacrifice of sixteen days of prayer and fasting was really a minor undertaking. I think that's the kind of attitude everyone should have, and it's an intelligent decision and wise attitude as well.

During practice some people may feel a little bit of hunger and thirst. But a little bit of hunger and thirst is absolutely worth going through when it's for the purpose of truly overcoming one's own future pain and suffering and that of all other sentient beings in the world. Consider how some people are willing to climb mountains and rocks for momentary exhilaration, and others are willing to go through all kinds of pain and suffering just for the purpose of survival. These are just minute and short-lived benefits, but still people are willing to go through such difficulties. My point is that the enormous benefits of the practice absolutely outweigh the hardships that you go through during the practice.

In the *Sutra of Great Liberation*, one of the most profound purification prayers, Lord Buddha mentions that if someone were to recite this sutra, such enormous purification could take place that even if they had the karma to be born in the hell realm, they might only experience a little headache instead. The benefits of Nyungne practice are very much like that, meaning that if you suffer at all, it goes a long way toward your own karmic purification.

One great Nyungne practitioner writing about Nyungne mentions that being able to complete eight sets of Nyungne should bring us more joy and happiness than receiving all the wealth in the entire world. I think he is quite correct, because the benefit of doing Eight Nyungne brings happiness in your future *forever*. As happy as you might be to receive all the wealth in the whole world, it would still be for a short period of time. The benefit of true practice has no limitation.

Generally speaking, every practice has a certain set number of practices that must be completed in order to have genuinely accomplished the practice. With the four foundation practices, for example, one hundred thousand prostrations are performed as well as one hundred thousand repetitions of the other three practices; when you have completed those you can say, "I have *done* the Four Foundations." For our Nyungne practice, to complete eight sets is to really *do* the Nyungne practice. Certain qualifications come with that. For example, if you wanted to lead others in the practice, you would be able to do so.

Following an introduction to Thousand-Armed Chenrezig and a commentary on the benefits of Nyungne practice, topics in Sections One through Three are arranged in the same order as our Nyungne practice text. Section Four includes specific information useful to the Nyungne practitioner, from preparation to samaya commitments. Section Five contains a thorough discussion of vegetarian diet and fasting, the suffering of sentient beings, and questions and answers about Nyungne practice. Section Six contains the complete Nyungne text in Tibetan, phonetic rendering, and English.

Throughout the commentary I often make a point by saying, "It has been said." When I use this phrase, I am indicating that the source is Lord Buddha, from sutras or tantras, or great enlightened masters of the past.

Section One

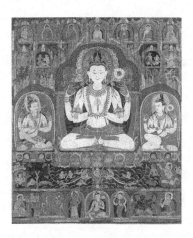

Eleven-Faced, Thousand-Armed Chenrezig 1

CHENREZIG (Tib.) is referred to as Avalokiteshvara in Sanskrit and as Quan Yin in Chinese. This deity is one of the most important deities in the mahayana and vajrayana Buddhist traditions because of what it represents. It is the embodiment of all the buddhas' loving-kindness and compassion combined together. For anyone who wishes to be connected with the enlightened power of love and compassion, it is essential to rely on this supreme manifestation of the buddhas. For those who wish to be on the true enlightened path, pure love and compassion are essential parts of spiritual growth.

There are, in fact, several different manifestations of Chenrezig, including Four-Armed White Chenrezig, Four-Armed Red Chenrezig, Two-Armed White Chenrezig, Two-Armed Red Chenrezig, Standing Chenrezig, Sitting Chenrezig, and many others. There is one associated with our practice called Triple Manifestation of the Six-Syllable Mantra. Among all the manifestations, Eleven-Faced, Thousand-Armed Chenrezig is the primary manifestation.

The Tibetan word, Chenrezig, literally means gazing with the eyes of compassion. Just as Chenrezig is the manifestation of all the buddhas' loving-kindness and compassion, similarly all the buddhas have infinite enlightened qualities and they manifest in the forms of wisdom, compassion, purification, etc. For example, Manjushri Bodhisattva is a manifestation of wisdom, Vajrasattva is a manifestation of all the buddhas' power of purification, and there are many others with specific enlightened qualities. While absolute Chenrezig is the embodiment of all the buddhas' loving-kindness and compassion, Chenrezig is also the inherent potential of the love and compassion of all sentient beings. In other words, all sentient beings are inherently Chenrezig in nature.

THE HISTORY OF THOUSAND-ARMED CHENREZIG

As a bodhisattva being, Chenrezig had the incredible enlightened aspiration to liberate all sentient beings. His powerful aspiration led him to the bodhisattva vow to not attain enlightenment if any single sentient being still remained in samsara. The understanding here is that a true bodhisattva is a completely pure being who cares only for the welfare of others. Therefore, as a bodhisattva being, Chenrezig worked tirelessly for the good of all. His commitment was, "No matter what happens, if I ever break my vow to save all fellow sentient beings, may my body fall into a thousand pieces."

Then, the story goes, Chenrezig worked tirelessly for eons and eons. Having worked for so many eons, he thought, "Now the number of sentient beings must be dramatically reduced." Using his wisdom eye's ability to see sentient beings in samsara, at the very time that the collective karma in the world was not very good, he saw that the world of samsara was experiencing a particular decline; neurosis and conflicting emotions were at their peak. There was tremendous confusion, illusion, and suffering in the world. The number of sentient beings in samsara appeared not to have declined. Chenrezig was very disappointed and began to feel it was an impossible task to save all sentient beings. As soon as he gave rise to that thought and doubted his own commitment to liberate all sentient beings, he broke his vow and his body fell into a thousand pieces. Chenrezig's guru, Amitabha Buddha, immediately knew what had happened, and he came right up to Chenrezig and said, "It's unfortunate that you gave up your vow like that. Now I must ask you to make an even greater commitment to liberate all sentient beings." Chenrezig accepted this command and Amitabha Buddha blessed his body which had fallen into one thousand pieces, and his body transformed into eleven faces and one thousand eyes and arms.

Through the manifestation of eleven faces and one thousand arms, Chenrezig works for the benefit of all. One thousand eyes are the representation of the one thousand buddhas that are to appear in this particular fortunate eon. This is to take place right here during the lifespan of our planet Earth. Lord Buddha Shakyamuni was the fourth Buddha. Maitreya Bodhisattva will be the fifth Buddha. According to prophecies, the sixth Buddha, the Buddha of the Lion's Roar, will be Karmapa, supreme head of the Kagyu lineage. It is believed that Jamgon Kongtrul the Great will be the manifestation of the one-thousandth Buddha, the last Buddha.

My supreme enlightened guru, Lord of Refuge Kalu Rinpoche, is the direct incarnation of Jamgon Kongtrul the Great.

The *Sutra of Great Fortune* is a biography of the one thousand buddhas. In it Lord Buddha states that the last buddha will have the collective activity of all one thousand buddhas combined together. In addition, he will live the combined life span of all the buddhas. This sutra is actually in our Tibetan Kangyur, which is the direct speech of the Buddha and is composed of 103 volumes. The volumes are in alphabetical order, and the *Sutra of Great Fortune* is in the first volume, called by the first letter of the Tibetan alphabet, Volume Ka.

The 103 volumes of the Tibetan Kangyur are definitely not all of the teachings of the Buddha. It is the amount of teachings the great Tibetan translators were able to translate. The Chinese, for example, have many more sutras than we do in Tibet. And of course, there are even more of Buddha's teachings in India. Lord Buddha taught eighty-four thousand volumes of teachings. The great fourth-century Indian Buddhist master Vasubandhu said, "If you have a big elephant, and the elephant carries as much ink as it can carry, it will take all that ink to write just one volume of the Buddha's teachings." One can only imagine how vast the perfectly enlightened Buddha's teaching really is.

One thousand arms are the symbolic representation of how Chenrezig performs his enlightened activity as a universal monarch in a thousand different ways. A universal monarch is someone who rules the entire world. The eleven faces represent his completely treading the path of the eleven bhumis. The eleventh bhumi is the buddha level, so this means completing the path to the level of the enlightenment of the Buddha.

Benefits
of the Practice 2

ACCORDING TO THE *Great Benefits of Nyungne* text,

> Oh, sons and daughters of noble family, if you practice Nyungne
> just one time, you will purify negativities of forty thousand kalpas
> (eons) and will be born as either supreme among men or have a
> godlike birth. The spiritual achievement of those who complete
> eight continuous Nyungne practices will equal the stage of a
> stream-enterer,[1] and they will be able to be born in the pure land
> of Amitabha Buddha. If one completes twenty-five Nyungne
> practices, this equals the spiritual achievement of the stage of a
> once-returner and the purification of eighty thousand kalpas.
> If one were to do fifty Nyungne practices, this is the equivalent
> of achieving the path of no more returning and the purification
> of eight hundred thousand kalpas of negativities. If one were to
> complete 108 Nyungne practices, it is equivalent to achieving
> arhathood; one hundred million kalpas of negativities are purified,
> and one will definitely be born in the pure land of Great Bliss in the
> presence of Buddha Amitayus (Long Life Buddha).

OBSCURATIONS OF BODY, SPEECH, AND MIND

Unenlightened beings are unable to experience real, pure body, speech, and
mind because of many levels of obscuration, all the way from obstruction

---

1 In general, on the path of buddhadharma, individual practitioners develop certain spiritual qualities of insight. They are then referred to as stream-enterer, once-returner, nonre-
turner, and arhat.

to omniscience to latent conditioning, afflictive emotions, and the most gross of all, karmic obscurations. This means that due to these obstacles we, as ordinary beings, cannot experience pure manifestations of the Buddha, either physically or mentally. At this point we are experiencing our form as a human body, but an impure human body. We are stuck with this form body because of the karmic obstacles and so forth. This experience is considered a relatively fortunate one, considering other possible form body experiences such as hell beings, hungry ghost beings, and animal beings. These are all form body experiences as well that are absolutely due to karmic obstacles and defilements. Sometimes the term "veil" is used to describe these obstacles. The understanding here is that the levels of obscurations are like layers, or veils, covering our pure nature of mind, which is buddha nature, with one obscuration after another. When the layers of obscuration are purified, we are able to experience our true nature, which is manifesting our own pure buddha nature completely.

How Purification Works

During our Nyungne practice, true purification is possible primarily because of the power of Chenrezig's compassion and blessing, as well as our faith, devotion, and correct motivation to do the practice. When such causes and conditions come together, a result inevitably occurs, and this result is understood as the interdependently-arising nature of all phenomena. For the most part, enlightened and unenlightened phenomena all arise due to this interdependently-arising nature. As a spiritual practitioner, the basic qualities one must bring to the practice are faith, devotion, and a trust in the power of the practice and Chenrezig. These qualities stem from our own pure nature of mind, a purity that is identical to Chenrezig's heart, that is, unceasing love and compassion. When these two things are combined together, our devotion and faith and Chenrezig's love and compassion, one could say miracles happen; a true purification takes place.

It has been said that when one is sitting before the mandala of Chenrezig, one should believe that although Chenrezig is not physically visible to us, in fact he is really there in front of us. Just as we would be very careful of our thoughts and behavior if we were in the presence of a powerful and clairvoyant enlightened guru, in the same way we must generate vigilance so that we don't act shamefully in front of this great being. If we develop such vigilance and noble habit, then our negativities will automatically decrease.

In the history of the Nyungne tradition, many practitioners have been able to overcome incurable disease through the practice of Nyungne. We could say miracles like this literally do take place, although in the Buddhist understanding, overcoming great obstacles and disease would be considered blessings. A miracle is something else. It is the enlightened power that is demonstrated by enlightened masters. A true miracle in the Buddhist sense would be like the miracle of Milarepa entering into a little horn while his student, Rechungpa, sees him in his usual size yet he is inside the horn. Or like the miracle of Milarepa sitting on a lake and people seeing that he hasn't become any larger nor has the lake shrunk in size, yet he is completely covering it. These are real, enlightened miracles. And then there are also common siddhis (accomplishments) that can be achieved by ordinary, accomplished practitioners. I stress ordinary practitioners, because in order to receive these siddhis one does not necessarily have to be an enlightened, accomplished being.

PURIFICATION OF BODY, SPEECH, AND MIND

During Nyungne practice, physical fasting purifies the negative karma of killing, stealing, and sexual misconduct, and overcomes obscurations of the body. Therefore, you will never be born in the preta (hungry ghost) realm and, when born as a human, you will not suffer from illness nor be harmed by evil spirits. Also, you will be born with a beautiful body and a striking presence. Ultimately one will attain the supreme body of the buddhas with major marks and minor marks of perfection.

Abstaining from speech and remaining in silence purifies the negative karma of lying, slandering, harsh words, and idle talk, and purifies obscurations of speech. You will not be born in the animal realm, and when born as a human, you will automatically have proper and gifted speech, and your words will carry weight. Ultimately one will attain the melodious, enlightened speech of the buddhas.

One-pointed concentration on practices during Nyungne purifies the negative karma of greed (as in covetousness), evil thoughts, and wrong view, and purifies obscurations of the mind. You will not be born in the hell realm and will have spiritual realization and satori (spiritual experience). As a human, you will always be bright and have integrity and a great understanding of dharma. Ultimately one will attain the five wisdoms of the buddhas.

Remember that negative deeds or karma of the mind are related to hellish experience, and that tells us that the actions of our mind are the most important, and the intentional wrong deeds of our mind are the worst of all possible deeds. I say this is because the scriptures mention that wrong deeds of body, such as stealing or even killing, in the absence of intention and hatred in the mind, are only a cause for the experience of the hungry ghost realm. We know for a fact that the worst of all realms is hell, and hell is connected with wrong deeds of the mind. The act of killing alone cannot be the cause of birth in the hell realm, but the act of killing with malicious intention has to be.

Here is an example of killing without intention. Imagine that you are driving and you become involved in an accident in which you are the cause of another's death. Because you did not intentionally mean it, and you did not enjoy it, and you regretted that it happened, even though someone died, your karma, in the absence of intention, cannot be that bad. You have some karma, definitely, but not a major karma causing you to fall into the hell realm.

STORY OF THE WOMAN WHO KILLED MANY PEOPLE

At one time the great Nyungne master Bodhisattva Dawa Gyeltsen was in the southern part of Tibet, where an old, infirm woman came for blessing. Bodhisattva gave her blessings and made dedication prayers on her behalf, and he told her that her illness was due to past life karma and that she should practice patience and develop bodhichitta. He gave her many instructions. She was very moved and devotion arose within her. With tears in her eyes, she told Bodhisattva, "I'm sure I have done lots of wrong deeds in the past, but even in this life I have committed terrible acts." Bodhisattva replied, "Well, wrong deeds can be overcome if you confess them sincerely." The old woman then told him her story.

"In a place called Kyi Dong, I was the wife of a rich businessman and had one son. When my son was seven years old, my husband went on a business trip to Nepal. He was gone for about three years. During that time I had an affair with another man and bore a daughter with him. I killed the daughter so that my husband wouldn't find out. I also wasted a lot of our fortune. My son told me, 'When father comes back, we'll see what will happen to you.' I was very angry and I grabbed a stone and hit him, saying, 'What did I do?' Then he bled to death. I was making up all kinds of stories about what had happened, but we had an old monk living in the house who said prayers for us. He knew everything, so I poisoned him. One day my husband came back with lots of wealth, and our maid told him everything. I was listening to them, and I heard my husband say, 'Tonight I will pretend that I don't know anything, but tomorrow I will punish her by gouging out her eyes.' I was so afraid that I put a lot of poison in the chang (Tibetan barley beer), and I gave it to my husband along with eight of his people, two of our neighbors, and two maids. The next morning, they were all in a coma and within two days they all died. So I ran far away to the south, and my parents and other family members suffered a lot because of what I had done. In addition to all this, in my life I have done many other despicable deeds."

Hearing this story, with tears in his eyes Bodhisattva thought, "What a poor woman, with so much negative karma. Nyungne is the solution for her since Lord Chenrezig has vowed to protect any sentient being who does one set of the practice from falling into the three lower realms." Then he gave her teaching and empowerment and instructed her to do eight sets of Nyungne practice.

After having received the blessing, the old woman felt better immediately, and during the month of Saka Dawa she participated in an Eight Nyungne practice. One day she was very thirsty and she drank a little bit of chang, and then another day she was very hungry and she ate two of the four torma offerings. So she did six perfect sets of Nyungne and two broken sets. Soon after that she died.

Many years passed and one day someone remembered the story of this old woman and asked Bodhisattva what happened to her. Bodhisattva, being completely clairvoyant, smiled and told everyone that even though this Nyungne practice of Thousand-Armed Chenrezig is extremely beneficial, very few people are able to do it. The woman was born in a wealthy, Brahman family in east India. Although she managed to obtain a human birth, because she violated one Nyungne by drinking, it caused her to have some mental problems. And because she ate the food, she had an ugly physical appearance. But she was very devoted to Chenrezig practice, and he could see her going to Amitabha Buddha's pure land after this life.

Bodhisattva further said, "Those who do Eight Nyungne properly will absolutely be able to go to the pure land of Amitabha Buddha, and they will eventually attain complete enlightenment; doing the practice once will protect them forever from falling into the lower realms. Therefore, this is the teaching and practice of all the buddhas and bodhisattvas, and everyone should try to practice it."

Since this is a truly powerful purification practice, I strongly recommend that people do at least eight consecutive practices if they are suffering from incurable disease or any forms of obstacles and defilements. If someone is suffering from a serious, ripening karmic illness, such as cancer, in order to counter and prevent further ripening of the karma they should do at least 108 Nyungne practices. If someone were to do 108 Nyungne practices, I believe with complete confidence that they would be able to overcome whatever karmic disease they might have, but those 108 Nyungne practices must be done consecutively.

I can describe some of the benefits that a few of my students have experienced. One woman had a heart problem that prior to doing the practice required surgical treatment. After the practice, the problem was no longer there. Another woman had a small breast tumor that disappeared after she did eight Nyungne practices. Another student was a cancer patient. I encouraged her to do eight sets of Nyungne, but she was only able to participate in two. After finishing the two practices, she told me that before the practices she had felt terrible, mentally and physically; and after the practices, she felt much better, as if a huge burden had been lifted. Another woman commented that she never knew what happiness was until she practiced Nyungne.

These are a few examples of the immediate, relative benefits of Nyungne practice. Additional great stories of overcoming karmic illness can be found in the biographies of Gelongma Palmo and the lineage holders of the practice in the next chapter.

It has been said that this practice is so great that even offering a meal to a Nyungne practitioner is like offering a meal to an eighth-bhumi bodhisattva, which is obviously a deed of considerable merit. It is also believed that if you offer a meal to a Nyungne practitioner on the day the practice ends, the merit is equal to offering a meal to five hundred solitary realizers (pratyekabuddhas). The merit of offering a meal to someone who merely took the eight precepts equals making such an offering to an arhat, so the merit of the offering in itself is extraordinary. One of the lineage holders of Nyungne told his disciples to use his possessions just to support Nyungne practitioners when he died; nothing else would be needed.

In conclusion, just by supporting Nyungne practitioners one will receive tremendous benefit. Through such deeds one will not fall into the lower realms, one will be able to develop bodhichitta, in all future lives one will have abundant wealth and, eventually, one will be able to completely perfect the practice of generosity.

Importance of Lineage and Guru 3

THE LINEAGE of this precious practice comes from Gelongma Palmo, an Afghani princess who became a completely enlightened being through the practice of Nyungne. She transmitted the teaching to her disciple, and so this precious lineage began.

For a lineage to be considered an enlightened lineage tradition, it must be founded by a completely enlightened being. This is essential. The importance of an authentic spiritual lineage derives from the fact that in the secret mantrayana tradition, one can only become enlightened through the blessings of a true guru who comes from a true enlightened lineage. Furthermore, without such a precious spiritual lineage, enlightenment cannot be reached. This is from the point of view of the ultimate promise of the secret tantric path, enlightenment in one lifetime. Of course, if one performs many correct, spiritually related virtuous deeds, one can become enlightened in future lives, but if one wishes to be a completely enlightened being in this form body, the only possibility is through a guru who comes from an enlightened lineage. There is no other possibility. For this reason, in all of our prayer texts you will always find that the first prayers are to the guru and to the precious spiritual lineage holders.

I personally think one of the truly precious treasures that comes from the Tibetan Buddhist tradition is the up-to-date teaching that is being passed on by enlightened beings who hold the lineage. They are enlightened and the teaching is alive, as much alive now as it was in the very beginning. At the present time, this is unique to the Tibetan Buddhist spiritual heritage. In other words, the blessings and the lineage are up-to-date, alive today. I don't know about the future, but right now it's as wonderful as it was over a thousand years ago. I hope and pray that the lineage will remain a pure and enlightened lineage for many centuries to come.

GELONGMA PALMO'S BIOGRAPHY

The founder of the Nyungne lineage, Bhikshuni Lakshmi (Tib. Gelongma Palmo), is believed to have been the daughter of the King of Oddiyana, an area of what is now modern-day Afghanistan. Oddiyana was a great Buddhist country where vajrayana Buddhism flourished a long time ago. Padmasambhava, who is considered second only to Lord Buddha, came from that part of the world. A sign of buddhadharma being a part of that country's historic culture was evident until recently when, as we all know, the Taliban destroyed the tallest Buddhist statue in the world at Bamiyan.[2]

Gelongma Palmo probably lived during the tenth or eleventh century. Due to her exceptional spiritual karma and past life spiritual habit, early in her life she understood the shortcomings of a samsaric, household lifestyle. She saw no possibility of true happiness in such a life, and she decided to give up the life of a princess to become a nun. She was very learned, in fact knowledgeable in all the five sciences,[3] as well as very strict in her discipline.

However, from some past-life karmic residue, she suffered from the debilitating condition of leprosy. In those days it was considered *the* incurable disease, and since it was contagious, society cast out such people. So, Gelongma Palmo was forced to live in isolation. Lepers were known to accidentally lose their limbs due to lack of sensation. This happened to her, and she lost her hands. Without the use of her hands, she had to eat like an animal. She suffered physically and mentally very much. Since prayer is the only solution, she certainly must have prayed intensely and with a great deal of sincerity during this time. Her prayers were answered one night in the form of a dream in which King Indrabodhi blessed her and prophesied that, if she genuinely practiced and prayed to Lord Chenrezig (Avalokiteshvara), she would achieve supreme siddhi (accomplishment) in this life. The next morning, she felt some mental peace right away and she started to recite the mantra OM MANI PEME HUNG during the daytime and the long dharani during the night.

Although this is the most widely accepted version of the story, there is another version in which Gelongma Palmo went to see a mahasiddha

2 Muslim extremists destroyed the Buddha statue from the belief that idol worship is stupid and wrong. According to this doctrine, someone who does this will go to hell because it is so wrong to make and worship such a statue.

3 The five major sciences are: art, medicine, linguistics, valid cognition, and the inner science of Buddhist philosophy.

of Avalokiteshvara known as Glorious Lion (Skt. Shri Sing Ha, Tib. Pal Gyi Senge) where he lived in a jungle called Khasarpani. From him she received teachings and the practice of Chenrezig.

In any event, Gelongma Palmo practiced diligently for about sixteen months, but she became a little bit discouraged because she didn't see much result. Early one morning, feeling depressed and with her mind in turmoil, she thought, "I really need a deity practice which is easy to accomplish. I'm not going to be successful doing this one, and I don't think I will be able to find another practice. There's no hope and I might as well be dead." Right after thinking these thoughts, she fell asleep and then woke to see a light shining in water, which totally captured her attention. In the light she saw a young boy riding a lion. He told her she should go to the east, to a place called Pundravardhana. "There you will find Thousand-Armed Chenrezig, who is the essence of all the buddhas of the three times," he said. "This is the deity practice which is easy to accomplish. You should go there and practice and pray. If you do, you will achieve Lord Tara's state of realization in five years." Speaking thus, he put a small blessing pill on her tongue. She asked this boy, "Who are you?" He replied, "I am Manjushri." Then she said, "Well then, I wish to make a request that you give me the ultimate siddhi." "That siddhi is what I have already given to you," Manjushri answered, and he disappeared.

From that morning on Gelongma Palmo was able to develop great bodhichitta and, with an enormous devotion to Chenrezig, she started off toward the east. After seven days of travel, as she was taking a rest under a tree, she fell asleep. She began to hear the fearful sounds of wild beasts. Terrified, she prayed to Chenrezig with intense devotion, and all her fear went away. In that same place, she met seven red-colored dakinis with wreaths of flowers on their heads. They told her, "When you achieve supreme siddhi, we would like to be your retinue and protectors." Gelongma Palmo asked them, "What family of dakinis are you and where did you come from?" They answered, "We are Lotus Family dakinis. Just now we came from Oddiyana, and tomorrow we would like you to go to Pundravardhana and become the chief dakini." She responded by saying, "Well, in that case I would like to have a siddhi to get there quickly." They lay down a piece of beautiful, silklike cloth and asked her to sit on it. The next thing she knew, it was evening and she was in Pundravardhana in the presence of the self-arisen statue of Thousand-Armed Chenrezig.[4] She

4 Several years ago when I was in Lhasa, I saw the statue in the Potala Palace, where it now resides. The konyer (Tibetan for caretaker of the temple) explained to me that this

vowed to remain in that spot until she achieved siddhi, and to practice Nyungne continuously.

Within a year, she was able to overcome her illness, and she achieved many different kinds of samadhis. Her hands were also restored. While she practiced, many demons tried to create obstacles to her practice; she was able to subdue them through her practice of creation and completion, and her increased bodhichitta. As a result of her practice, eight naga kings vowed to protect Nyungne practitioners.[5]

When Gelongma Palmo was twenty-seven, on the first day of the fourth lunar month (Saga Dawa), she had a vision of Tara, and she attained the level of a first-bhumi bodhisattva. Tara prophesied that Gelongma Palmo would perform activities of the buddhas of the three times. On the eighth day of that same month, she had a vision of all the deities of kriya tantra, and she attained the eighth bhumi. Again there was a prophecy, this time that she would liberate all sentient beings to buddhahood through Chenrezig practice.

On the fifteenth day of the same month, Gelongma Palmo had a vision of Thousand-Armed Chenrezig, and she saw entire mandalas of the Four Tantric Deities inside Thousand-Armed Chenrezig's body. Further, she saw innumerable buddha realms in each pore. She said to Chenrezig, "I have been praying to you for twelve years, waiting for you to appear." Chenrezig replied, "I was with you all along, from the time you started praying to me. It was due to your own obscurations that you were unable to see me." Then he gave her many teachings and blessings. She achieved the level of a tenth-bhumi bodhisattva, and she became inseparable from Lord Chenrezig. It is said that her body even became a golden color.

Gelongma Palmo began to engage in the conduct of a siddha, untraditional behavior that to the uninformed may appear to be unscrupulous activity. In order to dispel any doubt, during a Buddhist celebration of Khasarpani, in the middle of the crowd she danced and cut off her own head with her small ritual knife and placed it on top of her ritual staff.

---

statue came from Pundravardhana, and that it was the true, self-arisen statue of Eleven-Faced Avalokiteshvara. He said that, among all the precious spiritual items and statues, this was the single most valuable thing that existed in the Potala Palace. It is a small sandalwood statue. If you did not understand its importance, you would not be able to tell that it is the most valuable thing in the palace, because there are so many other elaborately ornate, beautiful statues and other spiritual items there. In the sutras, Lord Buddha mentions the importance of having a sandalwood statue as part of your shrine when you do the Nyungne practice.

5 These are the naga protector kings that we make torma offerings to during our practice.

She levitated into the sky, then came back to earth and replaced her head. Everyone there was greatly inspired, and she gave teachings on the practice of Chenrezig. All the men and women present went on to achieve siddhi and were able to go to the dakini realm.

GELONGMA PALMO'S DISCIPLES

Gelongma Palmo's lineage-holder disciple was **Dawa Shonnu**, Youthful Moon (Skt. Pandita Chandra Ku Mara). He was born in West India to a Brahman family. At the age of thirteen he became a monk. He studied the Tripitaka and became very learned in all five traditional Buddhist sciences. He was especially well versed in the logic of valid cognition and linguistics. His fame spread far and wide in India. At the age of twenty-one he was fully ordained, and at about that time he began to suffer from a condition similar to schizophrenia. In Tibetan, we call it a heart-wind problem; one's heart becomes very constricted and one is paranoid and easily bothered.

Dawa Shonnu tried everything to overcome this problem and was unsuccessful until he met Gelongma Palmo. Gelongma Palmo blessed him and he was cured. Further, she told him, "The cause of your illness is that in your past life you offended a great teacher, but you confessed to him. That's the reason that in this life you suffered from this illness, but in the end you were able to come to see me." She gave him teaching and instruction on Thousand-Armed Chenrezig practice, and through it he became a completely accomplished Mahamudra master.

The next lineage holder was **Yeshe Zangpo** (Skt. Pandita Jnana Bhadra), meaning Excellent Wisdom. He came from a royal family, but he became a monk and studied very well and was knowledgeable in all the five sciences. Like Dawa Shonnu, the lineage-holder master, he also suffered from a past-life karmic illness. In his case, it was a burning abcess on the lower part of his body. He tried medical remedies for relief and nothing worked. Thinking it was a condition caused by spirits, he went to a mahasiddha and received a practice to subdue the spirits. After that, his condition became three times worse. The abcess covered his entire body. He was in such extreme pain, he had to sit in cold water just to cool off. The heat was so intense that even the water became hot, and it had to be continuously changed. He went to see many great masters but no one could help him.

Finally Dawa Shonnu was asked to help. Right at the moment Dawa Shonnu was about to go to help Yeshe Zangpo, he had a vision of Tara.

Tara told him, "You really cannot help this monk. This is a condition of past-life karma caused by breaking samaya with a guru. Ask Gelongma Palmo to help him." So he prayed to Gelongma Palmo and invited her to come; then guru and disciple both went to see the poor monk where he was sitting in the lake. Yeshe Zangpo prayed to Gelongma Palmo from the lake, and she blessed him. Immediately he was cured. Gelongma Palmo gave him the Chenrezig practice and advised him to receive more instructions from her disciple, Dawa Shonnu. Yeshe Zangpo practiced Nyungne for three months and became a completely accomplished being.

The next disciple in the lineage was **Pandita Penyawa**, who is believed to have been Nepali. He too was born into a royal family and was very learned. His parents were continually telling him to get married and have royal offspring. He asked them, "Will that make me immortal and benefit other beings?" They answered, "No, it won't do that, but you will be able to carry on the royal tradition." "In that case," he answered, "I want to engage in activities which benefit many sentient beings, and I think that is superior to all family traditions."

Pandita Penyawa then engaged in Manjushri practice until he had a vision of Manjushri. He beseeched Manjushri, saying, "I would like to receive supreme siddhi to accomplish enlightenment in this lifetime." And Manjushri instructed him to go to India to meet Yeshe Zangpo and to receive the complete teachings and instructions for Thousand-Armed Chenrezig practice. "If you do that, you will achieve supreme siddhi in this lifetime," he said.

So Pandita Penyawa ran away from his parents and, taking some of his gold jewelry, went to India. There he met his gurus, Dawa Shonnu and Yeshe Zangpo. Both masters were very pleased with him and they took him as their disciple. He was given the teaching and practice of Thousand-Armed Chenrezig, which he practiced for five years, sustaining himself by begging. At the end of that time, he had a vision of Thousand-Armed Chenrezig and, just as prophesied, he became a completely accomplished being. He was able to benefit many beings in India. Then he returned to Nepal where he benefited many more beings. When he died, his body disappeared into a rainbow body.[6]

6 At death, the body of someone who has attained ultimate insight and realization is said to transform into the wisdom body, a body of rainbow light. Literally, the physical form body shrinks and eventually disappears. For such beings, sometimes only fingernails and hair are left behind.

Pandita Penyawa's disciple was the first Tibetan master in this lineage. His name was **Bodhisattva Dawa Gyeltsen**, meaning Victory-Banner Moon.[7] He was revered by all as being *the* Chenrezig, the Lord of Love and Compassion himself. Many learned and accomplished teachers had visions and prophecies about going to see Chenrezig, Bodhisattva Dawa Gyeltsen. There are four such stories that are very well known.

The first story happened while Bodhisattva was visiting Nepal. One evening a yogi saw many dakinis coming to make offerings at the very holy temple where he lived. The yogi asked them, "Where are you all coming from?" And they replied, "We're from Pundravardhana, a place in eastern India where Thousand-Armed Chenrezig resides. The Manifestation of Six Syllables also resides there. Its incarnation is Bodhisattva Dawa Gyeltsen, and we have come here to make offerings to him." This yogi had never heard the great Bodhisattva's name before, but because of this story, he searched for Bodhisattva until he found him and invited him to his temple. There the yogi received teachings and empowerments from Bodhisattva Dawa Gyeltsen.

The second story occurred in Tibet in a place called Mang Yul Kyi Drong. Another great teacher and devotee of Chenrezig was praying to him and circumambulating day and night for seven days. As he was doing this, he became very tired and fell asleep for a few moments. Just then he had a dream in which Chenrezig appeared. Chenrezig said to him, "If you are that devoted to me, then you should be devoted to Bodhisattva Dawa Gyeltsen. He and I are inseparable." When the teacher woke up, he remembered having met Dawa Gyeltsen in the past but not being devoted to him. Realizing this, he was filled with regret and developed a great deal of faith in Bodhisattva. The teacher became Bodhisattva Dawa Gyeltsen's disciple and offered service to him. He received teachings and empowerments, and from then on he was known to pray only to Dawa Gyeltsen.

The third story occurred in Tibet in a place called Ding Ri. A great practitioner called Hung Drag Pa, meaning Famous as the Syllable Hung, did Chenrezig practice for twenty-five years. One night a white man appeared in his dream and told him that Chenrezig's incarnation was Dawa Gyeltsen, and that he should be devoted to him. So he searched for Dawa Gyeltsen and received empowerments and instructions from him and became his student.

The fourth story happened in Tibet with a teacher named Ma Ja Jang

---

7 The story of the woman who killed many people in Chapter 2 comes from the time of this teacher.

Chup Yeshe, meaning Peacock Bodhi Wisdom. This teacher was quite an accomplished being, and he was able to communicate directly with his protector deity. The night before he was planning to go to see Bodhisattva Dawa Gyeltsen, he had a dream in which his protector told him that if he wanted to go to see Chenrezig, he should proceed immediately, and that he would clear all the obstacles on his journey. Replying to his protector, the teacher said, "How can I go to see Lord Chenrezig? I am going to see Bodhisattva Dawa Gyeltsen." The protector answered, "He is Chenrezig."

For all these reasons, Bodhisattva Dawa Gyeltsen is considered a true emanation of Chenrezig. He was also known to have had incredible spiritual activity, such as building a hundred temples and saving hundreds of people sentenced to death or sentenced to having their eyes gouged out. He provided food and lodging for about 1200 monks and made roads in dangerous areas safer for people.

One day Bodhisattva Dawa Gyeltsen was giving bodhisattva vows and teachings to a group of disciples. Right at that moment a mundane spirit being named Tsi Mara appeared to everyone and said to Bodhisattva, "Show some signs of your spiritual attainment." In response to that, Bodhisattva Dawa Gyeltsen revealed an eye in the middle of his palm openly staring at everyone, just as Chenrezig has eyes on all the palms of his thousand hands. Everybody saw this. Some people also saw his body in the form of Eleven-Faced Chenrezig, some saw him as Four-Armed Chenrezig, and some saw him as Two-Armed Chenrezig. When the spirit Tsi Mara saw this, he was very inspired and promised to protect the teachings of Nyungne.

Bodhisattva Dawa Gyeltsen's disciple was **Mahasiddha Nyi Phukpa**, meaning Sunny Cave Being. He was from Lhamo Oh Tro (Light Rays Dakini), in western Tibet. This place was believed to have been well-blessed spiritually, and he was born into a family of noble heritage. He was so adorable when he was born that he captured everybody's heart, and his childhood nickname became Yi Trog (Heart Capturer). By the time he was nine, he already knew how to read and write very proficiently, and he took ordination from a great abbot named Lion of Dharma (Skt. Dharma Sing Ha). Then he studied the scriptures very well and by the time he was twenty-six, he was well known for being noble, disciplined, and learned.

One evening Nyi Phukpa dreamed of a blue-colored woman who was supposed to be Tara's emanation. She told him, "Son of a noble family, you should not stay here but go to a place called Mang Yul Chu Gang. There you will find Chenrezig's emanation. Go to see him and you will receive

supreme siddhi, and you will be able to benefit many sentient beings."
As prophesied, Nyi Phukpa went to see Bodhisattva Dawa Gyeltsen and
offered him a piece of gold and three bolts of cotton. He made a request
to receive a teaching and practice that would quickly liberate him and
others from the pain and suffering of samsara. For a moment Bodhisattva
did not say anything, and then with a smile he said, "You are going to be
the great Lord Protector of many sentient beings." Bodhisattva was very
happy to take him as his disciple and gave him the complete teaching of
the Thousand-Armed Chenrezig practice. Bodhisattva told Nyi Phukpa
that he should not stay in that impure area but rather should go to the west
side of the mountain to the cave called Door of Horse Mountain. There he
should practice and he would receive a prophecy.

So, with no more than a limited supply of tsampa for food, Nyi Phukpa
went to the cave and he practiced without seeing anyone for seven years.
He had signs of spiritual accomplishment over all the five elements. For
example, he could make sun rays appear at will in the palm of his hand.
Initially, a local deity tried to harm him by performing all kinds of mischief
to create obstacles for him, but with his unconditional love and compassion, and the power of the Chenrezig practice, he was able to overcome all
the obstacles. One day he saw five white men with white headbands riding five white horses followed by five white dogs. They came to him and
said, "You are a great practitioner. The other day we tried to create mischief, but now we ask for your forgiveness, and we five brothers would
like to receive some teaching. We would also like to be your protectors
and offer service to you." So he gave many teachings related to the law of
karma, which they were all very happy to receive, and they took a solemn
oath to be his protector.

From that time on they came every day to receive teachings. Then Nyi
Phukpa thought that since he'd been practicing for many years and his
body felt weak and he was out of supplies, it was about time for him to go
somewhere where someone would offer him provisions. The local deity
came and requested that he remain, saying, "I will supply you with provisions." Soon the local spirit brought the body of a dead deer and left it
for him, and assured him that he would bring more supplies. The master
was upset and said, "You know, if you hurt sentient beings like this, I will
not stay in this place." Then another time the local god caused a nomadic
woman to become sick and call on the master to help her, so that he would
be served. The master again scolded him, saying, "Don't do that." Another
time he brought hail on the local farmers so they would offer grain to the
master for his help. Again Nyi Phukpa was upset and scolded him.

Finally he thought, "If I stay here, it just brings a lot of harm to sentient beings," and he wanted to leave. The local deity cried and requested again and again that he stay. But the master would not agree. In the end the local god told him where to go. On the north side, about one day's walking distance, was a beautiful cave called Nyi Phuk that would be a nice place to be. The master miraculously flew there, and he accomplished a great deal of spiritual activity in that area. With his own miraculous power and the help of others, he built a temple and statues, and the place became his spiritual seat. So he was called Nyi Phukpa (Sunny Cave Being).

This great being endured many experiences during his Nyungne practice. One night he had severe pain in his eyes, almost like his eyes would pop out, and a white man told him that five hundred lifetimes before he had been a fisherman in the south of India, and at that time he had killed a giant fish by crushing its eyes. "This is the final karmic residue of that." Another day he had a swollen jaw and a great deal of pain. Again he was told that some nine hundred lifetimes before he had broken the jaw of a buffalo with a stone. "This is the final karmic residue of that."

In any event, this great being had incredible spiritual activity and did Nyungne practice almost all the time. Even when he was sick or not feeling well, he would do Nyungne at least three times a month. He was known to have received the prophecy that he would be born in Amitabha Buddha's pure land and after that, Amitabha Buddha would prophesy his complete enlightenment. At the age of seventy-seven, on a half moon day, while he was doing Nyungne, on the afternoon of the silent day, with extraordinary signs, Mahasiddha Nyi Phukpa passed away.

Mahasiddha Nyi Phukpa's principal disciple was **Supa Dorje Gyalpo**, which means Vajra King from Suyul. He was known to have been born with a beautiful face and the extraordinary scent called "morality odor." They offered him the name Tsultrim Konchog, meaning Morality Sublime and Rare. At the age of seven his karmic spiritual connection was awakened and he met Mahasiddha Nyi Phukpa. The mahasiddha was very delighted to see him and told everyone that this young boy would hold the lineage of the victors and their sons (buddhas and bodhisattvas).

Supa Dorje Gyalpo received monastic ordination from the great mahasiddha, and he gradually became extremely learned in the three vehicles. He was particularly well versed in the vinaya, and he was known to be highly disciplined. At the age of twenty he became fully ordained. He went to see Mahasiddha Nyi Phukpa and asked him for teaching in order to do practice. Nyi Phukpa was delighted to hear the request and told him, "I shall give you one practice of dharma that is all-sufficient. You do not need to do many different things." Saying that, he gave him the empowerment and instructions for Nyungne. In response, Supa Dorje Gyalpo promised to continue doing Nyungne practice for the rest of his life. Mahasiddha was so delighted to hear his commitment that he gave him the only crystal Chenrezig statue that he had and prophesied that he would become an accomplished being.

After receiving the teachings, Supa Dorje Gyalpo did one Nyungne after another in the same location for five years. At the beginning of his sixth year of Nyungne practice, at the age of thirty-six, on the half moon day in the third month of the lunar calendar, he had a vision of Chenrezig. Chenrezig blessed him, and his body, speech, and mind became indistinguishable from those of Chenrezig. At that time he achieved tremendous supercognition and attained miraculous abilities. From that time on he was able to benefit sentient beings tremendously.

For the duration of his life, Supa Dorje Gyalpo sustained himself by begging and practiced mainly Nyungne. He was known to have visited all kinds of buddha fields in his dreams. One night he dreamt that he was in the presence of Amitabha Buddha, Medicine Buddha, and an assembly of various buddhas and bodhisattvas. He could hear the bodhisattvas talking together about him. They were saying, "We should adopt him as our son." One of the beautiful bodhisattvas, who had five-colored light rays coming from his body, said, "I have seventeen lifetimes of connections with him, and I want to make him my son." As Supa Dorje Gyalpo heard this, all the colored light rays came toward him and as they dissolved into him, he woke up. He later asked a thangka painter to make a painting of his vision.[8]

Supa Dorje Gyalpo had many miraculous activities which benefited beings. Throughout his life, he tasted neither liquor nor meat, and he continually practiced Nyungne until the end of his life. After he passed away, many images of Chenrezig were found on his bones, and many small, pearl-shaped relics were found among his remains. These relics were enshrined in a stupa. Up to the time of the writing of this text, the relics were known to produce additional relics that would be emitted from the stupa when supplicated or venerated.

Supa Dorje Gyalpo's principal disciple was known as **Shangton Drajig,** which means Enemy-Terrified Teacher from Shang. He was born in the region of Trophur. An earthquake and thunderstorm occurred at the time of his birth, which frightened an enemy of the family so much that he gave

---

8 I don't know for sure whether this thangka painting survives, but it did exist.

up his evil ways and no longer threatened them. For this reason, they gave the newborn the nickname Drajig.

By the time Shangton Drajig reached seven years of age, he knew how to read and write very well. He received monk vows from Supa Dorje Gyalpo and went to the great Sakya Monastery, where he studied extensively and became very learned. By the time he was twenty-nine, his scholarly fame had reached the entire region of Central Tibet. He was particularly well-versed in the vinaya, which he had memorized in its entirety and taught to others. He became an abbot to no less than five hundred monks, and he followed a lifestyle of extremely precise monastic discipline in the great Kadampa tradition. During this time his main practices were Medicine Buddha and Tara. A prophecy from Tara led him to go to meet Supa Dorje Gyalpo, and from him he received the instructions and empowerment of Thousand-Armed Chenrezig.

For three years and four months, Shangton Drajig continually did Nyungne practice. Then, in the beginning of the night on a full moon day, he had a vision of the Twenty-one Taras. In the middle of the same night he had a vision of Medicine Buddha with a retinue of seven buddhas. In the third part of the night, which is early morning, he had a vision of Chenrezig himself surrounded by many other kriya and charya tantra deities, and he received empowerment and blessing directly from these deities, particularly from Chenrezig.

Chenrezig instructed Shangton Drajig, "My dear son, do not rely on the food offerings of people who ask you for prayers for the living or the dead. Rely upon solitude, live in retreat, and, if possible, rely upon yogic sustenance or rasayana (a special practice of taking nutrients from space). If you cannot do that, then at least rely on begging for your food and benefit beings as much as possible." Shangton Drajig went to his guru and told him about his experience and said that he wanted to go into retreat. His guru instructed him to remain as a teacher for three years and gave him the crystal Chenrezig that he had received from his own guru.

After three years, Shangton Drajig gave away all of his fine robes, religious articles, and other belongings. Then he quietly disappeared into a hidden valley where for three months he continued to do one Nyungne after another, until he developed a terrible fever that lasted for seven days. The fever got so high that he thought he was going to die. Early one morning when he was half asleep, he had another vision of Chenrezig. Chenrezig said to him, "Many lifetimes ago you were a fisherman in India, and you cooked many live fish in boiling water and ate them. Because of that you spent many hundreds of millions of years in the Hell of Boiling Water, and while you were there I was able to hit you with a ray of light, causing you to be reborn as a human being. After sixteen lifetimes you were able to make a connection with me. Now you have actually met me face-to-face, and this fever is the experience of the last remnants of that karma." Saying that, Chenrezig placed his hand on him. The fever broke, and he recovered.

For three years, Shangton Drajig continued to persevere in his practice of Nyungne. During one period, because of the intensity of his austerity and the deprivation he endured, he developed an imbalance of winds that left him almost unconscious for seven days. After that he became desperately hungry and ate whatever he could find. Sometimes he ate wood ashes boiled in water, at other times nettles, and at times garbage left by shepherds. During one period he went for seven months without so much as a drop of water. In that way Shangton Drajig engaged in tremendous austerity, and he continued to meditate on the generation and completion aspects of the Chenrezig practice. At the end of three years, he became a mahasiddha and was known to often fly to the mountaintop to observe the sunrise and sunset, and he was able to reverse the currents of rivers. In short, he came to possess all sorts of miraculous abilities.

When Shangton Drajig passed away, there were many extraordinary signs. After the cremation, large quantities of little white relics were found, and his tongue and heart were not burned by the fire. These were all placed in two reliquaries.

Shangton Drajig's major disciple was called **Jangpa Khenchen Tsidulwa**, meaning Great Abbot Tsidulwa from the North. From an early age he exhibited special qualities. When he was eight he dreamed that the entire mountain in their area was covered with upala flowers, and he saw Tara sitting on top of each and every one of those flowers. At the age of nine, while he was playing with many children, a tiny louse[9] dropped from his body. He felt very bad for that louse and looked for it so he could put it back on his body. The other children also helped in the search, but when they couldn't find it, they said, "Let's go home." But Jangpa Khenchen Tsidulwa refused to leave, and he remained there for the whole night. The next morning he found the dead louse. Crying, he picked it up and placed it on his forehead. "This is my parent," he said.

---

9 Lice are tiny insects with six legs and are actually harmless. They are quite common in Tibet, probably because people there don't take showers and don't wash their clothing very often. We all had lice when I was in the monastery, because we didn't have the luxury of modern conveniences.

He would cry a lot when he was studying and reading sutra texts that described all the many shortcomings of samsara. When he heard others talking about dharma, he would say, "I want to practice the dharma," and he would make a wish to be able to do so. When he saw others experiencing pain and suffering, he would genuinely wish that he could take on their suffering and let them practice the dharma. On many occasions he dreamed of becoming a monk.

One night a white man came into Jangpa Khenchen Tsidulwa's dreams and told him, "Don't feel bad, you'll get to be a monk, and you will become a great leader and liberator of many, many sentient beings." Another time he dreamt about the Potala Pure Land and saw everything very clearly.

Jangpa Khenchen Tsidulwa regularly felt tremendous compassion for those who were suffering, and he increasingly developed his renunciation of the world. At the age of twenty-one he became a monk and began to study primarily the teachings of Maitreya. He soon became famous for achieving nobility of conduct and learning, and he was referred to as Tukje Jangchup (Unceasing Compassionate Bodhi). He is said to have been so pure in his discipline that the perfume of morality emanated from his body.

One night in the valley where he was staying, Jangpa Khenchen Tsidulwa dreamt that a blue-colored woman was striking a gendi.[10] He saw the entire population coming together in response. Then he woke up. He thought the dream was auspicious and a sign that if he were to establish a monastery, it would be beneficial. So he established a great monastery called Pal Den Dok Tho, and because of his great spiritual fortune, his monastic institution housed more than one thousand monks and he was able to serve the buddhadharma and benefit many sentient beings.

Jangpa Khenchen Tsidulwa's main practice was tonglen (taking and sending), and his personal deities were Medicine Buddha and Tara. One night in a dream, he received a prophecy from Tara that he should go to receive the Thousand-Armed Chenrezig empowerment and instruction from Lama Shangton Drajig. There he made the commitment to his guru to do one thousand sets of Nyungne.

When he had finished three hundred Nyungne practices, on the full

---

10 Sanskrit for an ancient wooden gong that monks have used from the time of the Buddha to call a gathering. The Tibetan monastic tradition uses this specific wooden gong during the rainy season retreat in summer, because it is a vinaya tradition to do so. This is the only time it is used. There exist also the *Sutra of the Gendi* (Wooden Gong) and the *Sutra on the Occasions for Use of the Gong*.

moon day of the fourth month (Saga Dawa), he had a vision of Thou-sand-Armed Chenrezig who gave him his blessing. At that moment he attained realization. On another occasion he had a vision of Tara, who dis-pelled all his obstacles to bodhichitta practice, and on another he dreamt of being in Victorious Palace where he received four empowerments and many auspicious omens from the Dakinis of the Five Families. He was consequently able to liberate and deliver many sentient beings to a state of freedom.

At the age of eighty-four, Jangpa Khenchen Tsidulwa died with many auspicious signs, and it is said that immediately after he passed away he was reborn in Sukhavati in the presence of the bodhisattva Maitreya. There-after he was known to have gone to the pure land of Amitabha Buddha.

The next lineage holder was **Chogyal Dewachenpa** (Dharmaraja of Sukhavati). He was born in a place called Dok Me, and his personal name was Shakya Jangchup. At the age of seven, he became a monk and was diligent in study. By the time he was fifteen, he had become very learned in the perfection of wisdom sutras and the vinaya, and he had become a teacher.

His personal deities were Medicine Buddha and Tara. One day in a vision of three emanations of Tara from the sandalwood forest, she advised him to go to see Jangpa Khenchen Tsidulwa. From him he received the empow-erment and instructions for Nyungne practice, and he performed the num-ber of mantras required to complete the practice twenty-one times. After doing so, he returned to his birthplace, where he built a monastery. He remained there and taught a continuous series of courses on the prajna-paramita and the vinaya twenty times. Then he made a commitment to his guru to perform one thousand Nyungne practices.

Like his guru, after he had done Nyungne practice three hundred times, on the half moon day he had a vision. He experienced a white light bring-ing him to the Potala Pure Land of Chenrezig, and he saw it exactly as it is described in the sutras. He saw the entire pure land made out of pre-cious jewels, with trees and flowers and beautiful lakes, and all kinds of beautiful things. In a precious palace right in the center, he saw Chenrezig sitting on top of a lotus and moon disk, surrounded by the buddhas and bodhisattvas of the ten directions. From Chenrezig he received prophe-cies and empowerment in the form of light. As a result Jangpa Khenchen Tsidulwa was able to generate many different samadhis. From that time on, he possessed spontaneous supercognition and miraculous powers that enabled him to benefit innumerable sentient beings.

At the end of his life, Jangpa Khenchen Tsidulwa died with many auspicious signs and was known to have gone to the Potala Pure Land of Chenrezig.

The next lineage holder was **Khenchen Chuzangwa**, which means the Great Abbot of Chuzangwa. He was born in a place called Mu Kyi Tong Kar. His ordination name was Jangchup Bar (Blazing Enlightenment). He too became very learned and through his dharma knowledge was able to serve the buddhadharma extensively. He always enjoyed living in retreat houses in the mountains. At the age of twenty, he became a fully ordained monk and dedicated himself one-pointedly to practice.

One night Khenchen Chuzangwa dreamt of a white man who told him that they were connected, and that he should go to see Chogyal Dewachenpa. According to prophecy, he went to see the master and from him received the entire teaching on Chenrezig practice and the Nyungne sadhana. In accordance with his guru's command, he immediately began to perform sets of Nyungne one after another. And like his guru and his guru's guru, after three hundred successive sets of Nyungne practice he attained realization. On the evening of the full moon day, which coincided with the main day of his Nyungne practice, he had a vision of Thousand-Armed Chenrezig surrounded by the gurus of the Kadampa tradition.

At that moment he lamented to Chenrezig, "I've been meditating and praying to you for so long. Why have I never seen you until now?" Chenrezig responded, "I have never been separate from you for even an instant, but when I first instructed you to go to meet your guru, you had a doubt about whether I was genuine or a deception of mara, and that small doubt has prevented you from seeing me until now."

Saying that, Chenrezig gave Khenchen Chuzangwa his blessing along with the instruction to benefit beings on a vast scale. From that time onward Khenchen Chuzangwa experienced himself as inseparable from Chenrezig and was never without his constant guidance. Relying solely upon begging as a means of sustenance, he was able to sustain a monastic sangha of three hundred monks. In this way he greatly benefited the teachings and sentient beings.

Many miraculous events occurred during Chuzangwa's life. When he performed Medicine Buddha practice, he had a vision of the Eight Medicine Buddhas and was given divine ambrosia by the yaksha chieftains, who are the attendants of Medicine Buddha. When he performed the ceremony of the Sixteen Arhats, he had a vision in which the Sixteen Arhats actually appeared.

Once when he was teaching, Chuzangwa made the prediction, "Three hundred years from now, at this place which I have founded, three signs will occur and when they do, it will be an indication that this dharma of Nyungne will be easy to practice and therefore should be especially emphasized. This teaching is the broom with which we sweep away our bad karma."

Before he passed away he told his disciples, "I'm going soon. There's no need to take the remains of my provisions and use them for any other purpose than Nyungne practice.[11] Just use them to support as many people as possible. If you can, use them to feed those who practice." By this he referred to the meal on the first day of Nyungne practice. "If the offerings are not enough to provide the meal, then use them for the soup or gruel that is served on the morning after the second day. If it is not enough for that, use them for salt and milk. If you can't do that, then use them to buy wood to feed the fires with which the gruel is cooked. In short, I have heard directly from Chenrezig himself that this will be far more beneficial and meritorious than anything else you could do. This is quite different from any ordinary statement, because it comes from Arya Chenrezig, who never lies."

Having given them these and many other instructions, Khenchen Chuzangwa passed away. If his body had been left alone for a week, it would have started to dissolve into the rainbow body; after three days it had shrunk to the size of a seven-year-old child. This was witnessed by one of his disciples who thought, "Before it disappears altogether, we'd better cremate it so we can have relics to pray to." They cremated what was left of the body, and it became a mass of shariram or relics.

Khenchen Chuzangwa's principal disciple was the Lord of Dharma **Sherab Bumpo**, who was born in the central Tibetan region called Dok To Zarong. Many remarkable events occurred at the time of his birth, and his childhood name was **Zangpo Pal**. At the age of eleven he became a monk, and his ordination name was **Sherab Bumpo**. He showed a natural, profound devotion to the buddhadharma, and in the same year he studied and taught Maitreya's teachings on prajnaparamita entitled *Abhisamayalamkara* and *Sutralamkara* . Everyone was amazed at the sharpness of his intellect at such a young age. He completed all his studies by the age of twenty, and from that time on he practiced the pure vinaya tradition, and he was known to be endowed with the twelve qualities[12] of the vinayas.

---

11 It is a tradition for devoted disciples to make sure all their guru's belongings are used for spiritual purposes, such as sponsoring special ceremonial prayers, building stupas, etc.

12 Much learning, great wisdom, renunciation of possessions, great compassion, the spirit of awakening, endurance of hardship, lack of fatigue, great practical advice, liberation from

Because of his profound karmic connection, he met the great Jonang Kunpong from whom he received teachings on many other sutras and tantras, and particularly the complete teaching on the Kalachakra Tantra and the teaching on Chenrezig. He practiced the six unions very diligently,[13] the completion stage practices of the Kalachakra Tantra, and he perfected all ten signs of accomplishment of the six unions.

He was also known to have attained five types of supercognition and many other miraculous powers. Just as his guru, the great Jonang Kunpong, commanded, he established a monastery in a place called Mu Shu Gu Tsal. There he was very prosperous, spiritually and otherwise, and he benefited many humans and nonhumans.

Sherab Bumpo had a vision of Red Manjushri and also a vision of Tara in which she instructed him to go to Chuzangwa, the previous lineage holder, from whom he received the Thousand-Armed Chenrezig empowerment of the Gelongma Palmo tradition and many other Chenrezig and Nyungne teachings. He began to do Nyungne practice, and after three months he had a vision of Thousand-Armed Chenrezig surrounded by manifestations of Tara. From that time on he became inseparable from Chenrezig. His major disciple, Thogme Zangpo, and others were known to see him in the form of Forty-Armed Chenrezig, Four-Armed Chenrezig, and so on.

Sherab Bumpo was extremely intelligent, and his ability to serve the dharma and benefit beings in the capacity of a teacher and practitioner was beyond measure. As with his predecessors, many miracles occurred when he passed away, and from the cremation of his body there were many, many relics.

The next great lineage holder was **Bodhisattva Thogme Zangpo Pal** (Skt. Shri Asanga Bhadra), who is referred to as the embodiment of the unceasing loving-kindness and compassion of the buddhas of the three times. He is best known for being the composer of a very famous text, *The Thirty-seven Practices of a Bodhisattva*, which is revered by all practitioners in the bodhisattva tradition. Most people know him by the name of **Ngulchu Thogme**. The word *ngulchu* means "mercury," and the place where he spent the latter part of his life was called Ngulchu Cho Dzong, meaning Dharma Fortress of Mercury. Thogme is from Bodhisattva Thogme.

Bodhisattva was born in a place called Drak Kya Chu Sho, which is

---

the mundane path, possessing knowledge, erudition, and comprehension of the signs of warmth.

13 *Jordruk* (Tib.) literally means "six unions." Some translators use the terms "six limbs of union," others say "six-branched yoga" or the "yoga of six limbs."

near the glorious Sakya Monastery. His birth coincided with the auspicious signs of the earth gently shaking and a rain of flowers. Initially he was named Kunchok Sangpo. As a result of a spiritual habit of practicing bodhichitta for many, many lifetimes, from the time he was first able to speak others were far more important to him than himself. He was particularly kind and compassionate toward those in the most pitiful circumstances. His behavior was very honorable and respectful in the presence of the Three Jewels and other honorable beings. And even during childhood play, his games always related to dharma teaching and practice.

Bodhisattva was a shepherd boy, like most Tibetan boys, and one day, at the age of fourteen, he went to the monastery and became a monk. He was given the ordination name of **Zangpo Pal**, and again on that day there was a shower of flowers. From that time on he studied and became extraordinarily learned in the teachings of the sutras, the middle way school, the prajnaparamita, the vinaya, the abhidharma, and so forth. While still quite young, his fame spread far and wide. He settled in a place called Bhodung and established his seat there.

Ngulchu Thogme studied with a great number of teachers, many of them famous. These included the Omniscient Dolpopa, the supreme lineage holder of the Jonang tradition; Buton Rinpoche, one of the greatest masters of the Kalachakra tradition; Sakya Palden Lama, a lineage holder of the glorious Sakya tradition; Sangye Won, a lineage holder of the Shangpa Kagyu tradition; terton Rinchen Lingpa, a great hidden-teaching revealer; and the great Pang Lotsawa, translator of dharma from Sanskrit into Tibetan; and other great masters such as Khenchen Cho Je Pal, Cho Je Sonam Pal, and many others. In total he studied with some fifty different teachers and studied practically every teaching available that was translated from Sanskrit into Tibetan.

Ngulchu Thogme's main practice was mind training practice, and he was able to generate the full attainment of both relative and absolute bodhichitta as they are described in the mind training teachings. His realization was such that he could actually take onto himself the illnesses of others. This meant that whenever he saw someone with problems such as wounds on their skin, a particularly virulent infestation of lice, or other types of chronic pain, mental problems, and so on, simply through the power of compassion they would get better and he would temporarily exhibit the symptoms of whatever had been afflicting them. He was able to make a connection with anyone he saw, such that they benefited immediately in this life and were placed on the path to ultimate liberation.

When Ngulchu Thogme took the precious bodhisattva vow from his guru, there were again many extraordinary signs, such as an earthquake and rainbow light appearing in the sky. From the Lord of Dharma Sherab Bumpo, he received the Six Unions of the Kalachakra Tantra, among many other teachings. Like his master, by meditating upon these six unions he perfected the ten signs and the eight qualities, and thus displayed the signs of accomplishment. However, his teacher told him that in fact his karmic yidam throughout many lifetimes was Thousand-Armed Chenrezig, and he gave him the empowerments, transmissions, and instructions of Nagarjuna, Chanda Gomen, Gelongma Palmo, and several other lineages of the deity.

At the age of forty-three, Ngulchu Thogme asked one of his teachers, the great Pang Lotsawa, to take over his position. He then went to the cave called Ngulchu Cho Dzong, Dharma Fortress of Mercury. From that time on he did not interact with anyone except his one attendant. For the next twenty years, his main practices of Nyungne and mind training were combined with one hundred prostrations and an incredible number of sutra and tantra prayers every day. The things that he did each day would have been inconceivable for an ordinary being to imagine.

Within six months he had a vision of Thousand-Armed Chenrezig surrounded by the five members of his mandala and many other forms of the deity. Ngulchu Thogme received Chenrezig's blessing and from then on he became inseparable from Chenrezig, and he generated a realization of emptiness and compassion that was indistinguishable from Chenrezig's.

A great contemporary master called Trewo Tokden, who was one of the primary disciples of the Third Karmapa, Rangjung Dorje, was well known for saying about Ngulchu Thogme, "When we refer to the Great Compassionate One (meaning Chenrezig), we are not really talking about the white figure that we paint on the walls of our monasteries. We are talking about someone who loves all beings as if each were his only child—someone who has mastered both emptiness and compassion like Bodhisattva Thogme."

He was someone who never looked into others' faults and shortcomings; rather he took them onto himself. No matter who it was, he spoke only about their virtues. He was never affected by the eight worldly dharmas.[14]

Because of the power of his loving-kindness and compassion, humans and nonhumans that came close to Ngulchu Thogme immediately calmed

14 The eight worldly dharmas are: gain and loss, praise and criticism, happiness and unhappiness, fame and disgrace.

down. This happened not only with domestic animals but also with wild animals and even predators; the watchdogs that attacked beggars became docile in his company, and the beggars who hated and feared them lost their fear. People who were involved in a dispute, or predators and their prey like cats and birds and sheep and wolves, would get along in his presence.

He continually perfected the six paramitas by giving away everything he owned, including the rug that he sat on and the clothing that he wore. In short, as the scriptural saying goes, "The genuine signs of bodhisattva beings are compassion, kind speech, dependability, generosity, profound wisdom, and the ability to explain the dharma in a definitive and authoritative way." Ngulchu Thogme exhibited every one of these qualities.

Whenever Ngulchu Thogme gave the bodhisattva vow, there were miraculous signs such as showers of flowers. On one occasion he made the following remark to his disciples: "During the days of Atisha and his spiritual son, Dromtonpa, the bodhisattva vow was bestowed somewhat restrictively and, as a result, since that time there have been very few who could bestow it and very few who have had the opportunity to generate bodhichitta. Now I shall lift that restriction, and henceforth those of you who are able to transmit the vow should do so."

His room and his clothing always bore the fragrant scent of moral discipline, and Ngulchu Thogme's disciples frequently saw him in the form of Chenrezig. He had complete control over dream yoga, mastery of the illusory body, and great supercognition. He gave monk vows and bodhisattva vows so often, he gave so many teachings, he wrote so many manuscripts, he spent so much of his life in isolated retreat, and so many of his disciples became siddhas, you would think that he had spent his entire life accomplishing any one of these things.

During his lifetime, all of the most renowned teachers of all the lineages throughout Tibet studied with Ngulchu Thogme. People from the Himalayan region, who spoke many different languages, came to learn from him. All those who came in contact with him, who saw him, heard him, thought of him, or touched him were ripened and brought to the state of liberation.

In the Year of the Bird, on the evening of the twentieth day of the ninth month, and in the midst of many miracles, Ngulchu Thogme dissolved into the heart of Chenrezig.

We will conclude the biographies of the masters of the Nyungne lineage with the life story of Ngulchu Thogme, who is probably the most famous holder of the lineage aside from Bhikshuni Lakshmi herself. This incredible, great bodhisattva had many disciples. He was the source of most of the popular Nyungne lineages which exist in Tibet today. We consider him the last member of the lineage not because it ended with him, but because he propagated it so widely that it is now part of all the lineages of Tibetan Buddhism.

One of his great lineage holders, Jo Den Konchok Zangpo, was the source of the Nyungne practice in the Karma Kagyu tradition. The author of the practice in another great tradition, the Jonang tradition, is Je Rigpa Dzinpa, and the original source of this tradition is the great bodhisattva Drakar Sonam Rinchen. His lineage eventually came down to Jamgon Kunga Drolchog and to Taranatha and so on. In this tradition all the biographies of the great masters are beyond description, and the blessings of the traditions are alive and unimpaired down to this day.

Those of you who want to know all the lineage holders can read the biographies of the individual masters. Many are difficult to find, therefore I have omitted biographies of the lineage holders after Bodhisattva Thogme.

KHENCHEN TASHI OZER

Khenchen Tashi Ozer is the author of our Nyungne text. Although I have never personally seen a biography of this great being, I will write something about him based on oral teachings and stories I heard from my precious enlightened guru, Dorje Chang Kalu Rinpoche.

Khenchen Tashi Ozer was a very great being. He lived in the nineteenth century, and he was still alive during the first decade of the twentieth century. He was very learned and a great master and a principal disciple of the completely enlightened nineteenth-century master Jamgon Kongtrul the Great. One can tell his greatness from Kongtrul the Great's writings. Every time he mentions Khenchen Tashi Ozer, he refers to him as the one who holds and preserves the three baskets.

Khenchen Tashi Ozer and Dorje Chang Kalu Rinpoche's father were spiritual siblings. They were both disciples of Jamgon Kongtrul the Great, and they had a very pure spiritual relationship. When Dorje Chang Kalu Rinpoche was born, Khenchen Tashi Ozer was in Kalu Rinpoche's father's home. He performed the traditional ceremony at birth, which involves hair cutting and water blessing similar to baptism.

The great Lama Norbu was the guru of my own enlightened guru, Dorje Chang Kalu Rinpoche. Khenchen Tashi Ozer was the principal guru of this completely enlightened teacher. Although the great Lama Norbu was known to have received teachings and empowerments directly from Jamgon Kongtrul the Great, he considered Khenchen Tashi Ozer to be his root guru.

Khenchen Tashi Ozer was an eminent lineage holder of the monk vow in the glorious Kagyu tradition. He was very much loved and respected by spiritual masters of his time. Furthermore, he was considered one of the greatest monks in the history of Tibet. Receiving vows from him was regarded as the same as receiving vows in a direct line from the Buddha; that means he had actually received the vow from Lord Buddha in the form of a vision.

Many different and illustrious lineages exist in our tradition, from the lineage of Mahamudra to the Bodhisattva lineage and the Monk lineage, as well as the Mahayana Eight-Precept lineage and the Nyungne lineage. For example, Jamgon Kongtrul the Great received his lineage of the mahayana eight-precept vow from a great Shangpa master, one of his root gurus, Karma Shenphen Ozer. This master was a true mahasiddha. He was even known to miraculously fly on occasion.

In addition to being a distinguished lineage holder of the monk vow, I think Khenchen Tashi Ozer should be in the lineage of Nyungne as well. In our Nyungne text, the "Lineage Prayer" is not up to date, and several lineage holders following the writing of the text are missing. I think we must add the names of those lineage masters. In my opinion, Khenchen Tashi Ozer, the great Lama Norbu, and Dorje Chang Kalu Rinpoche should be included; that will bring the lineage up to date.

AN INSPIRATIONAL STORY

I will tell you another story, which actually has nothing to do with Nyungne; a story about Khenchen Tashi Ozer that I think is very inspiring. He was known for living the life of a wandering yogi, traveling from place to place with no particular aim. This is called the natural, uncontrived act of a yogi. He had a companion, and on their journey they sometimes had difficulties because they ran out of provisions. When they met people, Khenchen was always modest and humble; when people asked who they were, he would always say, "Oh, we're just old folks from somewhere."

On one occasion when they were having difficulties, they came across some people and as usual he told them that he was nobody. His companion became very upset and said, "Why are you not telling the truth? That's a lie. If you would tell the truth, people would help us and make some offerings." Supposedly his companion fought with him like that, and then that evening his companion had swollen balls and he had some pain, and that was that.

The next day they met some people, and again the people asked who they were, and Khenchen said, "Well, my name is Khenchen Tashi Ozer, and he's my companion, and his name is so-and-so, and we came from so-and-so, and last night we stayed in such and such place, and during the night he had a ball problem, and his balls were swollen and he had lots of pain. Today we're here, and from here we're going to such and such place." So he told the whole story. His companion became very angry and said, "Why do you have to tell all those stories?" And he replied, "You told me to tell the truth, so I told the truth."

I felt like sharing this story with you because to me it is quite wonderful and illustrates the natural behavior of a great master, and I heard it from my enlightened guru.

Section Two

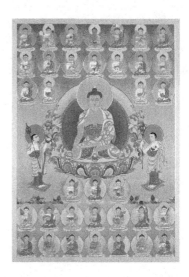

Praises to the Buddha, The Twelve Deeds 4

"THE TWELVE DEEDS of the Buddha" is the first prayer we recite during Nyungne practice. The twelve deeds are the twelve major activities of Lord Buddha:

- Descending from Tushita Heaven
- Entering into his mother's womb
- Birth in the garden of Lumbini
- Training in the sciences
- Achievement in sports competition
- Enjoying the palace and marriage
- Renouncing the life of a prince
- Practicing austerity for six years, then renouncing that
- Obtaining victory over the maras
- Enlightenment under the bodhi tree
- Turning the wheel of dharma
- And passing into parinirvana

Without a doubt, the coming of Lord Buddha was an extraordinary event. Such extraordinariness, of course, only occurs once in a while. An understanding of how such an event takes place is beyond ordinary comprehension. Only a completely enlightened being can understand the magnitude of such an event. Different Buddhist traditions have different understandings of this extraordinary activity of the Buddha. From the point of view of the mahayana tradition, Lord Buddha came to the world as a tenth-bhumi bodhisattva. He simply had to make the final transition to perfection, which is the eleventh bhumi, complete buddhahood.

Although, biographically speaking, Buddha seemed to experience all the events of normal samsaric life, actually all those activities were for specific enlightened reasons. "The Twelve Deeds of the Buddha" is an explanation of these activities from the mahayana perspective.

Prior to coming to the earth, our Lord Buddha is said to have been preaching to the gods in the heavenly realm of Tushita, a realm where fortunate beings are able to receive precious dharma teachings and practice. Our only Lord, Shakyamuni Buddha's, spiritual aspiration and accumulation of countless lifetimes of spiritual merit all came to complete fruition for him to become the perfect Buddha. As the time approached, buddhas of the ten directions inspired him to take the final step in order to benefit all sentient beings. It was heard in the form of music in the sky, which was the sound of the original prophecy made by Buddha Mar Me Dze (Skt. Tathagata Dipamkara) that he would become Shakyamuni Buddha.

In the *Perfection of Wisdom Sutra in Eight Thousand Lines*, the prophecy is recalled by Lord Buddha as follows:

> So it is, O Gods! So do I, when I met a tathagata, Dipamkara, in the bazaar of Dipavati, the royal city, possess the fullness of this perfection of wisdom, so Dipamkara, a tathagata, predicted one day I am to be fully enlightened, and said to me, "You, young Brahmin, in this future period, after incalculable aeons, become a tathagata, Shakyamuni by name, endowed with knowledge and virtue, Well-Gone, a world-knower, unsurpassed, tamer of beings to be tamed, teacher of gods and people, a Buddha, a Blessed Lord!"[15]

Lord Buddha was reigning in Tushita Heaven as spiritual leader and crowned prince, so he gave the spiritual responsibility and crown to Maitreya Bodhisattva and prophesied that he would be the next Buddha. He then decided to descend to earth from the heavenly realm. His descent took place with five specific observations regarding the location, the caste, the father, the mother, and the time. All five aspects were correct and appropriate, so he came down to the world and entered into the mother's womb. While his mother was observing the sojong vow and dreaming of a white baby elephant with six tusks, the Buddha entered her womb.

The entire pregnancy was an extremely pleasant experience for his

---

15   Translated into English by Richard Babcock (Copper), http://www.fodian.net/world/0228.html.

mother, and her mind was filled with tremendous joy. It is believed that Buddha's own experience in the womb was none other than that of dwelling in a precious palace. He spent ten months in the womb as a symbolic representation of completing the tenth-bhumi level of a bodhisattva. When the time came, his mother traveled from the palace toward her parent's home, the traditional place to give birth. On the way, she stopped in a forest in Lumbini and spontaneously placed her hand on the branch of a tree. The time was right and Buddha miraculously came out from under her right arm without causing her the slightest discomfort.

As soon as Buddha was born, gods and heavenly beings offered him special baths. As a symbol of a great bodhisattva leaning always toward the four immeasurables,[16] he took seven steps in each of the four directions. With each step a natural lotus flower spontaneously arose. In addition, the time of Buddha's birth coincided with the rising of a special star named Gyal (Skt. Tisya, Lat. Cancri). Then Lord Buddha was known to have pointed his finger up toward the sky and say, "I am the supreme being in the world." At that exact moment, all kinds of flowers blossomed in the forest of Lumbini, the earth gently shook, and the sky lit up in a golden color.

It is recorded in the Tibetan history book *The Blue Annals*[17] that the Emperor of China and his wise men were looking toward the west at that time, and they saw an unusual, golden color in the sky. Amazed by the sky's appearance, the Emperor consulted a wise man who was a great astrologer. The astrologer did a chart that indicated a perfect being had been born in the west, and the sky's golden color was the aura of that perfect being. According to *The Blue Annals*, this occurred in the Year of the Male Wood Tiger.

It is also known that Buddha's father consulted an ascetic wise man who told him, "This child is a remarkable child. If the child renounces the kingdom, he will become a buddha, and if he remains in the royal kingdom, he will rule the world." Buddha's father, not knowing the complete implication of what it means to be Buddha, hoped his wonderful

16 The four immeasurables are: May all beings have happiness and the cause of happiness, may all beings not have suffering and the cause of suffering, may all beings never be without supreme bliss which is free from all suffering, and may all beings live in the great equanimity which is free from all attachment and aversion.

17 *The Blue Annals* is a famous history book written by a great master, Geu Lo Shun Nu Pal.

son would become the ruler of the world. Seven days following the birth, Buddha's birth mother passed away, and he was nursed by thirty-two surrogate mothers.

Buddha studied a wide range of subjects such as the arts, letters, and sciences with many teachers. He was known to have surpassed all of them. At the proper time, his father consulted his advisors regarding a suitable partner for his son. They unanimously recommended that he marry one of the Shakya clan. However, Buddha stated that he was going to marry a very special woman, one who was free from the five defects and possessed the eight qualities. The father was concerned that he might not be able to find such a woman. Nevertheless, he sent a search party to look for a woman who fulfilled these requirements, and they finally found one. She was the daughter of a skilled archer. Buddha's father asked for her hand and, amazingly, the daughter's father refused saying, "My daughter shall marry someone with talent in archery, and since your son is a royal prince who has no such skill, the marriage will not work."

The king was very disappointed at this refusal to comply with his request. Buddha saw that his father was sad and came forward to ask him the cause. The father then told him what had happened. Buddha assured him there was no problem; he would compete with everybody in all areas of sports. Hearing him speak with such confidence, his father was very proud and he organized a huge competition to take place. During the competition, Buddha competed in every sport and was hugely victorious in them all. Archery was the final event. All the skilled archers placed their targets at a certain distance. The daughter's father placed his target farther than anyone, and everyone hit their target. Then it was Buddha's turn, and he placed his target even farther away, right in front of a line of nine sandalwood trees. When he shot his arrow it hit the target, penetrating through all nine sandalwood trees, and then disappeared into the ground. Spring water came out of that spot in the ground and became a small pond. There was no question as to who was the victor.

Buddha then married the archer's daughter as a skillful means to silence those heretics who might accuse him of being a eunuch. His wife later gave birth to Buddha's son. In this manner he dwelled in the royal palace and enjoyed marriage and his life as a prince.

Celestial sound in the form of music reminded him to completely abandon ordinary life, and he understood it to be the result of his former resolve to seek enlightenment. As a consequence, Buddha went outside the palace and saw the suffering of birth, old age, illness, and death. Finally he saw a perfectly peaceful monk meditating, and he said, "That's what I want to be." He made a solemn commitment to renounce his present life and to seek a solution to all suffering.

His father was afraid Buddha would leave the kingdom, so he ordered guards to guard him day and night. On the last day, Buddha went to his father and honorably asked his permission to leave the kingdom. His father would not give his permission. This being the case, it became obvious that he had no choice. That evening, Buddha blessed the guards and they all fell asleep. Accompanied by one of his attendants, he flew from the palace upon a horse with the help of four guardian kings. In the presence of Nam Da Stupa, he shaved his own hair and ordained himself by abandoning all ordinary clothing and putting on the robes of a monk.

Initially he followed two great ascetics and practiced austerity for six years. At the end of the sixth year, although he had achieved the highest meditative stabilization possible in samsara, he realized that he still remained *in* samsara. He knew that he had to go beyond. At that precise moment, buddhas and bodhisattvas encouraged him to move on from the inferior path to the path of complete enlightenment, so he rose out of his six years of practicing austerity, demonstrating to his ascetic teachers that they too were still bound by samsara.

When Buddha renounced his practice of austerity, his five followers were all disappointed in him for having given up, and they decided to go to Varanasi. Buddha went toward Bodhgaya as he had been encouraged to do. On the way, two girls named Nanda and Nandabala offered him milk and honey that they had prepared from the milk of one thousand cows. After partaking of this drink, the Buddha turned a golden color.

In Bodhgaya, Indra incarnated as the grass merchant Svastika. Buddha took some grass from him and prepared a mat for himself. He sat on the mat at the foot of the bodhi tree and promised to sit there steadfastly until reaching complete enlightenment. At dusk, he entered into a meditative absorption called "destruction of the forces of maras."

As his power of meditation reached everywhere, the king of the maras came in the form of a messenger and told him, "The town of Kapilavastu has been captured by Devadatta and the palace has been ransacked and all the Shakyas were murdered. What are you doing here?"

Buddha answered, "I'm here in order to attain perfect enlightenment."

And then Mara replied, "In order to attain perfect enlightenment, you must have enormous accumulation of merit. You, a prince who just enjoys the royal life, how can you attain such an accumulation?"

Buddha said, "You know, you have merely done some ritual prayers and practices, and because of that you've been born as a powerful mara in the god realm. I have accumulated two types of merit for countless numbers of eons; why wouldn't I become a perfect, enlightened being?"

Mara responded by saying, "If that is so, then there has to be a witness to such accomplishment. Where is your witness?"

And the Buddha touched his extraordinary hand to the ground: "The earth is my witness." As soon as he said that, the Goddess of the Earth, gold in color, rose halfway out of the ground. Holding a handful of miniscule particles, she told Mara, "I could count each and every one of the particles in my hand, but I could not count how many times this great being has sacrificed his head and limbs for the benefit of others. It is certainly the time for him to become a completely enlightened being." So saying, she disappeared.

Mara was very upset, and he went back and brought a whole army to attack Buddha. Since Buddha was a completely realized being, none of the attacks could affect him; and since not even the slightest trace of hate existed in him, with his enormous power of compassion all the weapons were transformed and came to him in the form of flowers, and all the horrific sounds came in the form of music. Again Mara tried to seduce Lord Buddha by appearing in the form of seven beautiful women. Since Buddha had overcome all desire, Mara was not able to cause even the tiniest speck of desire to arise in him. On the contrary, those beautiful female apparitions all transformed into seven hags and made confessions before him. Buddha forgave them all.

At midnight it was time for him to enter into meditation, and at dawn Buddha became a perfect, enlightened being. At that moment, the earth gently shook again and a lunar eclipse occurred. It was the full moon day of Vaisakha, the fourth month of the lunar calendar.

Immediately after his enlightenment, Buddha began to preach but nobody understood; the time was not right, therefore nobody could hear his teaching. He decided to go into silence for seven weeks. After seven weeks, Brahma and Indra made a special request that Buddha teach. Brahma offered Buddha a thousand-spoked golden wheel, and Indra offered a special white conch shell that spiraled clockwise. Buddha then saw that it was time to turn the wheel of dharma. At that exact moment, the sound of Buddha's preaching could be heard throughout the entire universe.

Buddha walked toward Varanasi knowing that because of aspiration prayers and virtuous karma coming together, his five followers were to become his first disciples. These five had originally been sent to accompany and look after him, three of them being from his father's side and two of them from his mother's side. They were disappointed when Buddha gave up his austerities, and they thought he had failed. Now they told themselves that since he had lost his courage, they were not going to show him any respect. As Buddha was approaching them, because of his enormous power they couldn't help but go to receive him. Once they had received him, they couldn't help but bow to him and ask for teaching.

Together with the five disciples, some eighty thousand gods came to listen to the Buddha teach. Then Lord Buddha gave the first sermon, which was on the Four Noble Truths. Upon hearing the teaching three times, all five disciples became arhats. This was the first turning of the wheel of dharma.

The second turning of the wheel of dharma, on the doctrine of emptiness, took place on Vulture Peak Mountain in Rajgir. Among the disciples were some five thousand arhats, five hundred fully ordained nuns, and many, many lay practitioners, in addition to celestial beings such as gods, nagas, and gandharvas. These were common disciples. The extraordinary disciples were the many, many great bodhisattvas.

The third turning of the wheel was primarily on the tantric doctrines, but there were numerous sutra teachings included in these sermons as well. They took place in southern India and several other realms such as the god realms, the naga realms, and so on. In the audience were great bodhisattvas, monks, nuns, gods, nagas, and many, many other fortunate beings.

Buddha was thirty-five when he attained enlightenment, and altogether he taught for forty-five years. At the age of eighty, knowing that his time here on earth was coming to an end, he said to Ananda, "If there are those who wish to truly practice, I would live for eons and eons." Buddha repeated that three times. But because of the influence of maras, Ananda was unable to hear and so he never thought to make requests for Buddha to live a long life. Buddha could see that there was nothing more he could do. Then an emanation of Mara appeared and requested him to leave. Buddha promised to leave in three months.

During this period of time, those beings who were to be tamed by Buddha were tamed, and those who were to be benefited, he benefited. Then he went to Kushinagar. There he told his fellow disciples to look at this perfect form of a tathagata, it is as rare as the udumbara flower;[18] and he told them that all composite phenomena are subject to decay. There, in order to inspire those beings who are lazy, he demonstrated that even the perfect

18 The udumbara flower is said to bloom only when Buddha is in the world.

body of the Buddha also passes into nirvana. He lay down in the posture of a sleeping lion. At that very moment the entire trichiliocosmic system shook. For seven days, offerings were made by gods and men. Afterwards Buddha's body was prepared for cremation by his fellow disciples, and it spontaneously burned and innumerable round relics appeared. Those relics were divided into eight portions and distributed to eight regions to be put into stupas.[19]

Those who lived at the time of the Buddha were so fortunate. Usually, just by hearing the Buddha's teachings they were liberated. He cannot be compared to any historical human. The extraordinariness of Buddha is only really understood by enlightened beings. From the point of view of the vajrayana, tantric tradition, Buddha was already a completely enlightened being when he came to the world. The tantric definition is difficult to understand for an ordinary being. Nevertheless this understanding is considered the ultimate understanding.

Lord Buddha is without a doubt the greatest being ever to walk on the face of the earth. No beings even come close to his level of perfection. My point in saying this is to properly convey the magnitude of the event of the Buddha coming to the world, so that those who have faith will perhaps appreciate this fact a little more and become less complacent with life, practice diligently, and make their human life meaningful.

19 It is still possible to see these relics today.

Thirty-five Buddhas
Confession Prayer 5

THIS CONFESSION PRAYER is very well known in the Tibetan Buddhist tradition. Among English-speaking Buddhist followers, it is commonly referred to as the "Thirty-five Buddhas Confession Prayer." The Thirty-five Buddhas (Fig. 1) are special confession buddhas who, while bodhisattvas, made special vows to assist others to overcome their negativities. Its actual title is the *Sutra of Three Heaps*. This sutra can be divided into three different sections; these three sections are referred to as three heaps. The first heap is homage by prostration to the Thirty-five Buddhas. The second heap is confession. The third is the heap of dedication. The four powers and the "Seven-Branch Prayer" are also included in the sutra.

THE THREE HEAPS

First Heap: Homage by Prostration

The heap of homage by prostration is done by imagining each and every one of the Thirty-five Buddhas and then physically or mentally bowing to them. Although the prayer starts with the words "I and all sentient beings perpetually take refuge in the Guru," and then "take refuge in Buddha, Dharma, and Sangha," taking refuge in the guru is not part of the original sutra. It was added by Tibetan masters because of their tantric Buddhist influence. The guru is key to very directly reaching all the buddhas, therefore this spiritual understanding is cherished by tantric masters very much.

While sincerely prostrating physically or mentally, you imagine and recite the names of each of the Thirty-five Buddhas. The main focus of your prayer is the Thirty-five Buddhas, but you must also visualize these buddhas surrounded by the buddhas of the ten directions.

Second Heap: Confession

The second heap of the confession prayer begins right after the homage to the Thirty-five Buddhas. When you begin to recite these words of confession, you must think and speak the prayers while openly admitting that these wrong deeds are your faults in your own samsaric history. These lines of prayer perfectly help us to express all our shortcomings. By saying these lines and identifying with them, you will have made a complete confession. Without these perfect prayers, even if we knew that lots of things must have been wrong in our past and we wanted to do something about it, we wouldn't know how to do it. The prayer clearly defines all the wrong deeds, in which we were directly involved, and those that we influenced others to do, as well as those that we rejoiced in from time without beginning, in all our previous lives. You will want to completely confess all the major deeds, from the five deeds that ripen immediately to the ten unvirtuous deeds, and all other deeds which may be obstacles to your spiritual progress, so that you can overcome them once and for all. By the way, according to bodhisattva doctrine, those who took bodhisattva vows are supposed to recite the "Thirty-five Buddhas Confession Prayer" three times each day.

All of our wrongdoings are basically caused by the three poisons. In the sutra, Shariputra asks Lord Buddha whether or not bodhisattvas[20] could be damaged by the three poisons. In response, Lord Buddha tells him that bodhisattvas could have two major violations and one minor violation. Hatred and stupidity are considered major, and desire is considered a minor violation. Although desire is considered minor, it is harder to overcome, whereas hatred is considered major but is easier to overcome. Stupidity on the other hand is both major and difficult to overcome. There is further teaching by Lord Buddha. If a major violation through desire occurs, then one must confess in the presence of ten bodhisattvas. Mediocre violations should be confessed in the presence of five bodhisattvas. A minor violation should be confessed in the presence of one or two bodhisattvas. With respect to violations by hatred or stupidity, the object of confession has to be doubled, meaning four bodhisattvas. Lord Buddha continued, a major

20 Bodhisattvas who are discussed here are basically those who took bodhisattva vows, not necessarily enlightened bodhisattva beings.

violation of a combination of all three poisons together, such as the five sins that ripen immediately and so on, can be overcome by confession to the Thirty-five Buddhas and buddhas of the ten directions.

Furthermore, anything and everything can be overcome by sincerely reciting the confession prayer and imagining that the Thirty-five Buddhas and all the buddhas of the ten directions are really there, and by being completely present yourself with total faith, devotion, remorse, humility, and complete conviction in wanting to overcome everything for the benefit of all sentient beings.

Third Heap: Dedication

The third heap is the heap of dedication. Right after the promise to never commit the wrongdoings again is a request for all the glorious, victorious buddhas to be gracious to you. That is the beginning of the dedication prayer. The first part of the dedication prayer is dedicating whatever conditional merit you have accumulated in this life and all lives from time without beginning, such as the virtuous deeds of generosity, morality, patience, rejoicing at the virtuous deeds of others, etc. Next we dedicate the deeds associated with bodhisattva virtue: aspiration bodhichitta, which is motivation to liberate all sentient beings, and application bodhichitta, such as engaging in the practice of the six perfections and all the other bodhisattva practices of the Great Vehicle. The practice of unsurpassable wisdom is also dedicated, which is the result of meditation.

Although dedication sounds like a simple spiritual idea, actually it is a very profound subject. As much as you have an enlightened intention to help all sentient beings and to attain perfect enlightenment, you would still not be able to do a perfect dedication on your own. Therefore it is very important to emulate all the enlightened buddhas of the past, present, and future and dedicate as they do. This Thirty-five Buddhas prayer has a perfect dedication prayer in it, and our responsibility is to recite the prayer with heartfelt sincerity.[21]

The last part of the prayer is in verse form; it was added by Tibetan masters and was not part of the original sutra. These lines of prayer are to reiterate your confession, and in addition to that there is a short seven-branch prayer.

---

21 For a more complete discussion of dedication, see "The Seventh Branch Prayer, Dedication of Merit" in Chapter 7.

THE FOUR POWERS

Power of Reliance

For true purification to take place, the most important aspect is to make confession with the four purifying powers, all of which are included in this confession prayer. The first power is referred to as the power of reliance. In order to overcome any wrongdoings you must have help, but this must be an ultimate help. Such help comes only from completely enlightened beings. The buddhas are the sources of purification, and you must completely believe in them and take refuge in them and develop bodhichitta. If you do that, then you have a correct power of reliance.

Power of Remorse

The second is the power of remorse. This power is essential for overcoming negativities, because without remorse there is no sincerity or serious intent to overcome the wrongdoings. Some who lack a proper understanding of the entire situation of samsara may feel they haven't done anything wrong. Others would like to reject the idea of being a sinner. Actually the Buddhist understanding is that there's nothing wrong with you fundamentally; as a matter of fact you have a perfect nature. Through confusion and illusion some mistakes have been made, and as a result they are causing you lots of unpleasant pain and suffering. You regret all those karmic mistakes very much, and you truly wish to overcome them. Jamgon Kongtrul the Great writes that just like the person who swallows poison and deeply regrets his mistake and desperately tries to get rid of it, similarly we should feel great remorse for our wrongdoings. That's what the power of remorse is all about.

Power of Remedy

The third is the power of remedy. Many different remedies for overcoming our negativities exit in tantric Buddhism. The general remedy is Vajrasattva practice and recitation of the One-Hundred-Syllable Mantra. Another method is Niguma's purification with the letter AH, which is an extraordinary and powerful practice. In this case, the "Thirty-five Buddhas Confession Prayer" is a remedy, and Nyungne practice as a whole is a very powerful purification practice.

Power of Commitment

The fourth is the power of the commitment to never engage in wrongdoing again. This power of commitment is necessary because without such commitment you will engage in negativities again. The main reason for not being able to overcome negativities is lack of seriousness and sincerity; the commitment must be a really powerful one from the bottom of your heart, otherwise all the other powers will be lacking as well. It has been said that you must make a vow that you will not commit wrongdoings again even at the cost of your own life. If you make such a commitment, then you can absolutely overcome any wrongdoing.

If you apply these four powers correctly, and you say the "Thirty-five Buddhas Confession Prayer" properly and do Nyungne practice sincerely, you can absolutely overcome all the karma and become completely free and liberated beings like the buddhas of the past, present, and future.

The Vows of Nyungne 6

THE EIGHT-PRECEPTS VOW

THE GENERAL eight-precepts vow is for lay people, and Buddhists of all traditions customarily take the vow every month on new moon and full moon days. Some lay practitioners take the vow on half moon days as well. The basic vows are taken for a twenty-four-hour period and, according to scripture, this period should be from sunrise to sunrise. There is also mention in a sutra of the precepts being taken for life; taking it for periods of months or years is therefore automatically understood. Taking all eight precepts is the highest vow possible for lay people. The novice monk and nun vows, all the way to the fully ordained monk and nun vows, are actually further elaborations of these eight vows.[22]

While the eight precepts are the same, there is a slight difference between taking the general eight precepts and the mahayana eight precepts, which is referred to as the Restoring and Purifying Ordination. The mahayana eight-precepts vow is taken by spiritual practitioners on the path of the Great Vehicle (mahayana). Taken in the context of the mahayana tradition, you are not only making a commitment to abide by the vow, but you are also making a completely enlightened commitment, meaning a bodhisattva commitment. This vow is aspiration bodhichitta, meaning generating the enlightened aspiration to benefit all sentient beings, and you must receive it from an authentic teacher within the lineage of the vow. Once you have received it from an authentic teacher, you can take the vow by yourself from then on. Although the commitment of preserving the eight precepts is only for a period of twenty-four hours, the aspiration bodhichitta

22 See "The Eight Vows of the Restoring and Purifying Ordination" later in this chapter.

associated with it will remain until your enlightenment; that is, if you do not violate the aspiration bodhichitta.

There are two ways of violating aspiration bodhichitta: first, by adopting an attitude that is contrary to bodhisattva principles, and second, by abandoning sentient beings. Adopting an attitude that is contrary to bodhisattva principles means that, for whatever reason, you somehow come to the conclusion that you cannot take on the responsibility of helping all sentient beings. "I would rather work for my own salvation," is your thinking. This is adopting an attitude according to the Lower Vehicle. If you do this, you violate the vow. Abandoning sentient beings means abandoning any single sentient being. For whatever reason, you exclude and abandon a particular person by saying, "I will never ever help this person, even if there comes a day that he or she needs my help." That is all it takes to violate the wonderful bodhisattva vow, because nobody abandons all sentient beings; it is always that one single being that everybody so easily singles out.

THE SOJONG VOW

In the context of Nyungne, the vow obviously involves much more than either the general eight-precepts vow or the mahayana vow; Nyungne practice includes twenty-four-hour fasting and silence as well. The vow at the Nyungne level, called the Sojong Vow, is supremely extraordinary because the benefits are compounded. You have the benefit of taking the eight-precepts vow in general, which is already a very, very special vow; it is the vow to abstain from harming other sentient beings. And then, when you take these eight precepts in the context of the mahayana Restoring and Purifying Ordination, it becomes a truly great vow; in addition to abstaining from harming others, one's commitment is to benefit others. When you take this vow in the context of Nyungne, it becomes supremely extraordinary, because you are showing true spiritual commitment by engaging in the superior tantric practices of creation and completion and recitation of the supreme mantra, and by being willing to fast and so on, for a supreme purpose. That is why the eight-precepts vow, in the context of Nyungne practice, is an extraordinarily superior vow. Finally, an important point to remember is that all the great benefits of the vow derive not just from taking the vow, but more importantly, from keeping the vow.

Now we will go through the actual vow taken at the beginning of our Nyungne practice, the Sojong Vow. Before taking the vow, you must visualize Chenrezig in the sky right in front of you, and think that he is the embodiment of the Three Jewels and Three Roots, surrounded by all the buddhas and bodhisattvas. In their presence, you must prostrate three times with the thought of making the seven-branch prayer offering. Prostration is performed by folding your hands in front of your heart while thinking you have a precious jewel between them, and then raising your hands to touch the crown of your head, your throat, and your heart area. You bow down by touching your knees, hands, and forehead to the floor. This is called "five points touching the ground."[23]

After the prostrations, you should kneel with your right knee down and your left knee up and fold your hands. Kneeling with hands folded is a symbolic posture to demonstrate your utmost respect and sincerity. Then you recite the actual prayer, following your teacher:

ཕྱོགས་བཅུ་ན་བཞུགས་པའི་སངས་རྒྱས་དང་བྱང་ཆུབ་སེམས་དཔའ་

CH'OK CHU NA   SH'UK PEI   SANG GYE DANG   JANG CH'UB SEM PA

the ten directions   residing in   buddhas and   bodhisattvas

ཐམས་ཅད་བདག་ལ་དགོངས་སུ་གསོལ།

T'AM CHE   DAG LA   GONG SU SOL

all   to me   be gracious

*All the buddhas and bodhisattvas residing in the
ten directions, please be gracious to me.*

Your teacher as well as Chenrezig and all these buddhas and bodhisattvas are your witnesses, and when you kneel down and make a commitment to abide by the eight precepts in their presence, it becomes something extremely precious. All the enlightened beings will be delighted because, as far as virtuous deeds are concerned, you are doing something exactly correct. It has been said that the buddhas and bodhisattvas will take a great deal of joy in your doing something truly right, just as parents are extremely happy if their child, who does so many things wrong all the time, finally does something right!

---

23 See "Benefits of the Prostrations" in Chapter 10 for further discussion of prostration.

ཇི་ལྟར་སྔོན་གྱི་དེ་བཞིན་གཤེགས་པ་དགྲ་བཅོམ་པ་

JI TAR   NGON GYI   DE SH'IN SHEK PA   DRA CHOM PA
just as   previous   tathagatas   arhats

ཡང་དག་པར་རྫོགས་པའི་སངས་རྒྱས་

YANG DAG PAR   DZOK PE   SANG GYE

perfectly pure complete   buddha

Just as the previous tathagatas, arhats, perfectly pure
and accomplished buddhas,

Tathagatas is a Sanskrit word for "ones thus gone." The meaning of "thus" is "thusness," which has to do with the essence of phenomena being of the nature of emptiness, the dharmata. "Gone" has to do with having arrived at the place of completely pure wisdom. Arhats are conquerors and foe destroyers. Here the idea of conqueror is from an ultimate sense, and does not refer to the insight of an arhat level of being; "conqueror" because afflictive emotions are the source of all negativities. The foe is ignorant ego-clinging, and this is overcome by the wisdom understanding the nonexistence of ego. This understanding is vajralike wisdom, which destroys all the foes and therefore is an ultimate conqueror. "Perfectly pure" refers to perfect accumulation of merit and wisdom. Perfect accumulation of merit and wisdom is complete accomplishment; therefore, buddhas are completely accomplished beings who possess all the qualities mentioned above.

རྟ་ཆང་ཤེས་ལྟ་བུ།

TA CHANG SHE   TA BU

the heavenly steed who are like

who are like the Heavenly Steed

The example of heavenly steed is taken from a mythical spiritual story. Long ago there was a captain named Senge (Lion). Captain Senge, with five hundred of his fellow men, went out on the mighty ocean and they became lost. They found themselves on an island full of flesh-eating demons. While there, all these men inbred with the demons and had many offspring. One day Captain Senge wandered off and came upon an area entirely encircled by black iron walls, and he saw a man who was an emanation of a god from the thirty-three gods realm. This emanation told the captain, "The beings here are flesh-eating demons, and they will put all of you inside this iron circle, and then you will be eaten." The captain asked him, "Is there any way out of this?" And the god's emanation said, "Yes, there is. In the middle month of spring, on the full moon day, a horse named Wise Heavenly Steed will come from the thirty-three gods realm, and with his wings he will fly like a bird to this island to eat the grass and drink the water and to roll around in the precious gem-sand beach. Then he will speak and make an announcement, saying "Oh, those who wish to go to the mainland, you should ride on my back and hold on to the hair on my body, mane, and tail, and if you do not look back, through my miraculous power you will be free." Having heard this story, the captain told it to his fellow men, and they all gathered around the lake where Heavenly Steed was supposed to arrive. He arrived as foretold and most of the men managed to ride this horse, and through the horse's miraculous power they made it to freedom. While this was happening, all the demons ran after them, crying, and those who looked back because of their attachment to them didn't make it out of there and were eaten.

Just as the wise heavenly steed liberates beings, Buddha the Conqueror liberates beings from samsaric pain, suffering, fear, and all kinds of turmoil.

 གླང་པོ་ཆེན་པོ

LANG PO   CH'EN PO

the elephant   great

and the Great Elephant,

The great elephant is an example of a conqueror. There is a story that a supreme elephant known as Sala Rab Ten supposedly exists in the thirty-three gods realm. This elephant has a gargantuan body, many miles long, and thirty-three heads. With this elephant, the gods are able to defeat the demi-gods. When they go to battle, the story goes, Vishnu, the king of the god realm, rides on the main head, and all the other leaders of the god realm ride on top of the other thirty-two heads. Many, many ordinary gods ride on its body like soldiers. The elephant's trunk is in the form of a weapon, and when they are at war with the demi-gods, the gods are always victorious and successfully defeat the demi-gods because of this powerful elephant, as well as because of their superior karma.

Similarly, victorious buddhas are successful in defeating all the foes. These foes are the four demons: the demon of afflictive emotions, the demon of skandhas, the demon of Deva Putra (the son of god), and the demon of death. Afflictive emotions are demons because they keep one constantly occupied within the realm of ego, attachment, and aversion. Skandhas are also demons, because as long as we experience skandhas we are stuck in samsara with a samsaric form body, feelings, and so on. This is an obstacle that prevents us from experiencing anything else. The demon of Deva Putra (son of god) is the temptation of attachment and desire which prevents us from freeing ourselves from the world. Death is a demon because as long as we exist in samsara, we are continually tormented by death, and death is unavoidable because in samsara, through karma, sentient beings take birth in one form or another and therefore experience death.

According to the hinayana tradition, even Shakyamuni Buddha had not relinquished the demon of death, which was believed to be the final demon, until he entered into mahaparinirvana in Kushinagar. This is not the understanding of mahayana or tantric traditions as to what Buddha is and how he overcame all the demons.

|བྱ་བ་བྱས་ཤིང་| |བྱེད་པ་བྱས་པ|

JA WA   JE SHING   JE PA   JE PA

action done   doer deed

accomplished in the past what had to be done,

This describes what buddhas in the past did, how they trained in moral and ethical principles, how they practiced meditative absorptions, and how they trained completely in wisdom awareness. Through this training, they accomplished the two bodies. The two bodies here refer to the dharmakaya attained for one's own purpose, and the rupakaya attained for the benefit of others. Rupakaya includes the sambhogakaya and nirmanakaya, which are both form bodies. The distinction between these form bodies is only the difference between subtle versus gross form, but they are both form bodies. Therefore, "two bodies" refers to 1) benefiting self and 2) benefiting others, and includes all the manifestations of various form bodies.

།ཁུར་བོར་བ།

K'UR BOR WA

load (burden) lay down

just as they laid down the burden,

"Burden" here refers to the skandhas, afflictive emotions, and so on. All these have been eliminated.

།རང་གི་དོན་རྗེས་སུ་ཐོབ་པ།

RANG GI DON JE SU T'OB PA

one's own   subsequently attained   welfare

subsequently attained their own welfare,

This means in the trainee stage of the path, a bodhisattva being takes complete responsibility to help others. Subsequently, at the stage of no more training, one achieves a dharmakaya buddha body, the perfect qualities of which benefit others spontaneously.

།སྲིད་པ་ཀུན་ཏུ་སྦྱོར་བ་ཡོངས་སུ་ཟད་པ།

SI PA KUN TU JOR WA YONG SU ZE PA

existence all bonds completely relinquished

and completely relinquished all bonds to the possibilities of existence;

Existence in samsara is due to a continuous chain of many causes and conditions. The root causes are desire, hatred, pride, ignorance, doubt, wrong view, holding on to supreme view, jealousy, and miserliness. ("Supreme view" means taking a theistic view as superior to all views.) All these have been overcome.

།ཡང་དག་པའི་བཀའ།

YANG DAG PEI KA

really pure speech   (command)

their speech is completely pure,

Completely pure speech is perfect speech, speech that liberates all beings to omniscient buddhahood. It is the verbal speech, blessing speech, and authorized speech.

།ལེགས་པར་རྣམ་པར་གྲོལ་བའི་ཐུགས།

LEK PAR   NAM PAR DROL WE   T'UG

excellent completely liberated mind

their minds are completely liberated,

Perfect liberation is the quality of Buddha's mind, the perfect relinquishment of all that needs to be relinquished; mind that is free from any stains of affliction or obstruction to omniscience.

།ལེགས་པར་རྣམ་པར་གྲོལ་བའི་ཤེས་རབ་ཅན་དེ་རྣམས་ཀྱིས།

LEK PAR   NAM PAR DROL WEI   SHE RAB CHEN   DE NAM KYI

excellent   completely liberated   possessing transcending   they   knowledge

possessing the completely liberated transcendental knowledge;

In the presence of complete relinquishment, there is a completely perfected wisdom understanding of the emptiness nature of self and phenomena.

།སེམས་ཅན་ཐམས་ཅད་ཀྱི་དོན་གྱི་ཕྱིར་དང་།

SEM CHEN   T'AM CHE KYI   DON GYI   CH'IR DANG

beings   all   reason purpose and

just as, for the sake of all beings,

"Just as" refers to buddhas of the past who have completely relinquished what needs to be relinquished and completely attained what needs to be attained acting for the sake of all beings.

།ཕན་པར་བྱ་བའི་ཕྱིར་དང་།

P'EN PAR   JA WEI   CH'IR DANG

benefit   work purpose and

to benefit them,

This has to do with how buddhas temporarily benefit sentient beings by liberating them from the pain and suffering of samsara, and how they ultimately liberate them from samsara.

ཁྲོལ་བར་བྱ་བའི་ཕྱིར་དང་།

DROL WAR   JA WEI   CH'IR DANG

liberate   work purpose and

to liberate them,

ནད་མེད་པར་བྱ་བའི་ཕྱིར་དང་།

NE   ME   PAR   JA WEI   CH'IR DANG

sickness   none   work   purpose and

to spare them from illness,

This means to liberate and spare beings from all kinds of illnesses.

མུ་གེ་མེད་པར་བྱ་བའི་ཕྱིར་དང་།

MU GE   ME PAR   JA WEI   CH'IR DANG

famine   none   work purpose and

to spare them from famine,

This is one of the specific wishes to eliminate a specific suffering, which in this case is famine due to impoverishment.

བྱང་ཆུབ་ཀྱི་ཕྱོགས་ཀྱི་ཆོས་རྣམས་ཡོངས་སུ་རྫོགས་པར་

JANG CH'UB KYI   CH'OK KYI   CH'O NAM   YONG SU DZOK PAR

bodhi (awakening) direction   dharma all   completely perfect

བྱ་བའི་ཕྱིར་དང་།

JA WEI   CH'IR DANG

work   purpose and

to perfect the aspects of the dharma directed towards awakening,

This refers to all the qualities of the bodhisattva, from the beginning stages of the path all the way to buddhahood, which need to be developed and perfected. They are, namely, the thirty-seven factors harmonious with enlightenment.

།བླ་ན་མེད་པ་ཡང་དག་པར་རྫོགས་པའི་བྱང་ཆུབ།

LA NA ME PA   YANG DAG PAR   DZOK PEI   JANG CH'UP

unsurpassable complete perfect bodhi (enlightenment)

རྟོགས་པར་བྱ་བའི་ཕྱིར།

TOK PAR   JA WEI CH'IR

realize   work purpose

and to realize the unsurpassable, perfect, and complete enlightenment;

Perfect and complete enlightenment is the ultimate wish, that which is an unsurpassable state of being. In order to attain such a state, one wishes to follow the path as a beginner in the trainee stage, and one wishes to take the vow of Restoring and Purifying Ordination, which is the mahayana eight-precepts vow.

།གསོ་སྦྱོང་ངེས་པར་བླངས་པ་དེ་བཞིན་ཏུ།

SO JONG   NGE PAR LANG PA   DE SH'IN TU

sojong vow definitely undertook in the same way

།བདག་མིང་འདི་ཞེས་བགྱི་བས་གྱང་།

DA MING ...   DI   SH'E GYI WE   KYANG

my name   this   referred to as   shall

།དུས་འདི་ནས་བཟུང་སྟེ།   །ཇི་སྲིད་སང་ཉི་མ

DU DI NE   ZUNG TE   JI SI   SANG NYI MA

time from now on until tomorrow sun

མ་ཤར་གྱི་བར་དུ་གསོ་སྦྱོང་ངེས་པར་བླང་བར་བགྱིའོ།

MA SHAR GYI   BAR DU   SO JONG   NGE PAR   LANG WAR GYI-O

not risen between sojong vow definitely   undertake

in the same way, I ...(name), from this moment until sunrise tomorrow, shall definitely undertake the Sojong vow,

The Sojong vow is the Restoring and Purifying Ordination; restoring as in restoration of the root virtuous deeds of the Great Vehicle, and purification of whatever mistakes, shortcomings, faults, and transgressions one might have committed.

The Eight Vows of the Restoring and Purifying Ordination:

ཌེང་ནས་སྲོག་གཅོད་མི་བྱ་ཞིང་།

DENG NE SOG CHOE MI JA SH'ING

1. *From now on I will not kill,*

གཞན་གྱི་ནོར་ཡང་བླང་མི་བྱ།

SH'EN GYI NOR YANG LANG MI JA

2. *I will not take the belongings of others,*

འཁྲིག་པའི་ཆོས་ཀྱང་མི་སྤྱད་ཅིང་།

TR'IG PEI CH'O KYANG MI CHE CHING

3. *I will avoid all sexual activities,*

རྫུན་གྱི་ཚིག་ཀྱང་མི་སྨྲའོ།

DZUN GYI TS'IG KYANG MI MA-O

4. *I will not lie,*

སྐྱོན་ནི་མང་པོ་ཉེར་བརྟེན་པའི།   ཆང་ནི་ཡོངས་སུ་སྤང་བར་བྱ།

KYON NI MANG PO NYER TEN PEI   CH'ANG NI YONG SU PANG WAR JA

5. *I will completely abandon intoxicants, which quickly lead to numerous shortcomings,*

ཁྲི་སྟན་ཆེ་མཐོ་མི་བྱ་ཞིང་།

TR'I TEN CH'E T'O MI JA SH'ING

6. *I will not use high and luxurious seats,*

དེ་བཞིན་དུས་མ་ཡིན་པའི་ཟས།

DE SH'IN DU MA YIN PEI ZE

7. *I will not eat at wrong times,*

ཁྲི་དང་ཕྲེང་བ་དང་ནི་རྒྱན།   གར་དང་གླུ་སོགས་སྤང་བར་བྱ།

DRI DANG TR'ENG WA DANG NI GYEN   GAR DANG LU SOK PANG WAR JA

8. *I will use neither perfume nor ornaments, and I will neither sing nor dance.*

To define each of the vows precisely, scripture mentions that any complete act of wrongdoing has four elements to it. So when one says, "From now on I will not kill," killing here means that, first and foremost, one understands that the other sentient being is a living being. Second, the intention to kill comes from afflictive emotions, the three poisons of desire, hatred, or stupidity. Third, the action is killing through the use of weapons or poison or even mantra power. Finally, one feels satisfaction in having accomplished what one set out to accomplish. And, when one makes a commitment not to kill, the commitment includes humans and all other forms of sentient beings, everything from big animals to tiny insects.

When one says, "I shall not take the belongings of others," first and foremost this means not stealing the possessions of others, meaning property that belongs to another individual. Then, as with killing, the intention to steal is inspired by any of the three poisons. And the action is carrying out that intention by actually taking the property, either by force or guile or other means of deceit. Finally, there is satisfaction in possessing the property. When one makes a commitment not to take others' belongings, the commitment includes all property, regardless of the value or size, from millions of dollars to nickels and dimes.

When one says, "I will avoid all sexual activities," although scripture assumes sexual activity is mainly on a heterosexual basis, today's world is so complicated and people's neurotic emotions are expressed in so many different ways, first and foremost this vow includes all objects of sexual activity. And then it includes the intention to have sexual activity that is inspired by one's lust or whatever. The action is carrying out that intention in whatever form it takes, and finally achieving some kind of satisfaction. When one makes a commitment to avoid sexual activity, it includes all forms of sexual activity.

The vow "I will not lie" first and foremost means knowingly deceiving others and intentionally causing harm, whether the subject matter is something one has seen, or heard, or understood. The intention is inspired by whatever ulterior motive one has. The act of lying includes lying oneself as well as influencing others to lie on one's behalf, and withholding information. The final result is that others accept and believe the untruths. So when one makes a commitment to avoid lying, it includes everything from grand spiritual misrepresentation to jokingly told fibs.

When one says, "I will completely abandon intoxicants," intoxicants include all substances, whether liquid-based, pill, smoke, gas, or whatever. So when one makes a commitment to completely abandon intoxication, it means not drinking even a drop of alcohol, or taking even a tiny speck of any other intoxicating substance.

When one says, "I will not use high and luxurious seats," high seats basically refer to thrones made out of precious stones and metals, and luxurious seats refer to cushions covered with all kinds of fur and animal skin. But when one makes a commitment not to use high seats, scripture mentions that a high throne also means one's bed, which should not be higher than a half-arm's length, measuring from the elbow to the fingertips. During Nyungne the tradition is that everyone sleeps on the floor.

The vow "I will not eat at wrong times" in the context of Nyungne means not eating at any time other than the one prescribed vegetarian meal on day one.

When one says, "I will use neither perfume nor ornaments, and I will neither sing nor dance," this basically means one will avoid any forms of self-adornment and entertainment during the two days devoted to Nyungne practice.

ཇི་ལྟར་དགྲ་བཅོམ་རྟག་ཏུ་ནི།

JI TAR   DRA CHOM   TAG TU   NI

just as foe destroyers always do

Just as the foe destroyers constantly abstain from

།སྲོག་གཅོད་ལ་སོགས་མི་བྱེད་ལྟར།

SOG CHOE   LA SOK   MI   JE TAR
killing and so on will not same way

taking lives and from doing these other actions,

།དེ་ལྟར་སྲོག་གཅོད་ལ་སོགས་སྤང་།

DE TAR   SOG CHOE   LA SOK   PANG
in the same way killing and so on abandon

in the same way, having abandoned all these actions,

།བླ་མེད་བྱང་ཆུབ་མྱུར་ཐོབ་ཤོག

LA ME   JANG CH'UB   NYUR T'OB   SHOK
unsurpassable enlightenment quickly obtain may

may I quickly obtain unsurpassable enlightenment.

།སྡུག་བསྔལ་མང་དཀྲུགས་འཇིག་རྟེན་འདི།

DUG NGAL   MANG DRUK   JIG TEN   DI
suffering   many shaken   world   this

།སྲིད་པའི་མཚོ་ལས་སྒྲོལ་བར་ཤོག།

SI PEI   TS'O LE   DROL WAR   SHOK
existence ocean from freed may

May we be freed from the ocean of existence,
the world of destruction, shaken by so many sufferings.

The commitment to attain enlightenment with an altruistic motivation and, thereafter, the wish to free all beings from the suffering of samsara is a crucial point. We must understand this point very clearly, and we must make a commitment precisely according to this understanding.

The list of eight precepts is basically clear as far as killing and stealing and so on are concerned. With respect to intoxication, drinking alcohol is obvious, and I believe smoking of any kind is included in it as well. As for high and luxurious seats, this vow is directed primarily at the kings and ministers who were disciples of Lord Buddha in ancient times. In traditional societies, kings and ministers sat on very high thrones made out of precious metals and stones, with animal furs and skins as well. People with power used to sit on those seats and dictate to others. When one takes vows, the basic idea is to practice humility and modesty, and to put one's ego aside. We are not supposed to put ourselves above other people and engage in abusive power.

This explanation is not to be confused with the spiritual teacher sitting on the throne and teaching the precious dharma. Scripture mentions that spiritual teachers sitting on thrones and teaching is not only okay, but it is an extremely virtuous activity; in fact, a true teacher teaching in this manner is giving all the devotees the opportunity to respect and honor the precious dharma teaching, and this is the buddhas' and bodhisattvas' way to benefit others.

Not eating at wrong times[24] means first of all, eating one vegetarian meal at noontime on the first day, which in our practice we schedule between 12:00 noon and 1:00 p.m. The meal is supposed to be eaten in one sitting as well. Drinks are permitted during the first day up until the time you go to sleep in the evening. The following day is a fasting day, so absolutely no drink and no food is taken at all.

Abstaining from perfume and ornaments, and singing and dancing, may sound like two different types of vows, but they are actually one vow, precept number eight. Sometimes there are questions regarding the use of moisturizers and lotions on your face. I think as long as it is free from perfume, a nonscented cream should be fine. Singing and dancing is clear, but it also includes such activities as listening to music and watching TV and movies.[25] I think reading material used for entertainment purposes only is wrong as well. In the old days one would not have seen these activities mentioned in the scripture, because the materials did not exist; but in the context of modern life, if we sincerely observe the vow, it is obvious that these are entertainment and therefore should be avoided.

The eight-precepts vow falls into three different categories of discipline:

24 For a complete discussion of eating and drinking during Nyungne, see "Pure Physical Action" in Chapter 13.

25 For further discussion of rules during Nyungne, see "Additional Rules" in Chapter 13.

1. The first four root vows are part of moral and ethical discipline.
2. The fifth vow regarding intoxication is part of conscientious discipline.
3. The last three vows are part of yogic discipline.

Among these three categories of discipline, I think moral and ethical discipline are obvious. The discipline of conscientiousness refers to the idea of preserving sanity and mindfulness, whereas yogic discipline has to do with austerity. This idea comes from one's willingness to undergo extreme hardship if that is what it takes to become enlightened.

The Powerful Benefits of the Sojong Vow:

- If one abandons killing, above all, in future lives one will experience longevity, freedom from sickness, and have a striking presence.
- By abandoning stealing, one will experience abundant wealth and prosperity.
- By abandoning sexual activity, one will experience a beautiful and properly developed body in future lives, and one will not experience sexual confusion.
- By abandoning lying, one will have articulate speech, words that carry weight, and one will not be deceived by others.
- By abandoning intoxication, one will be a conscientious and sane person, and very bright.
- By abandoning high and luxurious seats, one will be respected and praised by others, and have material comforts.
- By abandoning eating food at the wrong time, one will have pleasant body odor [26] and a beautiful complexion.
- By abandoning perfume and ornaments, and singing and dancing, one will have a stable and peaceful nature, and speech that delights in prayer recitation and chanting the dharma.

---

26 There are stories of perfect monks who abide by all the disciplines perfectly. They were known to have "discipline odor," which is a pleasing scent that can be detected at long distances. For example, Lord Gampopa, who was arguably the greatest monk of Tibet, had such discipline odor. It has been said that people could smell his beautiful scent all over the entire mountain where he lived. In the context of Nyungne practice, it is understandable that keeping these vows will be the cause of beautiful body odor and all the other qualities in future lives.

These are the specific benefits of each and every vow. The general benefits of the vows are that one will obtain a precious human birth and abandon the eight unfavorable conditions,[27] shut the door to the lower realms, continually be able to engage in the spiritual path, and ultimately attain buddhahood.

27 The eight leisures refer to freedom from the eight unfavorable conditions which prevent proper Buddhist practice and therefore the possession of a precious human birth: 1. the state of a hell-being; 2. the state of a hungry ghost; 3. the state of an animal; 4. the state of a long-living god; 5. living in a barbarous country where habits are contrary to dharma; 6. holding wrong views and doubts; 7. being born in a country where Buddhism is unknown; and 8. having nonreceptive senses. For additional information, see the chapter on precious human birth in Gampopa's *Jewel Ornament of Liberation*.

Seven-Branch Offering Prayer 7

IN GENERAL, the idea of an offering prayer is a very important part of spiritual practice. As long as we are deluded beings unable to experience complete purity, which is the perfection of wisdom mind, we need to accumulate merit. From the point of view of how reality works, we know for a certainty that all phenomenal experience is due to certain causes and conditions. The distinctions among these experiences are: pain and pleasure, positive and negative, enlightened and unenlightened. It is also clear that the vast majority of sentient beings are lacking good and pure karma and therefore their need to accumulate merit is obvious. Since we are imperfect beings, we have lots of work to do in order to become like the perfect buddhas. In other words, we need to accumulate and gather spiritual merit so that we can transform our ordinary experience into pure enlightened experience.

Virtue is of two kinds, merit and wisdom; one is gathered through numerous deeds associated with action, the other is gained through meditation. The former is the cause of rupakaya, the form body, and the latter is the cause for dharmakaya, the body of emptiness.

The "Seven-Branch Prayer" is one of the most skillful ways to accumulate merit. There are various means of accumulating merit, but if you practice this prayer, all methods are included in it. For this reason one finds it included in many practices. In fact, the "Seven-Branch Prayer" is used to accumulate merit by Buddhists of all traditions: hinayana, mahayana, and vajrayana.

THE FIRST BRANCH PRAYER: PROSTRATION

The first offering in the "Seven-Branch Prayer" is prostration,[28] the remedy for pride or ego. All Lord Buddha's teachings are remedies for our shortcomings, which are the cause of all our unfortunate experiences. Therefore it is important to apply the appropriate remedy for each specific negative shortcoming. Pride and ego are wrong states of mind which are connected to prejudice. Such states of mind create further bad karma, which leads to unfortunate experiences in this life and the next. In modern society, pride and ego are regarded as qualities or strengths in the name of individual rights and freedom. Pride and ego are misconceived as confidence and self-esteem, but these are all just fancy names for characteristics that actually do us a lot of harm. Therefore, spiritually speaking, such states of mind are incorrect mind-sets, and with them there is no chance of developing pure qualities. We're speaking about true spiritual qualities, and such qualities can only be developed in the absence of the afflictive mind-set of ego.

Ultimately our own pure mind is buddha nature, and the objects of prostration are also the buddhas and bodhisattvas of the ten directions; but because we have not been able to manifest the wisdom mind of the buddhas as our own mind, there is definitely a need to perform prostrations. A wonderful story about a very great, undisputed mahasiddha, Drukpa Kunleg, illustrates this point. He was actually known as a mad mahasiddha, because he had a unique way of teaching and giving messages to people through all kinds of crazy means. One of the things he did was go to the Jokhang Temple in Lhasa where the famous Buddha statue resides. Standing in front of this statue, he first looked at it rather strangely and then spontaneously said a prayer and bowed to the statue. His prayer was:

> You were very diligent in your spiritual undertaking,
> Therefore you became a perfect Buddha.
> I was lazy, therefore I wander around in samsara.
> I now bow down to you.

The actual prostration has three parts, related to body, speech, and mind. With our body we physically prostrate, with our speech we say prostration

---

28 Further explanation of prostration is found in Chapter 10. One of the main activities during the "Po Prayer" is praise to Lord Chenrezig through prostration. These explanations may be redundant, but I think it is an important topic that warrants repeating.

prayers, and with our mind we develop complete confidence and devotion and visualize a multitude of our own bodies simultaneously prostrating. While prostrating, we must also include all sentient beings and visualize them performing prostrations with us. It is very important to do the prostration one-pointedly through body, speech, and mind, without becoming distracted.

The proper way to prostrate is to stand with hands folded together in the heart area. Your hands should be gently touching, neither completely flat nor open, resembling the bud of a lotus. You then raise your hands to touch the top of your head, your throat, and your heart, and bow down to touch the five points of your body to the ground. The five points are your two hands, two knees, and your forehead. When you touch your hands to the top of your head, you purify obscurations of your body, and at the same time establish a connection that enables you to receive the blessings of the buddhas' body. When you touch your hands to your throat, you purify obscurations of your speech and establish a connection that enables you to receive the blessings of the buddhas' speech. When you touch your hands to your heart, you purify obscurations of your mind and establish a connection that enables you to receive the blessings of the buddhas' mind. When you touch your five points to the ground, you purify the obscurations of the five poisons and make a connection that enables you to receive the blessings of all the buddhas' body, speech, mind, quality, and activity.

The Benefits of Prostration

During the time of Lord Buddha, while a monk was sincerely doing prostrations to a stupa which had Buddha's hair and nails inside it, Ananda asked Lord Buddha about the benefits of doing prostration. Among many benefits, the Buddha said that whatever amount of minute particles of the earth your body covers when you perform a single, sincere prostration, from the surface to the bottom of the earth, one can become a universal monarch that many times and beyond. One of the major marks of perfection of the sublime nirmanakaya buddha body is the unique protrusion on the top of his head, and it is understood that this also comes about from demonstrating respect and honor through prostration. Of course another benefit is that when one displays respect and honor, one receives respect and honor and so on.

Prostration has its place even at the ultimate level. Ultimately speaking, prostration and bowing are to one's own true nature of mind as the root guru, buddha nature; one is respecting and honoring and bowing to that buddha nature.

THE SECOND BRANCH PRAYER: OFFERING

Offering is the second branch prayer, and it is the remedy for miserliness. Since the law of nature is that giving is receiving, offering definitely has its place in the mundane world, our world in samsara, as well as the super-mundane world, meaning the enlightened world beyond samsara.

General tantric offerings include external offerings, inner offerings, secret offerings, and ultimate offerings. During Nyungne practice we engage in external offerings of substantial substances and imaginary, visualized substances.

While making offerings, it is important not to hold anything back or to feign generosity through pretense or show. Whatever offering one makes must be a sincere, pure offering, and this forms the basis for one's imaginary offering. We visualize all of space entirely filled with all kinds of wonderful substances that please gods and men such as beautiful flowers, incense, lamps, perfumed water, food, and music. In terms of the mandala offering, we include Mt. Meru, the four continents, the seven possessions of a universal monarch, the eight auspicious signs, the eight auspicious substances, and so on.

In addition to these, we imagine making immense offerings like those of Bodhisattva Samantabhadra's offering clouds. This bodhisattva is the greatest example to follow, because his clouds of offerings were unsurpassable. Samantabhadra Bodhisattva visualized light coming from his heart and filling all of space. He further imagined additional Samantabhadra Bodhisattvas on the tip of every one of those lights. And then again he imagined light coming from their hearts doing the same thing. He repeated this process multiple times and in this way filled the entire universe with Samantabhadra Bodhisattvas making offerings to all the buddhas. Doing this, one accumulates inexhaustible merit.

It has been said that one can imagine all the many things that exist in the universe that don't belong to anyone and offer all of it to the buddhas. This is a perfectly appropriate offering as well as a skillful means to accumulate merit. Doing this is the same as making the actual offering; therefore those without much wealth need not feel they lack the means to accumulate merit. As long as one is willing to do the proper visualization and to sincerely recite offering prayers, there is no limit to what one can offer.

Whenever one receives something new, whether it's clothing, food, or whatever, it is the Buddhist practice to always first offer it to one's own guru and the Three Jewels by saying, "I offer this to my guru and to the Three Jewels." In this way, one has the opportunity to constantly accumulate merit. When I was a child, every time we saw a beautiful landscape, mountains, water, flowers, or vast city lights, my completely enlightened guru used to tell me, "You can make these things an offering."

Here I wish to stress another point. I have heard people make comments such as, "Why make offerings to spiritual teachers who might not suffer from poverty and to monasteries and temples that are prospering quite well? It is better to give to the poor and needy," or, "It is better to build schools than to build temples." Such people don't have a complete understanding of how offering really works. Of course, giving to the poor is a generous act, and building a school is a charitable act as well. Both activities, if done sincerely, undoubtedly have lots of merit. But I have personally known people who I could see had questionable motivation; people who were quite comfortable looking down on some poor guy while giving him something, whose egos felt good in doing so. On the other hand, humbly making offerings to the Three Jewels and Three Roots is something one does with humility and with gratitude for having the opportunity.

Another very important point needs to be understood. There's a big difference in the amount of merit we can accumulate by offering to the Three Jewels and Three Roots versus giving to the poor. The reason is that one object is completely pure and sublime and the other is merely ordinary. Any offerings to true spiritual causes and conditions are offerings to truly unsurpassable, enlightened causes, while giving donations for ordinary schools and so on are very limited causes. I do not mean to minimize the benefit of ordinary charities; however the issue remains that if we were to support the education of one thousand kids, as wonderful as that might be, it's still only for the duration of the lifetimes of those one thousand kids. This is the meaning of a limited cause. Planting some kind of spiritual seed in even one person is another way of giving, and that gift can become a supreme cause, which means providing benefit to that person's limitless future. This is the meaning of an enlightened cause. Supporting Nyungne practitioners, retreat centers, building stupas, etc. are all examples of enlightened causes.

Having said that, as good Buddhists, when someone asks for something we are not supposed let them go away empty-handed. I think in today's world, building schools and hospitals should also be part of Buddhists' activity.

We human beings can usually give gifts to one another quite easily because we anticipate being rewarded by generosity in return, which is very tangible and immediate, whereas making offerings to spiritual causes and conditions is often intangible and the reward is not immediate. We may only be able to expect it to happen in our future lives. Actually, if one accumulates enough merit, the results will happen even in this life. There are many examples of this. One such example is the story of the couple who lived during the time of one of the previous buddhas.

There was an impoverished old couple who only had one piece of cloth- ing between them. Whenever one of them went out they would put it on. All their lives they were extremely poor and one day a great arhat, who knew their condition, came to see them. He could see that they needed to accumulate merit, and the perfect way to do that would be to make an offering to Buddha. He encouraged them to make such an offering. They had nothing to offer except their one piece of clothing. The arhat told them to make that their offering. They had faith and they agreed to make the offering. Asking the arhat to please wait outside, they took the clothing and handed it out to him. The Buddha was preaching to a large gathering of people that included kings and queens, and the arhat carried the cloth to this place. As I recall the story, the piece of cloth was smelly and dirty, and some were appalled that such a thing would be offered to the Bud- dha. But Buddha said, "Oh no, no. This is an offering from old folks and I must accept it in order for them to accumulate merit." When the kings and queens heard the complete story, they all wanted to help and overnight the old folks became wealthy, received beautiful clothing, and so on. This is a perfect example of how things really work.

Ultimately, the ideal offering is offering free from attachment or clinging to the six sense fields. Lord Milarepa said, "When one no longer clings to ego clinging, there is no separate practice of offering or generosity." In other words, the ultimate offering is the offering of perfect understanding.

THE THIRD BRANCH PRAYER: CONFESSION

Confession is the remedy for ignorance because all negativities, defile- ments, and sins are basically created due to ignorance. Lack of under- standing causes people to engage in wrong action, which then leads to unfortunate results that further bring more confusion, pain, and suffering. It is ignorance that causes us to not know how to overcome all these wrong actions and results, and it is negativities and sins that prevent us from receiving blessings and siddhis. Therefore, confession is a very important spiritual practice.

When we recite confession prayers, we confess all the wrongdoings that we have engaged in from time without beginning, things that we remember and things that we don't remember. In the presence of Lord Chenrezig, buddhas, and bodhisattvas, we confess all the wrongdoings of our body, speech, and mind: negative deeds such as the ten unvirtuous deeds, the five deeds that ripen immediately, violations of the vows that are associated with individual liberation, violations associated with bodhisattva vows, and violations of tantric vows, injuring the Three Jewels, abandoning the dharma, disrespecting the sangha, disrespecting the teachers, disrespecting the parents, and so on. All these transgressions, which might obstruct our freedom from samsara and our achievement of buddhahood, we sincerely regret and, with hands folded in prayer, we confess from the bottom of our hearts. During this time you should imagine that rays of light are coming to you from Lord Chenrezig and the buddhas and bodhisattvas, and that all your negativities are being purified.

Many people like to think that they have done nothing wrong, that they are good human beings and have nothing to confess. But the only time you don't need confession is when you are a completely perfect, pure being. As long as you are in the world, it means you are an imperfect being with karma and limitations. Otherwise you wouldn't be here. Our real situation is that we've been living and experiencing things in samsara from time without beginning. Therefore we have engaged in all sorts of wrong deeds in the past, and this is the main issue. If you are a decent human being, you may not have engaged in extreme negative deeds during this lifetime. However, in terms of your spiritual growth, the major obstacle that prevents spiritual achievement is impure karma from your past life.

I would like to clarify one thing and that is, even though we may not have done any major wrong in this life, the truth is we engage in misdeeds all the time, all the way from the food that we eat[29] to our speech which is very imperfect and our minds that are filled with negativities. So we cannot be too proud and naively think that we are completely innocent of all wrongdoing.

Ultimately, confession is understanding the emptiness nature of phenomena. In that realm one transcends everything including confession, negative deeds, and ignorance. This understanding of emptiness has to be true realization. Conceptual understanding would not be sufficient to truly purify everything.

29 See "Pure Physical Action" in Chapter 13.

THE FOURTH BRANCH PRAYER: REJOICING

Rejoicing is the fourth branch prayer and is the remedy for jealousy. According to Lord Buddha, if we rejoice in others' good deeds instead of being jealous, we receive the same benefit as they do.

The proper way to rejoice is to rejoice in conditional virtuous deeds as well as nonconditional virtuous deeds. "Conditional" means virtuous deeds that are limited and occur within the bounds of samsara; the good deeds done by sentient beings, such as the ten virtuous deeds which lead to higher birth and to positive experiences in this life as well as future lives. Nonconditional virtuous deeds are limitless, the supreme deeds of the buddhas and bodhisattvas. In other words, one rejoices in any virtuous deeds, all the way from the ordinary deeds of sentient beings to the extraordinary virtuous deeds of shravakas, pratyekabuddhas, and the vast, profound activities of bodhisattvas. When doing so, one should not limit one's thoughts to this world alone. One should include all the virtuous deeds of sentient beings and buddhas and bodhisattvas who exist in the totality of vast and infinite space.

Rejoicing is a truly great virtue because it is hard to do. We know this for a fact from the common reactions of people to the good fortune of others, such as their material success, good looks, fame and fortune, or any good qualities they might have. Instead of being happy for them, the first thought that comes to most people's mind is, "Why do they get to have that?" It is pure jealousy. Obviously, spiritually speaking, this is an incorrect emotion, and the main reason is because it damages us.

The following story taken from a sutra is a great example of how rejoicing works. A devoted patron, King Kosala (Skt. Prasenajit, Tib. Sal Gyal), was offering meals to Lord Buddha and all his followers. Outside of his palace, an old beggar woman took great delight and joy in the king's virtuous deeds—delight in his good fortune from his past life and delight in his continuous accumulation of merit in this life by making offerings to the buddhas. Being omniscient, Buddha knew of her pure rejoicing and he asked his disciple, the king, "When doing the dedication of merit, should I dedicate in your name or in the name of another person whose virtue is greater than yours?" The king politely responded, "Please dedicate in the name of the other person whose virtue is greater than mine." So Buddha dedicated the merit that day in the name of the poor beggar woman. It went on like that for three days, and the king was not very happy. His ministers discussed the issue and one of them came up with a solution. He spoke to the people who gave the leftover food to the beggars and told them, when giving out the food, just beat up the old woman. And that day the beggar woman became very angry, and she didn't think at all about rejoicing. Again, Buddha knew, and on that day Buddha dedicated the merit in the king's name.

You may ask how a simple rejoicing can result in virtue equal to that of a deed, when another person is actually performing the deed and yours is just a thought. Here's how it works. Mental phenomena are primary among all phenomena. Therefore virtuous deeds associated with thoughts are the most powerful, and deeds associated with body and speech are less so. Thus having a pure heart is the most important thing, and the ability to rejoice is a demonstration of pure heart.

As I recall the story of the beggar woman, at that time Buddha was making prophecies about the future buddhahood of his fellow bodhisattvas and devoted kings and patrons, and that king expected to hear his name too. It was a long time before Buddha spoke his name, and this had something to do with his treatment of the old beggar woman.

Ultimately, to rejoice is to understand that there is a constant, unceasing flow of compassion by all the buddhas and bodhisattvas, and that unceasing flow of compassion is the source of all virtuous deeds in the world and the world beyond.

THE FIFTH BRANCH PRAYER: REQUEST TO TURN THE DHARMA WHEEL

Requesting that the dharma wheel be turned is the remedy for abandoning the dharma. Abandoning the dharma is a specific-cause wrongdoing which leads to a specific unfortunate result. Because of ignorance, people can easily abandon dharma, and that is the primary cause of not finding a true teacher and true teaching.

In today's world there are many examples of people looking for a true spiritual teaching and path, and although they may desperately want to find a pure teaching and pure path, many are unable to find them. Some find a wrong teaching and a wrong path, and others who may find buddhadharma might still not be able to find the right teacher and the right teaching. Because of that, they may become upset and turn away from the dharma altogether, creating the same kind of karma again that was the cause for their being lost in the first place. Then one never knows for how many lifetimes they may get caught in a vicious cycle like this. If done properly, requesting the dharma teaching will help one to overcome this unfortunate situation once and for all.

A true teacher and true teaching are absolute necessities. Without them, we have no way of learning anything. Every little bit of knowledge that anybody has comes from a teacher, and in the case of dharma teaching, all dharma knowledge also comes from the teacher. Therefore it is absolutely necessary to request that the buddhas and bodhisattvas teach the three vehicles so that we can overcome pain and suffering, and confusion and illusion, and experience the wisdom mind of the buddhas.

One of the important reasons for requesting the turning of the dharma wheel is to ask those great bodhisattvas who are on the tenth-bhumi level to quickly become perfect buddhas; to sit under the bodhi tree, like the historic Buddha Shakyamuni, and subdue the maras, and to turn the dharma wheel for the benefit of all sentient beings.

Another important reason is that buddhas and bodhisattvas are committed to helping fellow beings. However, when they actually take rebirth in the world in order to help others, through circumstantial reasons such as sentient beings engaging in excessive wrongdoings and disappointing them, many of these great beings might just peacefully sit there instead of actively engaging in teaching and propagating the dharma. The reason for this is the collective karma of these particular sentient beings. So, by earnestly requesting them to teach, one is trying to create depending-arising circumstances. That is, new, positive karma so that the teachings can benefit even such wrongdoers.

The proper way to supplicate is to visualize a multitude of ourselves throughout the universe who are humbly requesting in the presence of all the great buddhas and bodhisattvas that the wheel of dharma be turned.

Ultimately, to request the dharma wheel to be turned is to understand that all-pervading wisdom is the fundamental inherent quality that exists primordially, and because of it all the precious wisdom teachings become accessible.

THE SIXTH BRANCH PRAYER: BESEECHING BUDDHAS AND BODHISATTVAS NOT TO PASS INTO NIRVANA

Beseeching buddhas not to pass into nirvana is the remedy for wrong view. From the point of view of true dharma, those who hang on to the world with eternalistic or nihilistic views have wrong views. While there are many erroneous spiritual and philosophical views, they are all included in eternalism and nihilism.

One of the main reasons that sentient beings have wrong views is their inability, in the past, to develop faith in and devotion to enlightened causes. When we beseech the buddhas and bodhisattvas to remain with us in samsara, everyone is afforded the opportunity to eventually develop the right view. Beseeching sublime ones to dispel wrong views is for our own benefit as well as the benefit of others. Even though we are already on the path, we still have residual wrong-view karma. When true enlightened teachers remain with us, slowly, slowly their blessings will transform us and our view will mature. Eventually, it will become perfect.

It is understood that throughout the universe many buddhas and bodhisattvas have come to the world to benefit others and are about to pass into nirvana. We are asking them to remain in the world until samsara is emptied.

In the tantric tradition of Tibet, we have an elaborate long-life ceremony to request a great vajra master not to pass into nirvana. If the ceremony is an extensive one, long-life pujas will be performed for at least seven days. At the end of the seventh day, elaborate mandala offerings combined with seven-branch prayers, bathing water prayers, homage prayers, specially composed long-life prayers for the guru, and many other offerings are made. In addition to all these offerings and prayers, a special ceremony is performed that involves five virgin girls, symbols of the pure dakinis of the five directions: the Buddha Dakini, Vajra Dakini, Ratna Dakini, Padma Dakini, and the Karma Dakini. Symbolically these girls are dressed in five different colors, and they come to escort the great vajra master back to the dakini realm. Then, to convince them to go without the master, five different kinds of torma offerings are presented to them; they accept the gifts and leave without disappointment. In the monastery, usually young monks are chosen to dress as dakinis and perform the dances and rituals, and they recite invitation prayers that they have memorized to the vajra master.

There is enormous benefit in beseeching the sublime ones to remain, relative as well as ultimate benefit. Relatively, dependent-arising causes and conditions are established so that our own obstacles to longevity will be dispelled and we can enjoy long life and freedom from sickness; and good karma is created, enabling us to receive dharma teachings and to spend a long time together with great masters. The ultimate benefit is having the opportunity to intermingle our minds with the wisdom minds of the buddhas.

Ultimate beseeching is to request all the buddhas to remain in the supreme unchanging dharmakaya, the realm from which all nirmanakaya buddhas and bodhisattvas appearing in the world originate.

THE SEVENTH BRANCH PRAYER: DEDICATION OF MERIT

Dedication of merit is the remedy for doubts and skepticism in the sense that the obscuration of disbelief is purified when one dedicates without hesitation. In other words, mind's habit of obfuscating is eliminated.

Dedication is one of the very important spiritual practices. Without proper dedication, the result of any virtuous deed will come to an end once the fruit is enjoyed. On the other hand, if you do a proper dedication, you will be able to enjoy its result life after life, and the deed will be inexhaustible until you attain enlightenment. Without dedication there is a danger of the virtuous deed being destroyed by a subsequent powerful, aggressive deed; and if you brag about your good deed, without dedication there is a danger of the virtue being robbed altogether. In the case of virtuous deeds accumulated through offerings, the virtue will be diminished if, out of greed, you later regret these offerings. However, when one dedicates the merit for one's deeds, the power of anger, boasting, and greed cannot destroy it. It has been said in the scripture that nondedicated virtue will never increase, whereas dedicated virtue will double every single day. In this way we have the opportunity to make our little virtue into truly great virtue.

Knowing what constitutes a proper dedication is important. A correct dedication must be free from the three concepts of subject, object, and action (the meritorious deed). Conceptually-bound dedication is considered venomous dedication because it is not really a true dedication, therefore its effect can only be within the samsaric realm; it cannot become a truly enlightened cause. This is the hard part, because no ordinary being can do it. But there is a trick and that is to request all the buddhas and bodhisattvas to witness your wish to make a pure dedication prayer, free from the three concepts. Then you pray, "Just as buddhas of the past, present, and future have dedicated merit, similarly I wish to follow in their footsteps and dedicate the merit for the benefit of all beings." Another way to dedicate correctly is to pray to follow in the footsteps of Manjushri Bodhisattva and Samantabhadra Bodhisattva, and then to recite the "Resolve to Practice Excellence." According to Lord Atisha, ordinary practitioners can also make comparable dedication prayers by understanding that subject, object, and action are all illusion.

There is another important point to understand. When you wish to dedicate the merit to a specific being, whether alive or dead, there is no way that other being will be able to benefit from it unless you do a proper dedication prayer. And when dedicating, you can specify a particular being, but you must also include all sentient beings to make it a completely correct dedication.

Ultimate dedication is to dedicate the virtue that all sentient beings achieve the unsurpassable realm of dharmata, so that everyone has the opportunity to achieve trikayahood, the three bodies of the buddha.

ACCUMULATION OF MERIT AND WISDOM

In order to attain perfect enlightenment one has to accumulate perfect merit and wisdom. No buddha exists that did not accumulate perfect virtue, and therefore the accumulation of virtue through recitation of the "Seven-Branch Prayer" is a very important part of spiritual practice. In the tradition of the Great Vehicle, the path to perfect buddhahood is called the five paths. The first of the five paths is the path of accumulation. One enters into this path as a first step and the main focus of one's practice is to accumulate merit. That is why it is called the path of accumulation. Our spiritual progress depends solely on accumulating merit, and if we do this, we will be on the lesser path of accumulation, the beginner's stage. Then if you do well, you will enter into the mediocre path of accumulation, and eventually the superior path of accumulation. As spiritual practitioners we will never stop accumulating merit, no matter how advanced we are on our spiritual path; but if we are beyond the path of accumulation, it will not be our main focus, whereas if we are on the path of accumulation, accumulating merit is our main practice.

As practitioners, some may be more advanced than others, but in all likelihood most of us are in the beginning stages of the path of accumulation. Therefore accumulation of virtue through the recitation of seven-branch offering prayers, and all other means, is very important to keep in mind.

Lord Milarepa's famous words to Lord Gampopa illustrate exactly how things really work:

> Without merit there will be no siddhis,
> Just as there will be no oil from pressing a grain of sand;
> But if you press a sesame seed, you will have oil.

Then there are other well-known Tibetan sayings, which are also right to the point:

If you churn water, no matter how long you do it you get no butter,
Whereas if you churn milk, butter will appear.

It is better to accumulate merit, even a tiny bit,
Than to work very hard to gather a lot.

Another great quote, undoubtedly from one of the mahasiddhas, is found in many books:

Our absolute innate wisdom mind can only appear
Through having accumulated merit and purified obscurations,
And through the blessings of a truly realized guru.
To rely on any other means is foolish.

The great Lord of the Drikung Kagyu tradition, Kyobpa Jig Ten Sum Gyi Gompo, said the following:

Unless by offering aspiration prayers
You rub the wish-granting gem of the two accumulations of merit,
The results you wish for will never appear.
Therefore, do the concluding dedication wholeheartedly.

Visualization 8

VISUALIZATION of the yidam deity has two phases, the creation phase and the completion phase. The creation phase is self-generation of the deity, which is a part of the skillful means of tantric teaching, a profound method in which we instantaneously transform ourselves into a completely pure, divine, perfect being. We use this profound and powerful technique to transform all impure phenomena into pure phenomena, and deluded, ordinary form into a divine wisdom form. This technique absolutely works as far as transforming imperfection into perfection is concerned; doing so, we are able to overcome ordinary experiences through the power of transforming them into pure experiences.

Thousand-Armed Chenrezig, Avalokiteshvara, is a sambhogakaya buddha manifestation, a pure, subtle manifestation that is the union of prana and mind and not simply a fantasy form. Chenrezig represents the pure power of enlightened energy. Such form inherently exists in the pure nature of mind and can manifest to everyone, because pure buddha nature is the nature of all sentient beings.

The completion phase is equally important. This phase refers to the dissolution of the created deity form into emptiness. Since the deity arises from emptiness, it then must dissolve back into emptiness. Generation and completion must be united in our practice to overcome both the extreme, eternalistic belief in an inherently existing reality (theistic view) and our grasping after it, and the nihilistic, extreme belief that nothing whatsoever exists (atheistic view).

The arisal of the deity form body is possible because of the emptiness nature of phenomena. The fact is, whether pure or impure, all phenomena are possible because of their underlying nature being emptiness. In order to transform impure phenomena, one must rely on the skillful means of transforming it into pure phenomena, and this inherently pure phenomena is possible because of its emptiness nature. To further perfect the practice we must go back into emptiness by dissolving the deity into emptiness, because one cannot hang on to either pure or impure form. The true nature of all phenomena is neither existent nor nonexistent; it is simply beyond all conceptual fabrications and elaborations. So here one can understand how profound the technique of creation and completion deity practice is. It is perfect practice.

FIELD OF ACCUMULATION OF MERIT PHASE

During Nyungne practice the field of accumulation of merit phase follows the lineage and refuge prayers, during which one instantaneously visualizes oneself as Chenrezig. The visualization can be a two-armed, four-armed, or thousand-armed Chenrezig. The purpose of this visualization is simply to purify oneself enough in order to approach Chenrezig. This portion is not the actual self-visualization of the deity.

Further, you visualize the letter HRIH (ཧྲཱིཿ) in your heart; from it light radiates, inviting the deity from the pure land. Guru Chenrezig comes, accompanied by buddhas, bodhisattvas, dakas, dakinis, and protectors. You imagine Chenrezig in front of you on top of a thousand-petaled lotus and moon cushion surrounded by all the buddhas and bodhisattvas. You then make the "Seven-Branch Offering Prayer," the offering of prostrations, substances, confession, rejoicing, entreaty, supplication, and dedication. The "Four Immeasurables Prayer" follows. Finally, the field of accumulation of merit returns to its natural origin.

THE THREE ASPECTS OF DEITY YOGA: CLARITY, PURITY, AND STABILITY

Chenrezig's form body represents complete perfection; therefore, in order to do deity visualization and practice correctly, we must practice with what are called three aspects of deity yoga: clarity, purity, and stability. First is the clarity of the deity. This means we must engage in practice with as clear a visualization of the deity as possible. One must be able to visualize every aspect of the form body, and each aspect in precise detail. This is called clarity of appearance, being able to see ourselves in this completely pure manifestation. In addition, one must remember the perfection of the deity form body, meaning one must have recollection of each and every aspect of the manifestation and what it purely represents. This is called being mindful of purity. Finally, one must have proper stability, or vajra pride, meaning that one must be able to think that one is indeed the deity itself. Vajra pride does not mean pride from the point of view of thinking with conceit that one is greater than others. That is ordinary pride. Rather vajra pride recognizes that one indeed embodies all the perfect qualities of the perfect deity naturally and inherently. This is called stability of vajra pride.

THE THREE SATTVAS

There are three levels of deity: the samayasattva, the jnanasattva, and the samadhisattva. The samayasattva deity stage is the stage of one's own creation deity, *samaya* meaning "commitment." One perceives one's own body as a naturally divine body, and one is committed to that. Further, it means that one does not waver from this commitment by unclear visualization or any ordinary ego problems and ego clinging, which requires tremendous courage and strength. *Sattva* means "brave." So one is committed and brave; brave because one does not waver from the mind that clearly identifies the deity, and because one is not afraid of being influenced by ego clinging and so forth.

Jnanasattva is a wisdom deity that one invokes from the pure realm. *Jnana*, pristine pure wisdom, is inherently Chenrezig's and all the buddhas' nature, as well as one's own pure nature of mind, that manifests as a wisdom deity in order to benefit beings. It is also *sattva*, the brave, because it is not afraid of any extreme views, such as the views of eternalists, nihilists, and dualists, and all other views that are incorrect. It is completely free from fear.

Samadhisattva, the absorption sattva, is the letter HRIH (ཧྲཱིཿ) in the heart center of the wisdom deity, the thumb-sized Chenrezig in one's own heart. Absorption is in the sense that we one-pointedly focus our mind on the letter HRIH in the heart center; and it is *sattva*, the brave, because it is not afraid of mind being agitated and dull and all other defects of the practice of meditation.

We have made a chart to illustrate the relationship of the three sattvas in terms of deity yoga, and how through these three sattvas purification takes place (see next page).

COMPLETE STEPS OF THE CREATION PHASE (SELF-GENERATION)

We begin with the recitation of the mantra: OM SVABHAWA SHUDDHA SARVA DHARMA SVABHAWA SHUDDHO HAM (ༀ་སྭ་བྷཱ་ཝ་ཤུདྡྷཿ་སརྦ་དྷརྨ་

		SANSKRIT	TIBETAN
FIRST OBJECTS OF PURIFICATION	Five aggregates	skandhas	pung po
	Eighteen constituents	dhatus	kham
	Twelve sources[1]	ayatanas	kye che
Agents of purification	Commitment deity	samayasattva	dam tsik sempa
Purified result	Form-body deity, which is the union of emptiness and appearance		nang tong nyi me kyi ku
SECOND OBJECT OF PURIFICATION	Fundamental ignorance	avidya	ma rigpa
Agent of purification	Wisdom deity	jnanasattva	yeshe sempa
Purified result	Dharmakaya body, which is endowed with two purities, inherent purity (inherent buddha) and subsequent purity	dharmakaya	cho kyi ku
THIRD OBJECT OF PURIFICATION	Conflicting emotional thoughts	kleshas	nyon mong pa
Agent of purification	Absorption deity	dhyanasattva	tingdzin sempa
Purified result	All thoughts manifesting as none other than great wisdom		tok tsok yeshe kyi rolpa

1 Source of interaction: sense + sense field, for example.

སུ་བྲ་པ་རྫོ༹ཆེ་ཧོ༦) and imagine all phenomena, including our bodies, as completely dissolved with no residue. If this is difficult, because your body and other things around you are still there, concentrate on withdrawing your sense consciousness from them so that your attention is entirely focused on their imagined emptiness. Then focus one-pointedly on the elements you visualize as appearing from that emptiness. From emptiness, we visualize a green letter PAM (པཾ) that turns into a multicolored, eight-petaled lotus. Next we visualize a white letter AH (ཨ) above the lotus that turns into a moon cushion. A white syllable HRIH (ཧྲཱིཿ) appears on the moon cushion, and this HRIH is your mind. (The text describes the generation as beginning immediately with the white letter HRIH. This visualization is perfectly adequate, but the additional steps provide the visualization with greater stability.)

The letter HRIH (ཧྲཱིཿ) emanates light rays that purify the negativities and obscurations of all sentient beings in all realms of samsara, causing them to become Chenrezig. Then all the Chenrezigs dissolve into light and, together with the light which you have emanated, come back to you and dissolve into the letter HRIH.

The white letter HRIH transforms into a blazing golden HRIH (ཧྲཱིཿ) on a golden lotus, which remains on top of the original multicolored lotus and moon cushion. Light rays emanate from the golden letter HRIH and golden lotus in the form of hooks and lassos, inviting all the buddhas and bodhisattvas from the ten directions who appear in the form of Chenrezig. They dissolve into the golden letter HRIH, causing the HRIH to turn into an image of you as Thousand-Armed Chenrezig.

Since the seed syllable HRIH (ཧྲཱིཿ) is your mind, the image derived from the HRIH is your mental body with the characteristics of Thousand-Armed Chenrezig. Its nature is like the moon's reflection on water, or that of a rainbow, not solid like a material object.

Deity Meditation with Five Purifications and Perfections, Blessing Being the Sixth

A purification and perfection takes place in each step of the main visualization process. The main point of this profound skillful means is to transform every aspect of the impure phenomena of our existence into pure phenomena. For example, our existence as impure ordinary human form bodies came about from the seeds of the father and mother, and eventually a complete body resulted. In an elaborate form of visualization, there is a method to purify and perfect all these stages.

The first purification and perfection is through meditation on emptiness, which clears away the extremes of eternalism. One instantaneously imagines all appearing phenomena as emptiness.

The second purification and perfection is through benefiting others by clearing away the extremes of nihilism. One meditates with compassion on those who have no understanding of emptiness.

The third purification and perfection is from one's seat, the sun and the moon and the lotus. The letter P A M (པཾ) becomes the lotus, the letter A H (ཨ) becomes a moon, and the letter M A (མ) becomes a sun.[30]

The fourth purification and perfection is from the seed syllable. The white syllable H R I H (ཧྲཱིཿ) on top of the lotus and moon disk radiates and transforms into another symbol. In our practice it transforms into a golden lotus and golden letter H R I H.

The fifth purification and perfection is from the deity body. One transforms oneself from the symbols of the golden lotus and letter H R I H into the body of Chenrezig, complete with all the attributes.

The sixth is not referred to as purification and perfection, but the blessing of one's body, speech, and mind. By visualizing the white letter O M (ཨོཾ) on your forehead, the red letter A H (ཨ) in your throat, and the blue letter H U N G (ཧཱུཾ) in your heart, one imagines becoming inseparable from the body, speech, and mind of all the buddhas.[31]

ESSENTIAL ELEMENTS OF THOUSAND-ARMED CHENREZIG

A white, youthful body stands on a moon cushion and multicolored lotus; clear like a diamond, it both radiates light and allows light to pass through it. Eleven faces, in the colors white, green, red, and black, are arranged as follows (mirror image view):[32]

---

30 In our practice we only have the lotus and moon disk on which Lord Chenrezig stands. I mention sun disks here because I am basing these teachings on the *Mani Kabum* and they are included there.

31 This sixth step in our visualization happens right after the invited Wisdom Deities merge with us. See "Self-Generation Continued" later in this chapter.

32 There are recognizable patterns to help with the memorization of the arrangement of these faces, such as the order of the colors, and so forth. The principal or root face in the center of the lowest head is white. Imagine turning this head counterclockwise one face. This results in the look of the second head above it, whose center face is green. Give the second head an equal turn, and the result is the look of the third head above it, whose center face is red. In visualizing yourself as Thousand-Armed Chenrezig, think that you are both able to feel what you are and also to look at yourself from the inside out. For instance, you can feel that your second right hand is holding a rosary. Since you have a body of light, you can also look right through it and see your faces as if looking into a mirror.

Red

Black

Green—Red—White

White—Green—Red

Red—White—Green

Eleven faces are a symbolic representation of the complete accomplishment and realization of the tenth-bhumi bodhisattva's qualities, the eleventh bhumi being the bhumi of complete buddhahood, complete perfection, and complete manifestation of all the qualities combined together. Complete relinquishment of all obscurations and defilements combined with complete manifestation of all qualities equals perfect buddhahood, and that's what the eleven faces represent.

A further representation of the details of the colors of these faces and the other aspects of Chenrezig's body is as follows. The three white faces are a representation of all the buddhas' form bodies, and Chenrezig benefits all sentient beings through the essence of this form, and the blessings of this form, and the activities of this form. Similarly, the three red faces are a representation of all the buddhas' speech, and Chenrezig benefits all sentient beings through the essence of this speech, and the blessings of this speech, and the activities of this speech. The three green faces are the representation of all the buddhas' mind, and Chenrezig benefits all sentient beings through the essence of this mind, and the blessings of this mind, and the activities of this mind. The wrathful, black face on top represents how Chenrezig benefits sentient beings that are very difficult to subdue or to tame. Wrathfulness is compassion turned into anger, because it is compassion in its most powerful state. Therefore the meaning is that Chenrezig finds a way to benefit even the most difficult sentient beings. On top of the wrathful face is a red, Amitabha Buddha face. In terms of the mandala principle, this symbolizes that Chenrezig belongs to the Amitabha Buddha Family, the buddha of the western direction, or the Lotus Family.

One could understand the colors of the faces in terms of the four enlightened activities as well. White is for pacification, green is for enrichment, red is for magnetizing, and black is for subjugation.

White also represents purification, shamatha or calm-abiding meditation, and the overcoming of conflicting emotions. Green also represents wisdom, that is, improvement or increase of qualities, especially knowledge and wisdom (in other texts sometimes represented as yellow). Red also represents attraction and empowerment. Black also represents the wrathful mode of the deity; in this case it is the face of Mahakala, an emanation of Chenrezig. All except the wrathful face wear the usual sambhogakaya ornaments (see below).

Chenrezig has one thousand arms, of which 992 are in the gesture of supreme giving, and one thousand arms represent the one thousand chakravartins (universal monarchs). They also represent Chenrezig's wish to protect all beings in a thousand different ways. The thousand eyes in these hands represent the thousand buddhas of this virtuous eon.[33] Finally, the one thousand eyes and arms represent the activity of all one thousand buddhas combined together.

Chenrezig holds implements in the eight principal arms as follows (mirror image view):

- First two hands, palms joined with the wish-fulfilling jewel
- Second right arm, crystal mala (rosary)
- Second left arm, golden lotus with stem
- Third right arm, mudra of supreme giving (no implement)
- Third left arm, empowerment vase
- Fourth right arm, wheel of knowledge
- Fourth left arm, bow and arrow

You may see a thangka in which the third pair of hands appears to be the fourth and vice versa, but the gesture of supreme giving is the third right hand, and the empowerment vase is in the third left hand. The right hand holding the wheel and the left hand holding the bow and arrow may appear to be up in the air like a third pair, but they are actually the fourth pair.

Chenrezig wears thirteen different types of ornaments:

The eight jeweled adornments:

1. A jewel crown
2. Jewel earrings
3. A short necklace
4. Two long necklaces, one longer than the other
5. A bracelet on each wrist
6. A golden belt at the waist with loops of jewelry
7. Armlets on each arm
8. An anklet on each foot

---

33 One thousand buddhas are predicted to appear on planet Earth, and therefore the lifetime of planet Earth is referred to as the virtuous eon.

The five silks:

1. A silk ribbon hanging from the back of the head
2. An upper garment
3. A long scarf
4. A silk skirt
5. A lower garment

Chenrezig radiates white or crystal clear light and appears translucent and insubstantial. In his heart center is a white syllable HRIH (ཧྲཱིཿ) on a moon cushion.

ADDITIONAL ASPECTS OF THE VISUALIZATION AND THEIR MEANINGS

The two palms joined right in the heart area are a symbol of direct perception into the dharmata, the true nature of phenomena. The wish-fulfilling jewel symbolizes bodhichitta. Just as a wish-fulfilling jewel fulfills everybody's wishes, similarly bodhichitta, which is the completely pure enlightened mind of Chenrezig, fulfills the wishes of everyone who prays for it.

In general, the golden lotus flower is a symbol of wisdom; it is completely pure and clear, even though it grows in muddy water. Furthermore, there is the understanding that even though Chenrezig manifests in samsara, he remains completely pure and unstained by it. The golden color symbolizes the lotus' rich quality, just as gold is universally considered precious and valuable. The crystal rosary is intended to lead beings from samsara in the same way that one bead leads to another.

The gesture of supreme giving represents how Chenrezig gives ultimate siddhis to everyone, and in particular the nectar flowing from his fingers is directed toward the beings in the hungry ghost realm to whom it provides relief from their suffering. The hungry ghost realm is the primary focus of attention because, from the point of view of the mandala principle, Chenrezig is the manifestation of the Lotus Family, and the Lotus Family buddhas have special power to benefit beings in the hungry ghost realm. However, visualizing the nectar benefiting beings in all realms is also fine.

The empowerment vase with its nectar is a symbol of purification. Just as water washes away dirt, similarly nectar from the empowerment vase purifies all negativities, karma, obscurations, and defilements.

The wheel of knowledge implies that Chenrezig is turning the wheel of dharma throughout the universe, beyond time and space. It also represents how he provides common, mundane siddhis. The bow and arrow signify that Chenrezig is perfectly skilled at balancing and harmonizing skillful means and wisdom.

Chenrezig stands on the moon cushion with two feet to indicate that he abides in neither samsara nor nirvana. Chenrezig's ornaments and robes symbolize the abundance of his enlightened qualities. The lotus Chenrezig stands on represents renunciation, and the moon cushion above the lotus represents bodhichitta. The five colored silks symbolize the five wisdoms with which Chenrezig is endowed.

A *tenasera* (Skt.) deerskin covers his left shoulder. The symbolic understanding of this special deer is that it has natural-born compassion. Its skin covers Chenrezig's left shoulder over his heart area, which represents Chenrezig's unceasing love and compassion for all sentient beings.[34]

SELF-GENERATION CONTINUED

The letter HRIH (ཧྲཱིཿ) in your heart center radiates light, inviting the essence of the real wisdom Chenrezig to appear from the Potala Realm, the pure land of Chenrezig. He obliges and appears before you, standing on top of a one-hundred-thousand-petaled lotus flower, surrounded by all the buddhas and bodhisattvas.

Using the appropriate mudras, you make offerings with mantra prayers and visualize the eight offering goddesses emanating from your heart center and carrying the offerings to Chenrezig. You then recite the "Four-Line Homage Prayer" with hands folded.

Following the Homage Prayer, Chenrezig merges with you through the recitation of the mantra DZA HUM BAM HO (ཛཿཧཱུྃ་བཾ་ཧོཿ) and the use of the appropriate mudra. As a result, the syllables OM AH HUNG (ཨོཾ་ཨཱཿཧཱུྃ), white, red, and blue respectively, appear at your three places (forehead, throat, and heart). At that moment you become identical with all the buddhas' body, speech, and mind.

The letter HRIH (ཧྲཱིཿ) again radiates light, inviting the Five Dhyani Buddhas (Fig. 4: Five Dhyani Buddhas), who appear before you in the order of Akshobhya, Ratnasambhava, Amitabha, Vairochana, and Amoghasiddhi. You request that they empower you, and the Five Female Buddhas (Fig. 5) emerge from their heart centers carrying vases of nectar. They pour

---

34 If you wish to know more about the compassionate deer, see "Praise to Chenrezig's Body" in Chapter 10.

this empowering nectar into your body and it enters through your crown, causing it to fill your body and overflow on the top of your head. From this, the Five Dhyani Buddhas are formed and become a crowning formation in the center and four directions as follows:

- *Amitabha*, red in color with the mudra of meditation, is located above your crown. This image merges with the peaceful, uppermost face.
- *Akshobhya*, blue in color with the earth-touching mudra, is located in front of your crown, above your forehead, to the east. (East is always the direction we look toward in meditation.)
- *Ratnasambhava*, yellow in color with the mudra of giving, is located to the south, above your right ear.
- *Vairochana*, white in color with the mudra of turning the dharma wheel, is located to the west, behind your crown.
- *Amoghasiddhi*, green in color with the mudra of giving refuge, is located to the north, above your left ear.

In this way, we are crowned by the Five Dhyani Buddhas, and the Five Female Buddhas melt into us. Occasionally reexamining this crown of buddhas during the visualization enhances the feeling of vajra pride, pride of being the deity.

As you come to the recitation of the mantra, visualize a thumb-sized Thousand-Armed Chenrezig in your heart center. Chenrezig is an exact replica of you and is the very essence of the deities of supreme knowledge (jnanasattva). The syllable HRIH (ཧྲཱིཿ) appears in Chenrezig's heart center and is the entity of the state of absorption of the deity (dhyanasattva). Some texts mention that the thumb-sized Chenrezig should be visualized as Chenrezig Kasarpani. This Chenrezig is two-armed and is sitting in bodhisattva posture. Either visualization is fine.

During recitation of the short mantra that begins TAYATA (ཏདྱ་ཐཱ) 108 times, and the mantra OM MANI PEME HUNG (ཨོཾ་མ་ཎི་པདྨེ་ཧཱུྃ) recited as many times as possible, we imagine the letter HRIH (ཧྲཱིཿ) in the heart of the thumb-sized Chenrezig radiating white or clear light that purifies all beings in the six realms. They become Chenrezig and dissolve into light, which is reabsorbed into the heart center. This is meant to be a continuous process.

Alternatively, imagine the Six-Syllable Mantra continuously circulating around the letter HRIH with light radiating from the syllables. Another possibility is to visualize the mantra OM MANI PEME HUNG (ཨོཾ་མ་ཎི་པདྨེ་ཧཱུྃ) in your heart center and concentrate on it spinning, which is the main visualization during Four-Armed Chenrezig meditation.

Furthermore, to practice with body, speech, and mind, visualize one's own body as Chenrezig's body, one's speech as the Six-Syllable Mantra, while meditating with one's mind on emptiness nature. Visualizing one's body as Chenrezig's body is to completely abandon one's own ordinary perception of body and to meditate on the supreme deity body. This supreme deity body is appearing yet in essence, empty; emptiness, yet clearly appearing. Speech recitation of the Six-Syllable Mantra should be as a vajra melody, and it should be uninterruptedly recited without attachment to ordinary speech. Mind meditating on emptiness nature is to meditate on the state of being free from conceptual elaboration and fabrication, uninterrupted by ordinary thoughts, and to not follow whatever thoughts do arise; rather to see them as the self-arising, luminous nature of mind, and to dwell in this state without any clinging.

THE FRONTAL VISUALIZATION FOR THE PURPOSE OF WORSHIP

We begin by reciting the mantra of emptiness, OM SVABHAWA SHUDDHA SARVA DHARMA SVABHA WA SHUDDHO HUM (ༀ་སྭ་བྷ་ཝ་ཤུདྡྷ་ སརྦ་དྷརྨ་ སྭ་བྷ་ཝ་ཤུདྡྷོ་ཧཱུྃ༔). It dissolves all phenomena except oneself, Chenrezig, into emptiness.

In your own heart center is the thumb-sized Chenrezig and the letter HRIH (ཧྲཱིཿ). From this letter HRIH, the seed syllable DRUM (ཌྲུཾ)[35] appears in the space in front of you. DRUM (ཌྲུཾ) transforms into a precious mandala palace, a four-sided structure that is insubstantial and translucent as if made of light, with four gates and a throne made of gems in its center. This is the mandala to which you invite the deity for the purpose of worship and prayer. The shrine represents this mandala, which is understood to be present in its entirety.

In the center of the mandala palace, visualize a green letter PAM (པཾ)) that transforms into a multicolored, eight-petaled lotus. On top of the lotus, you visualize a white letter AH (ཨ) that transforms into moon cushions in the center and four directions of the lotus. In the middle of the central moon cushion, a white syllable HRIH (ཧྲཱིཿ) appears, which you visualize transforming into Thousand-Armed Chenrezig, identical to oneself.

On the moon cushion of the front petal, to the east, the blue-colored seed syllable HUNG (ཧཱུྃ) appears. It transforms into Buddha Akshobhya, who is

---

35 DRUM (ཌྲུཾ) is the seed syllable of the precious mandala palace.

blue in color in the form of a nirmanakaya buddha,[36] with the earth-touching mudra.

On the moon cushion of the petal to Chenrezig's right, the south, a yellow-colored seed syllable TRAM (ཏྲཱཾ) appears. It transforms into Buddha Ratnasambhava, who is yellow in color in the nirmanakaya form with the mudra of supreme giving.

On the moon cushion of the petal to the back of Chenrezig, the west, the white-colored seed syllable OM (ཨོཾ) appears. It transforms into Buddha Vairochana, who is white in color in the nirmanakaya form, with the mudra of turning the wheel of dharma.

On the moon cushion to Chenrezig's left, the north, the green seed syllable AH (ཨཱཿ) appears. It transforms into Buddha Amoghasiddhi, who is green in color in the nirmanakaya form, with the mudra of giving refuge.

In addition to visualizing Chenrezig in front of you, and the Four Dhyani Buddhas on lotus petals in each of the four cardinal directions surrounding Chenrezig, you must also visualize four vases placed on the four petals between the buddhas.

A white letter OM (ཨོཾ), red letter AH (ཨཱཿ), and blue letter HUNG (ཧཱུྃ) appear on the forehead, throat, and heart areas of all the buddhas and the central Chenrezig, whereupon they become the embodiment of all the buddhas' body, speech, and mind. Light radiates from these three letters to the buddhafields, invoking the Wisdom Deities to appear in the sky right in front of you. (Although it is not mentioned in our Nyungne text, during this segment one should continually make homage and offerings to Chenrezig and the buddhas with mantras and mudras, if possible.)

Then the Wisdom Deities merge into the frontal visualization of Chenrezig and the buddhas with the mantra DZA HUNG BAM HO (ཛཿཧཱུྃ་བཾ་ཧོཿ). Again, light radiates from the letter HRIH (ཧྲཱིཿ) in the heart center of the frontal visualization of Thousand-Armed Chenrezig and invites the empowerment buddhas, the Five Dhyani Buddhas, to appear. From their hearts, the Five Female Buddhas emerge and pour nectar on the crowns of Chenrezig and the buddhas. As a sign of this empowerment, Chenrezig is crowned by Amitabha Buddha, who merges with Chenrezig's peaceful upper face and each of the four buddhas surrounding the central Chenrezig is crowned by a miniature replica of himself.

Next comes the recitation of the long mantra 108 times, followed by the Six-Syllable Mantra recited as much as possible. During the recitation, one visualizes nectar flowing from Chenrezig's third right hand and from

---

36 The nirmanakaya buddha form is identical to the Shakyamuni Buddha form.

one's own hand. The nectar flows into a huge victory vase that we visualize is placed in front of Chenrezig, and then it flows out into the universe in all directions, satisfying the thirst and suffering of the hungry ghosts. Although it is not mentioned in our Nyungne text, one can also visualize a thumb-sized Chenrezig on a lotus and moon cushion in the heart center of the frontal Chenrezig.

Light radiates from the letter HRIH (ཧྲཱི༔) located in the heart center and invokes a multitude of Chenrezigs. They purify the negativities of sentient beings in the three realms and deliver all beings to the level of Chenrezig. Light returns and dissolves back into the letter HRIH. This visualization is repeated during the recitation.

At the end of the recitation, the thumb-sized Chenrezig, which is the representation of the essence of the deities of supreme knowledge (jnanasattva), leaves your heart center and merges with the frontal visualization of Thousand-Armed Chenrezig. (Wisdom or jnanasattva Chenrezig returns to you at the end of the "Po Prayer," when he is absorbed by you together with Gelongma Palmo.)

Next, in ordinary form you engage in the "Seven-Branch Offering Prayer." The first offering is the offering of prostrations, which are physically performed with the prayer. After that you sit down. The second offering is the five substances with their appropriate mudras (during the final session we add recitation of Shantideva's "Offering Cloud"), and we offer the mandala of the universe. The third offering is the confession prayer, fourth is the prayer of rejoicing, and fifth is the prayer to turn the wheel of dharma. The sixth offering is the prayer not to pass into nirvana, and finally the seventh is the dedication of merit.

The famous homage prayer to Chenrezig (the "Po Prayer") follows with actual prostrations. Prior to engaging in prostration, one visualizes Gelongma Palmo on top of one's head and imagines that she graciously introduces you to Chenrezig. One bows sincerely while saying the "Po Prayer" seven times, then one returns to one's seat and with folded hands makes the "Special Request Prayer." Right after it, one imagines that Gelongma Palmo, who was sitting on top of our head, becomes Chenrezig and dissolves into oneself. As soon as this happens, we imagine ourselves once again in the form of Chenrezig, just like before.

Section Three

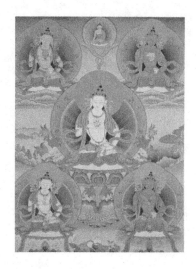

Mantras of Nyungne 9

IN GENERAL, a distinction is made between *dharani* (Skt.; Tib. *zung*) and *hridhaya* (Skt.; Tib. *nyingpo*). Both of these are mantras, however dharani relates to the body and speech of a particular deity whereas hridhaya relates to the mind. In this case dharani is the long mantra, and hridhaya is the short mantra, ༀ་མ་ཎི་པདྨེ་ཧཱུྃ། OM MANI PEME HUNG.

The long mantra is the main mantra recited during Nyungne practice. It has two parts, the long version and the short version, which is the second half of the long dharani.

BENEFITS OF THE RECITATION OF THE DHARANI

In the sutra *Thousand-Armed Chenrezig's Penetrating Mantra Power*, it mentions that if a connection is made to Lord Chenrezig, one will never be abandoned:

> Tathagata, any sentient being who recites and holds on to this awareness mantra of the Lord of Great Compassion, if they ever fall into the three lower realms, I, Chenrezig, vow to never attain enlightenment. If they are not born into the pure land of the Buddha, I vow to never attain enlightenment. If they do not develop great samadhi and tremendous spiritual confidence, I vow to never attain enlightenment. If their wishes in their immediate life do not come true, it shall not be called the mantra of the Great Compassionate One, unless they engage in wrong, unvirtuous activity, or recite the mantra without one-pointed concentration.

If there is a doubt in the power of the mantra, then the benefits will not come about. For those who commit the transgression of using offerings dedicated to the sangha, their deeds would only be completely purified through confession in the presence of a thousand buddhas; but if they recite the mantra of the Great Compassionate One, they will be able to completely overcome their misdeeds. The karma of misusing the offerings and possessions of the Three Jewels can be overcome by sincere confession in the presence of the buddhas of the ten directions. During the recitation of the mantra of the Great Compassionate One, the buddhas of the ten directions will automatically be present and, because of their power and blessing, one will be able to overcome all negativities. Furthermore, the ten unvirtuous deeds, the five sins which ripen immediately, and disparaging honorable beings, breaking vows, destroying stupas and temples, stealing possessions that belong to the sangha, etc., all such major transgressions will be overcome by reciting this mantra, unless you doubt the power of the mantra. If you doubt this power, there is no need to mention the major transgressions; even the minor ones will not be overcome. In the long run, however, it will still be an enlightened cause.

Furthermore, Chenrezig vows to liberate sentient beings from the prison of samsara, and he wishes to gaze on all beings with his eleven faces and touch them all with his thousand hands:

> Noble sons and daughters who practice Nyungne on auspicious days, full moon or half moon days, and bow down and recite the mantra 108 times, and hold me in their thoughts, even if they have the karma of the five sins which ripen immediately, I will bring such beings into the pure land of Great Bliss. If such beings ever fall to the lower realms, I shall never attain enlightenment.

Anything and everything in the universe may change, but not the power of the ultimate truth of the bodhisattva's vow; this is unchangeable.

Here is a passage from the sutra which basically summarizes all the benefits in this life and beyond:

> Those who always rise early in the morning and recite this mantra 108 times will receive ten benefits in this very lifetime:
>
> 1. They will be free from physical illness.
> 2. They will be protected by gods and buddhas.
> 3. They will have abundant wealth and food.
> 4. Their enemies will be subdued.

5. They will be respected and honored by their spouse.
6. They will be free from harm by poisons, ghosts, and demons.
7. The sweet smell of their body will please everyone.
8. They will be free from the ill thoughts and ill speech of others.
9. They will be free from contagious disease.
10. They will not suffer from untimely death.

In addition they will attain the following:

1. At the time of death they will see the Buddha and see a light in the sky and be worshipped by the gods.
2. They will not be born in the lower realms.
3. They will be born in the pure land of Great Bliss (Skt. Sukhavati).
4. They will inherit the attributes of al the buddhas and bodhisattvas.

This great mantra of Thousand-Armed Chenrezig is known to have been taught by eleven billion buddhas. If you have faith and recite this mantra you will undoubtedly receive all that you need and wish for, and be free from all obstacles. Whoever thinks about Chenrezig and recites this long dharani will receive immediate and ultimate benefits.

BENEFITS OF THE SIX-SYLLABLE MANTRA

ཨོཾ་མ་ཎི་པདྨེ་ཧཱུྃ།

OM MANI PEME HUNG

This precious mantra, supreme among all mantras, has a vast array of meanings. The mantra, OM MANI PEME HUNG, arises from the power of the compassion and activity of Lord Chenrezig, who is the embodiment of the combined wisdom of all the buddhas.

The letter OM (ཨོཾ) is all the buddhas' body. Here one can understand that OM (ཨོཾ) is the essence of all the buddhas of the past, present, and future, so whenever you say this supreme among all sounds, you are praying to all the buddhas as well as to the potential buddha within. This supreme syllable gives us the opportunity to become buddha. This possibility arises because of the next syllables, MANI (མ་ཎི) and PEME (པདྨེ), the jewel and the lotus.

The jewel represents bodhichitta, the enlightened heart, and only this enlightened heart can fulfill everybody's wishes. Just as a wish-fulfilling jewel fulfills the outer needs of all sentient beings, similarly bodhichitta, the compassion of Lord Chenrezig, fulfills the inner needs of all sentient beings. The lotus represents wisdom. Just as the beautiful and pure lotus grows out of muddy water, similarly wisdom born from mind is unaffected by the mind's ordinary thoughts; understanding of the true nature of phenomena is completely pure and clear and transcends mundane existence.

Last is the letter HUNG (ཧཱུྃ), which has the qualities of immutability and unity. Immutability is the quality of the vajra, and this vajra quality of mind demonstrates the union of compassion and emptiness, which is Lord Chenrezig's emptiness nature of mind. This means that the immutable quality of Chenrezig's mind never wavers and constantly benefits sentient beings. The completely perfected body of the Buddha exists in this final letter, the symbol of immutability and the unity of wisdom and compassion. From it the perfect form buddha body arises, which is represented by OM (ༀ).

Practically speaking, when we recite the mantra OM MANI PEME HUNG we are showing our faith and devotion to Chenrezig and the buddhas, taking refuge in them, seeking protection for all sentient beings, engendering bodhichitta, purifying negativities, shutting the door to the six realms, and so forth.

Padmasambhava said,

> The mantra OM MANI PEME HUNG is the embodiment of all the buddhas' heart, the root of the eighty-four thousand teachings of the Buddha, the essence of the Five Buddhas, and the essence of the secret holders. Each word is a pith instruction, the source of the qualities of all the tathagatas, the root of all goodness and siddhis, the great path to higher realms and complete freedom. To recite this supreme among all mantras, the six syllables, the heart of all the teaching, just once can put you onto a spiritual path of no-turning-back, and you can become a great liberator of other sentient beings. Even a small insect, if it were to hear the sounds of the mantra just before dying, would be liberated from that body and be born in the pure land of Amitabha. Just to think of it is like the sun shining on a snow mountain so brightly that bad karmic obscurations and defilements are eliminated, and one can be born in the pure land of Amitabha Buddha. Just touching the mantra OM MANI PEME HUNG is receiving empowerment from many buddhas and bodhisattvas. Meditating on it once equals the practices of listening, contemplating, and meditating combined together. In this way the entire experience of phenomena can be

transformed into dharmakaya experience, and great treasure gates of activity can be opened to benefit sentient beings.

The following speech of the Buddha is taken from the *Mani Kabum*:[37]

Sons and daughters of noble family, I can measure on a pound scale how much the entire Mt. Meru weighs, but I cannot measure the merit of reciting the mantra OM MANI PEME HUNG just one time. I can tell you it is possible to eliminate a solid vajralike rock by rubbing it with a silk cloth once every hundred years, but I cannot measure the amount of merit gathered by reciting the mantra OM MANI PEME HUNG just one time. One can eliminate this mighty ocean drop by drop, but one cannot eliminate the merit of reciting the mantra OM MANI PEME HUNG just one time. I can count each snowflake, every blade of grass, and every leaf in the entire world, but I cannot count the merit of reciting the mantra OM MANI PEME HUNG just one time. By removing one sesame seed every day it is possible to exhaust the sesame seeds filling a gigantic house more than a hundred miles high,[38] but it is not possible to exhaust the merit of reciting the mantra OM MANI PEME HUNG just one time. I can count every drop of rain that falls nonstop everywhere in the entire world for twelve years, but I cannot count the merit of reciting the mantra OM MANI PEME HUNG just one time. Thus it is, children of noble family; though it is not necessary to speak of many things, I can count the merit accumulated by praying and making offerings to a million tathagatas like myself, but I cannot count the merit of reciting the mantra OM MANI PEME HUNG just one time. This is the mantra that shuts the door to the six realms and that helps beings tread the path of the six perfections, and this is the one that helps purify obscurations of karma and afflictive emotions and purifies one's own future buddhafield of three kayas.

Listen, children of noble family, blessed by all the victors, the

---

37 The *Mani Kabum* is one of the first dharma books ever written in the Tibetan language. It is a two-volume work by the first Tibetan dharma king, Songtsen Gompo, who is believed to be an emanation of Chenrezig.

38 Although I translated this as "a hundred miles," a standardized American measurement, the actual measurement is according to Buddhist scriptural designation; therefore this is an approximation.

essential heart of everything, source of benefit and joy, root of
all the siddhis, ladder to the higher realms, this shuts the door
to the lower realms; vessel that crosses cyclic existence, beacon
that illumines the darkness, courageous subduer of the five
poisons, fire that burns sins and obscurations, hammer that
pounds suffering, remedy for conquering the untamed land,[39]
dharma fortune of the land of snow, sutras, tantras and shastras,
listening, contemplating and meditating, this is the essence all
in one; precious, victorious one that does all. So recite the six
syllables.

Here I wish to clarify one thing. One may ask, how could it be that the
merit of reciting the mantra one time is far greater than offering and praying to a million tathagatas and all these other comparisons? The reason is
the distinction between ordinary and supreme merit. The examples given
here are of ordinary merit, whereas the merit of reciting the mantra OM
MANI PEME HUNG is so vast because it is always supreme merit. It can
never be ordinary merit. To make a spiritual deed a supreme deed, usually one has to engage in such a deed with pure motivation and one must
conclude with a proper dedication prayer. In the case of reciting OM MANI
PEME HUNG, it is naturally perfect all by itself. Therefore, reciting this
mantra whenever you can is limitlessly beneficial.

According to the *Sutra Designed as a Jewel*,

This mantra is the essence of Lord Chenrezig, and he who
embraces this Six-Syllable Mantra is a karmically fortunate being.
When reciting this mantra, he will attract as many buddhas as the
grains of sand in the Ganges River multiplied ninety-two times.
He will further attract as many bodhisattvas as there are countless subatomic particles. Thus one will be able to enter the door
of the six perfections and will also attract gods of the thirty-sec-
ond realm. The four god kings will protect him, all the naga kings
and millions of other nagas will also protect him, and many other
spirit beings will offer protection as well.

One pore of Lord Chenrezig's body contains one million

---

39 Prior to the arrival of the dharma, the land of Tibet was considered wild and untamed.
Tibetan kings, who were believed to be incarnations of Chenrezig, spread the dharma and
particularly made the recitation of the mantra OM MANI PEME HUNG very popular.

buddhas, and you will be blessed to receive the wish-fulfilling jewel of enlightenment within seven lifetimes. All the beings that live in and on your body will also be liberated. The body of those who wear this mantra will become a vajra body; their body will be like a stupa with relics in it and will represent Buddha's wisdom. He who recites this mantra will gain tremendous confidence, will gain wisdom, and will develop enormous compassion; with each passing day he will be able to perfect the six perfections and become a Vidyadhara, a victorious ruler, and quickly attain perfect buddhahood. He who touches others will enable them to become bodhisattvas, as well as cause this to be their last samsaric birth. Even animals and others who see this person, or are in this person's thoughts, will end their suffering lives and become bodhisattvas, and that will be their last samsaric birth as well.

In addition to all the great comparisons of the benefits of the recitation of the mantra OM MANI PEME HUNG, Lord Buddha also mentions in the sutra that to write this mantra is to write the entire eighty-four thousand teachings of the Buddha. Another comparison is if you were to build as many statues out of gold from the god realm as the number of subatomic particles in the universe, they would equal in value one syllable of the mantra OM MANI PEME HUNG. This really is the heart of the doctrine, whereas others are like "window dressing."

Here is an excerpt from the writing of the Fifteenth Gyalwa Karmapa[40] on the mantra OM MANI PEME HUNG:

> The first syllable, OM (ༀ), is white in color; it is the display of Lord Chenrezig's five wisdoms and the essence of all his qualities. It is in the nature of the perfection of meditation. It purifies the karma of pride, the general result of pride, and in particular it purifies the suffering of change and falling of the god realms. It is also the inseparable union of the activity and body of the buddha of the god realm (Tib. Gya jin, Skt. Muni Zakra). The self-arisen form of the wisdom of equanimity, it liberates beings from the six realms to the Glorious Pure Land of the southern direction (Tib. Lho pal

---

40 The Fifteenth Karmapa wrote this commentary on a Four-Armed Chenrezig practice at the request of two of his female disciples.

tang den pa'i shing, Skt. Ratnaloka) and it enables everyone to achieve the buddhahood of Ratnasambhava.

The second syllable, MA (མ), is green in color and is the grace of Lord Chenrezig touching all sentient beings. It is the display of Chenrezig's limitless benevolence, the essence of all his activity, and is in the nature of the perfection of patience. It purifies the karma of jealousy, the general result of jealousy, and in particular purifies the suffering of the fighting and quarreling of the demi-god realm. It is also the inseparable union of the activity and body of the buddha of the demi-god realm (Tib. Thag zang ri tib, Skt. Vemachitra). The self-arisen form of all-accomplishing wisdom, it liberates beings from the six realms to the Supreme Perfected Realm of the northern direction (Tib. Chang le rab dzok pa'i shing, Skt. Karmaprasiddhi), and it enables everyone to achieve the buddhahood of Amoghasiddhi.

The third syllable, NI (ཎི), is yellow in color and is the grace of Lord Chenrezig effortlessly reaching out. It is the display of the combined body, speech, mind, and activity of vajra wisdom, the syllable of reversing samsara naturally into the realm of nirvana. It is in the nature of the perfection of morality. It purifies the ignorance of clinging to duality, and the general result of ignorance; and in particular it purifies the suffering of birth, old age, illness, and death of the human realm. It is the inseparable union of the activity and body of the buddha of the human realm, Shakyamuni Buddha. The self-arisen form of self-arising wisdom, it liberates beings from the six realms to the pure land of the Absolute Realm of Dharmadhatu (Tib. Og min cho kyi ying, Skt. Akanishtha Dharmadhatu) and it enables everyone to achieve the buddhahood of the sixth buddha, Vajradhara.

The fourth syllable, PE (པད), is blue in color and is the grace of Lord Chenrezig's limitless equanimity. It is the display of the syllable of form, and is in the nature of the perfection of wisdom. It purifies the karma of stupidity and its general result, and in particular it purifies the suffering of the tormented bewilderment of the animal realm. It is the inseparable union of the activity and body of the buddha of the animal realm (Tib. Sang gye rab ten, Skt. Shravasinha). The self-arising wisdom of dharmata, it liberates beings from the six realms to the central pure land of Densely Displayed (Tib. Tug po kodpa, Skt. Ghanavyuha). It enables everyone to achieve the buddhahood of Vairochana.

The fifth syllable, ME (མེ), is red in color and is the grace of reaching all with limitless joy. It is the display of the syllable of speech, and is in the nature of the perfection of generosity. It purifies the karma of desire and greed and their general results, and in particular it purifies the suffering of the hunger and thirst of the hungry ghost realm. It is the inseparable union of the activity and body of the buddha of the hungry ghost realm (Tib. Kha la me bar, Skt. Mukha Agni Valate). Self-arising discriminating wisdom, it liberates beings from the six realms to the pure land of Great Bliss (Tib. Dewachen, Skt. Sukhavati), the western buddhafield. It enables everyone to achieve the buddhahood of Amitabha.

The sixth syllable, HUNG (ཧཱུྃ), is black in color, and it is the grace of Lord Chenrezig gazing with limitless compassion on all beings as if they were all his children. It is the display of the syllable of mind and is in the nature of the perfection of mirrorlike wisdom. It purifies the karma of hatred and its general result, and in particular it purifies the suffering of the hot and cold of the hell realms. It is the inseparable union of the activity and body of the buddha of the hell realms (Tib. Cho kyi gyal po, Skt. Dharmaraja). Self-arising mirrorlike wisdom, it liberates beings from the six realms to the pure land of Obvious Joy (Tib. Ngon par ga wa, Skt. Abhirati), the eastern buddhafield. It enables everyone to achieve the buddhahood of Akshobhya.

When one recites the mantra OM MANI PEME HUNG, one must say it with one-pointed focus and attention on Lord Chenrezig. Each recitation is like saying, "Guru Chenrezig, think of me."

Another way of understanding this is that the letter OM (ༀ) is the condensation of the five wisdoms and the five kayas; MANI (མ་ཎི) is precious jewel and PEME (པདྨེ) means lotus, the jewel and the lotus, which is Chenrezig's name; and the letter HUNG (ཧཱུྃ) is Lord Chenrezig's activity to protect beings from the suffering of the six realms. In other words, when we recite the mantra we are saying, "Embodiment of the Five Kayas and Five Wisdoms, Jewel and Lotus, please protect all of us from the suffering of the six realms."

This is definitely a mantra that has been highly praised in the sutras and tantras. For mantra recitation, you cannot find a more profound one than this; therefore it is ultimately important for the serious practitioner to put a great deal of effort into reciting this mantra.

How the Six-Syllable Mantra Relates to the External, Internal, and Secret Aspects

The following information about the Six-Syllable Mantra is taken from the *Mani Kabum*:

> According to the sutra tradition, the correlation of the six syllables to the six perfections is the first of three external aspects:
>
> OM   to the perfection of generosity,
> MA   to the perfection of morality,
> NI   to the perfection of patience,
> PE   to the perfection of perseverance,
> ME   to the perfection of meditation,
> HUNG   to the perfection of wisdom.
>
> The second aspect is:
>
> OM   helps keep the hinayana vows,
> MA   helps keep the bodhisattva vows,
> NI   helps keep the eight-precepts vows,
> PE   helps keep the genyan vow,
> ME   helps keep the vow of celibacy, and
> HUNG   helps keep tantric vows.
>
> The third aspect is:
>
> OM   limitless benefit to others, purifies obscurations of body;
> MA   limitless loving-kindness, purifies obscurations of speech;
> NI   limitless compassion, purifies obscurations of mind;
> PE   limitless joy, purifies obscurations of afflictive emotions;
> ME   limitless equanimity, purifies obscurations of habitual tendencies;
> HUNG   limitless dharmata, purifies obscurations of knowledge.
>
> The internal aspects correlate with the secret mantrayana and also have three parts. The first six are:
>
> OM   connected to the buddha of the god realm, helps to purify the suffering of falling and changing;

MA   connected to the buddha of the demi-god realm, purifies
     the suffering of fighting and quarreling;
NI   connected to the buddha of the human realm, purifies
     the suffering of change: birth, old age, illness, and death;
PE   connected to the buddha of the animal realm, purifies
     the suffering of dullness and stupidity;
ME   connected to the buddha of the hungry ghost realm,
     purifies the suffering of hunger and thirst;
HUNG   connected to the buddha of the hell realms, purifies the
     suffering of heat and cold.

The second six are connected to the six fathers, mothers, and dakinis
that pacify the six afflictive emotions:

OM   All inclusive family, Father Lord Chenrezig, Mother Six
     Syllables, All-Dakini; pacifies all conflicting emotions.
MA   Father Buddha Vairochana, Mother Buddha Lochana,
     Buddha Dakini; pacifies the conflicting emotions of
     ignorance.
NI   Father Buddha Vajrasattva, Mother Buddha Samanta-
     bhadri, Vajra Dakini; pacifies the conflicting emotions of
     aggression.
PE   Father Buddha Ratnasambhava, Mother Buddha Mamaki,
     Ratna Dakini; pacifies the conflicting emotions of pride.
ME   Father Buddha Amitabha, Mother Buddha Pandaravasini,
     Padma Dakini; pacifies the conflicting emotions of desire.
HUNG   Father Buddha Amoghasiddhi, Mother Buddha Samaya-
     tara, Karma Dakini; pacifies the conflicting emotions of
     jealousy.

The third six are correlations of the six kayas and six wisdoms:

OM   Dharmakaya, wisdom of dharmadhatu;
MA   Sambhogakaya, mirrorlike wisdom;
NI   Nirmanakaya, wisdom of equanimity;
PE   Svabhavikakaya, discriminating wisdom;
ME   Abhisambodhikaya, wisdom of activity;
HUNG   Immutable Vajrakaya, wisdom born of itself.

The secret aspects correlate with the six dharmatas. The first six ultimate points of dharmata are:

OM   Uncontrived ground,

MA   Unobstructed path,

NI   Transformation of affliction into wisdom,

PE   The inseparability of wisdom and skillful means,

ME   Self-arising wisdom burning all thoughts,

HUNG   Magnetizing rigpa (awareness), self-arising from dharmata.

The second six ultimate meanings of the dharmatas are:

OM   Self-arising wisdom is the meaning of dharmata;

MA   The essence is the meaning of dharmata;

NI   The natural reverse of samsara is the meaning of dharmata;

PE   The union of dharmadhatu and wisdom is the meaning of dharmata;

ME   Burning all thoughts and habits into emptiness is the meaning of dharmata;

HUNG   Immutable heart is the meaning of dharmata.

The third six correlate with view, meditation, and action:

OM   View by way of the six senses, naturally without fabrication;

MA   Meditation, uncontrived mind without clinging;

NI   Action, naturally reversing from incorrectness;

PE   Result or fruit, self-arising dharmakaya free from extremes;

ME   Flawless samaya, self-purifying imprints;

HUNG   Self-arising dharmata, rigpa (awareness), and wisdom: in it everything is contained.

RECITATION OF THE MANTRA IS OF SIX DIFFERENT KINDS

The first kind of recitation of the mantra OM MANI PEME HUNG is referred to as sutra tradition recitation. The Six-Syllable Mantra should be recited like a talented person blowing a conch shell, continuously making a big or small sound. Imagining that whoever hears the sounds of the mantra has their obscurations purified is recitation in the sutra tradition.

The second, inner tantric recitation, is divided into two sections, jnanasattva and samayasattva. Imagining that light radiates from the samayasattva's heart and touches the jnanasattva's heart, one thinks all kinds of offerings are being made to please the body, speech, and mind of the jnanasattva. Light comes from the jnanasattva and touches the samayasattva's heart, by which one thinks one is receiving all the siddhis. In this way light continuously circles back and forth, and one recites the mantra like the sound of a flute, with high and low pitch.

Third is the secret dakinis' blessing-sign recitation. While reciting the mantra, multicolored light radiates from the letter HRIH (ཧྲཱིཿ) in one's heart and goes to the dakini realm. From there dakinis are magnetized and one imagines that they come right in front of you. In this way your body, speech, and mind, and those of others, are blessed by the dakinis. Recite the mantra like the sounds of a damaru, stronger and stronger.

The fourth, homage and prayer to guru and deity, is like children-calling-for-their-mother recitation. While reciting, light radiates from the letter HRIH in the heart center and it touches gurus, deities, and dakinis. Then, just as a mother will compassionately answer the call of a child, they will appear in the sky right in front of you. Imagining them blessing you and dispelling your obstacles, one recites the mantra like the sounds of a tambura, with changing melody.

Each syllable is itself a prayer and offering:

> OM   is the prayer and offering to the body of the buddhas;
> MA   is the prayer and offering to the speech of the buddhas;
> NI   is the prayer and offering to the mind of the buddhas;
> PE   is the prayer and offering to the qualities of the buddhas;
> ME   is the prayer and offering to the activities of the buddhas;
> HUNG   gathers the blessings of the body, speech, mind, qualities, and activities of the buddhas.

The fifth is purification practice recitation. Here one visualizes one's tongue as a six-petaled lotus, in the center of which is the letter HRIH. On each of the petals is a syllable of the Six-Syllable Mantra. One recites the mantra like a well-versed text reader, with clear and precise sounds that capture the attention. One should recite with devotion from one's body, speech, and mind:

> OM   purifies obscurations of the body;
> MA   purifies obscurations of speech;
> NI   purifies obscurations of mind;

> PE purifies obscurations of afflictive emotions;
> ME purifies obscurations of habitual tendencies;
> HUNG purifies obscurations of obstructions to omniscience.

The sixth, vajra recitation, is with meditative equipoise and samadhi. While reciting the mantra one rests one's body, speech, and mind and recites the mantra mentally, in complete silence. Speech is uninterrupted with ordinary words, and mind rests without any discursive thoughts, clear yet undistracted.

> OM mind and dharmata, free from conceptual fabrications;
> MA mind and dharmata, self-arising;
> NI mind and dharmata, self-clarity;
> PE mind and dharmata, clarity and purity;
> ME mind and dharmata, emptiness and clarity;
> HUNG mind and dharmata, inherent purity.

Such recitation could generate the experience of the union of bliss, clarity, and emptiness.

In general, the meaning of the Six-Syllable Mantra can be condensed into OM AH HUNG as follows:

OM (ཨོཾ) is the condensation of the five wisdoms. The letter AH (ས) in itself represents the wisdom of dharmadhatu. The sphere (°) is mirror-like wisdom. The moon sliver (˘) is the wisdom of equanimity. The vowel naro (˘) is discriminating wisdom. The long stroke (❙) is all-accomplishing wisdom.[41]

Between the letters OM and HUNG, the four syllables MA (མ), NI (ཎི), PE (པད), ME (མེ) are condensed into AH (ས). The letter AH (ས) is the essence of the unborn nature of reality, free from conceptual fabrications and elaborations.

HUNG (ཧཱུྃ) is the vajralike immutable syllable. Lord Chenrezig's dharmadhatulike emptiness nature of mind is like the vajra, and it is inseparable from compassion and emptiness. It is immutable in benefiting other sentient beings.

The three letters OM AH HUNG are naturally associated with our breath: inhaling is naturally OM (ཨོཾ), holding the breath is naturally AH (ས), and exhaling the breath is naturally HUNG (ཧཱུྃ). In tantra one can find statements

---

41 This stroke is seen more clearly in the Sanskrit OM (ॐ·). The long stroke is the wavy line on the right. In the Tibetan version the line was drawn straight down from the top (ཨ), to which a vertical line was also added (ཨོཾ).

such as, "If one dwells in nonconceptual mind, one is naturally dwelling in the deity and mantra." The reason we are saying this is because it describes the natural state of being, and when one is in such a natural state of being, one is automatically reciting the Six-Syllable Mantra.

> OM   is the foundation for body,
> AH   is the foundation for speech,
> HUNG   is the natural reverse of samsara, the meaning of
>   dharmata.

A sentient being's body, speech, and mind are naturally the three syllables; the enlightened body, speech, and mind are also the three syllables.

> OM   is the essence of all the buddhas' body, and it purifies a
>   sentient being's body and enables sambhogakaya bud-
>   dha body.
> AH   is the essence of all the buddhas' speech, and it purifies
>   a sentient being's speech and enables nirmanakaya bud-
>   dha body.
> HUNG   is the essence of all the buddhas' mind and it purifies a
>   sentient being's mind and enables dharmakaya buddha
>   body.

THE POWER OF MANTRA

Since mantras are just made up of words, people in modern society may have difficulty understanding that reciting mantras brings genuine beneficial effects. They don't see the potential effect of words on our minds, whereas in traditional Buddhist societies like Tibet everybody believes the recitation of mantras is beneficial, and they recite mantras such as OM MANI PEME HUNG continuously. I remember my enlightened guru teaching on the power of mantra and how words really work. He would say things like, some sounds are just sounds and once you utter them, there is no particular meaning and they may just disappear into space. Nevertheless, words can be very powerful, and everyday life experience illustrates this. For instance, if someone praises you with all kinds of flattering words, you feel good and great and so on, even though they are just words. On the contrary, if someone speaks about you in a derogatory manner, you feel upset, angry, sad, all the unpleasant emotions. My guru used to quote a famous Tibetan saying:

> Words do not have sharp points like arrows or spears,
> But they shatter the heart into many pieces.

This illustrates that there definitely is a power behind words and the question is, how do we tap into real, spiritually powerful, and beneficial words? That's where the benefits of mantra come in. My precious Lord Guru used to explain it in very simple terms. He said that when we recite the mantra OM MANI PEME HUNG, through Chenrezig we are praying to the body, speech, and mind of all the buddhas and invoking the power of loving-kindness and compassion.

He also spoke about how it is that we human beings are able to utter such words as mantras and all kinds of other sophisticated speech. It mainly has to do with some seventy-two thousand channels that exist in the body, and how they are in the form of letters: the Sanskrit vowels and consonants. Energy flowing through these channels gives us the ability to produce many varied sounds. Perhaps this is the reason thousands of languages exist in the world. Apparently animal forms lack certain channels and therefore their means of communication are limited. In addition to the five elements, intricate expression also requires the element of primordial awareness, which is a total of six elements. These six elements make our human body a vajra body. This body is the basis for expressing and understanding in a very complex manner.

My guru also said no ordinary person can make mantra, nor can they completely comprehend the depth of the meaning of mantra from the point of view of exactly how it works and so on. He said that one has to be at least on the level of an eighth-bhumi bodhisattva or higher to completely comprehend the effects of the mantra and to create a mantra. Although eighth-bhumi bodhisattvas and higher have the ability to create mantras, the mantras are always naturally present, and when and if there is a need, such beings can make them available.

Benefits of Practice

According to the *Mani Kabum*, the signs of the benefits of practice are:

> With respect to the body, negativities of the body are purified, blessings of the body are received, and visions of Chenrezig's body appear. With respect to speech, speech is purified, blessings of one's speech make it powerful, and prophecy through speech is received; and the sounds of the Six-Syllable Mantra are heard and

perceived. With respect to mind, one's mind is purified, blessings of the mind enable one to experience joy and realization, and a true state of mind of great bliss, clarity, and nonthought arises.

In conclusion, the true signs of spiritual improvement and benefit from the practice are an increased faith and devotion to the Three Jewels and Three Roots, loving-kindness and compassion towards fellow sentient beings, and sacred outlook toward one's spiritual siblings. These are the real measures of spiritual growth.

Songtsen Gompo's Verses on the Mantra om mani peme hung[42]

OM: If one recites this self-arisen primordial wisdom,
In the realm of the great wisdom awareness
There is natural purification of the stain of confusion;
The perfection of wisdom awareness is completed.

MA: If one recites this great compassion,
Through undistracted meditative absorption
There is natural purification of the stain of distraction;
The perfection of meditative concentration is completed.

NI: If one recites this source of everything,
All conflicting emotions are pacified and
There is natural purification of the stain of confusion;
The perfection of ethical discipline is completed.

PE: If one recites this stainless purity,
Through great effort one benefits others.
There is natural purification of the stain of laziness;
The perfection of perseverance is completed.

ME: If one recites this ripener of things,
Inexhaustible wealth abundantly arises.
There is natural purification of the stain of stinginess;
The perfection of generosity is completed.

---

42 Songtsen Gompo is a Tibetan king who is believed to be an emanation of Chenrezig. These verses are taken from *Mani Kabum*.

HUNG: If one recites this amasser of things,
Suffering will enter into the realm of joy.
There is natural purification of the stain of aggression;
The perfection of patience is completed.

This explains how the six syllables are the essence of the six perfections.

OM: Recitation of self-luminous primordial wisdom:
This realm of great wisdom awareness gloriously
Pacifies the change and falling of the god realm.
Taking rebirth in the realm of gods is blocked.

MA: Recitation of this unobstructed equilibrium:
Unceasing great compassion of meditative concentration
Pacifies the pain of quarreling and delivers joy.
Taking rebirth in the realm of demi-gods is blocked.

NI: Recitation of this union of everything:
Conflicting emotions are pacified and dharmata arises,
Suffering is pacified, one achieves the five kayas.
Taking rebirth in the realm of humans is blocked.

PE: Recitation of this stainless pure clarity:
Abandoning laziness, with faith and perseverance,
Confusion is overcome and pure awareness arises.
Taking rebirth in the realm of animals is blocked.

ME: Recitation of this great primordial wisdom:
In the absence of stinginess, great abundance;
Hunger and thirst are pacified, all wishes come true.
Taking rebirth in the realm of hungry ghosts is blocked.

HUNG: Recitation of this great magnetizing power:
Patience can greatly eliminate aggression,
Pacify heat and cold, and deliver joy.
Taking rebirth in the realm of hell is blocked.

This explains how the six syllables eliminate all the suffering of the six realms and shut the door to the six migrations.

OM: Reciting that which is the ultimate arising kaya,
Suffering from clinging is pacified, with
No attachment to the six sense-field objects.
This is the essence of dharmakaya.

MA: Reciting that which is freedom from dualistic fixation
And which cares with loving-kindness and compassion,
There will be no clinging to self and others.
This is the essence of sambhogakaya.

NI: Reciting that which is the essence of everything,
The power of kindness will capture all beings.
Thus is all-pervading compassion.
This is the essence of nirmanakaya.

PE: Reciting that which is the pure and stainless,
All wrong habitual tendencies are purified.
Such is the power of transformation manifestation.
This is the essence of svabhavikakaya.

ME: Reciting that which abandons attachment and clinging,
Abiding equilibriumly, free from the two extremes,
Not affected by desire and attachment.
This is the essence of pure manifestation.

HUNG: Reciting that which arises from within,
Firm in its fundamental, immutable quality,
It abides without time, beginning, or end.
This is the essence of vajrakaya.

Thus the six kayas are achieved through this precious Six-Syllable Mantra.

OM: To recite this self-luminous primordial wisdom,
There is no clinging to good or bad form.
The sense field of eye is nonattached to phenomena;
Form is liberated and dissolves in the realm of emptiness.

MA: To recite this unobstructed flow of thoughts,
There is no clinging to pleasant and unpleasant sound.

The sense field of ear is nonattached to phenomena;
Sound is liberated and dissolves in the realm of emptiness.

NI: To recite this self-arising primordial wisdom,
There is no clinging to good or bad smell.
The sense field of nose is nonattached to phenomena;
Smell is liberated and dissolves in the realm of emptiness.

PE: To recite this supreme self-luminosity,
There is no clinging to pleasant and unpleasant taste.
The sense field of tongue is nonattached to phenomena;
Taste is liberated and dissolves in the realm of emptiness.

ME: To recite this uncontrived dharmata,
There is no clinging to good or bad tactile sense.
The sense field of body is nonattached to phenomena;
Touch is liberated and dissolves in the realm of emptiness.

HUNG: To recite this immutable nature of phenomena,
There is no clinging to pleasant and unpleasant thought.
The sense field of mind is nonattached to phenomena;
The mind is liberated and dissolves in the realm of emptiness.

Thus, this precious Six-Syllable Mantra transforms the six senses into pure virtue and the six sense-field objects into phenomena of emptiness.

OM: To recite this subduer of stupidity,
Ignorance is cleared away in the field of awareness.
The nature of dharma is unchangeably self-reliant,
Pristine wisdom of dharmata manifest.

MA: To recite this destroyer of aggression,
Self-awareness is clear in the bodhi mind—
The realm of clarity and purity,
Mirrorlike pristine wisdom manifest.

NI: To recite this destroyer of pride,
The experience of suchness appears
Distinctively in the realm of self-clarity—
Pristine wisdom of equanimity manifest.

PE: To recite this destroyer of desire,
The sphere of suchness neither increases nor decreases.
Awareness of the three times is noncomposite—
Pristine wisdom of discrimination manifest.

ME: To recite this destroyer of jealousy,
The field of knowledge is primordially pure.
The sphere of the unchangeable is immutable—
Pristine wisdom of accomplishment manifest.

HUNG: To recite this destroyer of the five poisons,
From the three secret syllables one sees
Self-awareness of mind is luminosity—
Pristine wisdom of coemergence manifest.

By transforming the six afflictions, this supreme Six-Syllable Mantra is the source manifestation of the six wisdoms.

OM: To recite these five primordial wisdoms:
Five poisons eradicated and five wisdoms attained.
Unobstructed, anything and everything arises.
Great emptiness is the sphere of phenomena.

MA: To recite this uncontrived natural existence:
Nonconceptual, nondivided equality
With unceasing compassion pervading all.
The display of unobstructedness is self-arising.

NI: To recite this natural transformation of wisdom:
Realization clears away ignorance into wisdom
And liberates from the realm of samsara.
Clearly the bodhi realm is the realm of great joy.

PE: To recite this undivided wisdom: union free
From the extremes of eternalism and nihilism;
In the views of the boundless and dependentless,
The undivided unity exists uniformly.

ME: To recite this blazing fire of wisdom:
Conceptual thought-signs are burned in themselves.

Nonabandoned, the five poisons disappear into space;
Equilibrium is in the realm of bodhi mind.

HUNG: To recite this suchness of the mind:
Concealed suchness is exposed by realization;
Everything comes together in the bodhi mind and
Becomes clear in the realm of the unchangeable.

This precious Six-Syllable Mantra is the one which reveals the ultimate nature of suchness.

Thus the Six-Syllable Mantra, OM MANI PEME HUNG, is the source of all the good qualities of samsara and nirvana. This mantra is the supreme vajra sound, therefore one should recite it with faith and devotion while contemplating its profound meaning. It has been further stated that any other form of virtue carries the danger of being destroyed by the power of aggression or other emotions, whereas recitation of this precious mantra cannot be destroyed by any external, internal, or secret force; therefore the benefit of this precious mantra is unsurpassable.

ADDITIONAL DHARANIS AND MANTRAS

Following the recitation that accompanies the self-visualization, Jamgon Kongtrul the Great mentions that, in addition to the long dharani and the Six-Syllable Mantra, if possible one should recite the Essence Mantra and the dharanis of the Blue Neck One,[43] the Wish-fulfilling Chakra, the Ten Bhumis, and the Endless Gate. Although it is not absolutely necessary, one should recite the long dharani of the Blue Neck One, composed by Nagarjuna, three times in order to receive blessings and benefits.

The long dharani of the Wish-fulfilling Chakra should be recited twenty-one times. The Essence Mantra should be recited 108 times. As for the Ten-Bhumi Dharani, in total there are ten mantras which correlate with each of the ten bhumis. Although there are ten mantras in total, the recommended mantra to recite is the tenth-bhumi mantra, and it should be recited 108 times. It is also mentioned in the tantra that reciting each one of these mantras one hundred thousand times will enable one to achieve the first- to the

---

43 We have included in this book all the mantras mentioned in the text except the Long Dharani of the Blue Neck One, which is too long. However the shorter version is included.

tenth-bhumi bodhisattva levels, respectively. The Endless Gate Dharani should be recited once.

According to tradition, each time one finishes the recitation of mantras one recites the Sanskrit vowels and consonants, the Essence of Dependent-Arising Mantra, and the One-Hundred-Syllable Mantra three times.

མགྲིན་སྔོན་ཅན་གྱི་གཟུངས་ཐུང་།

Blue Neck One—Short Dharani

ཨོཾ་སྤུ་ལིང་གཀྐ་ཏ་ཧ་སཀྐ།

OM SAPHU LING KAK TA HA SAK KA

ཡིད་བཞིན་འཁོར་ལོའི་གཟུངས།

Wish-fulfilling Chakra Dharani

ན་མོ་རཏྣ་ཏྲ་ཡཱ་ཡ།   ན་མ་ཨཱརྱ་ཨ་ཝ་ལོ་ཀི་ཏེ་ཤྭ་ར་ཡ།

NA MO RAT NA TRA YA YA   NA MA AR YA AH WA LO KI TE SHVA RA YA

བོ་དྷི་ས་ཏྭ་ཡ།   མ་ཧཱ་ས་ཏྭ་ཡ་མ་ཧཱ་ཀཱ་རུ་ཎི་ཀ་ཡ་ཏ་ཡ་ཏ།

BO DHI SA TO YA   MA HA SA TO YA MA HA KA RU NI KA YA TA YA TA

ཨོཾ་ཙ་ཀྲ་བརྟི་ཙིན་ཏ་མ་ཎི་མ་ཧཱ་པེ་མེ་རུ་རུ་ཏིཀྟ་ཛོ་ལ་ཨཱ་ཀར་ཀ་ཡ་ཧཱུྃ་ཕཊ་སྭཱ་ཧཱ།

OM TSA KRA WAR TI TSIN TA MA NI MA HA PE ME RU RU TIK THA DZO LA AH KAR KA YA HUNG PHET SO HA

རྒྱག་རསྐྱང་དྲུ། དཔའ་བླུ་མི་ཀྲ་དྲིའི། བོད་སྐྱང་དྲུ། ས་བཅུ་པའི་གཟུངས།

Ten-Bhumi Dharani

ཨོཾ། ཡི་གེ་གཅིག་པའོ། ཨོཾ་བྷུཿ ཡི་གེ་གཉིས་པའོ

OM   One-syllable dharani   OM BHU   Two-syllable dharani

ཨོཾ་པདྨེ། ཡི་གེ་གསུམ་པའོ།

OM PEME   Three-syllable dharani

ཨོཾ་པདུ་ཧྲཱིཿ   ས་བཞི་པའོ།   ཨོཾ་པདྨ་བྷུ་ཛེ།   ས་ལྔ་པའོ།

OM PEMA HRIH   Four-syllable dharani   OM PEMA BHU DZE   Five-syllable
                                                                   dharani

ཨོཾ་པདྨ་ལོ་ཀི་ཏེ།   གཟུངས་སྟྭགས་ཡི་གེ་དྲུག་པ།

OM PEMA LO KI TE   Six-syllable dharani

ཨོཾ་པདྨ་ཛོ་ལ་ཧཱུྃ་ཧྲཱི་ཀ།   གསང་སྟྭགས་ཡི་གེ་བདུན་པ།

OM PEMA DZO LA HUNG DRHI KA   Seven-syllable dharani

ཨོཾ་ཨ་མོ་གྷ་མ་ཎི་པདྨེ།   གསང་སྟྭགས་ཡི་གེ་བརྒྱད་པ།

OM AH MO GHA MA NI PEMA   Eight-syllable dharani

ཨོཾ་པདྨོ་ལོ་ཙཱ་ཎི་ཧུ་རུ་ཧཱུྃ།   གསང་སྟྭགས་ཡི་གེ་དགུ་པ།

OM PEMO LO TSA NI HU RU HUNG   Nine-syllable dharani

ཨོཾ་པདྨོ་ཀྲ་ཎའི་ཀ་བི་མ་ལེ་ཧཱུྃ་ཕཊ།   གསང་སྟྭགས་ཡི་གེ་བཅུ་པ།

OM PEMO KHANI KA BI MA LE HUNG PHET   Ten-syllable dharani

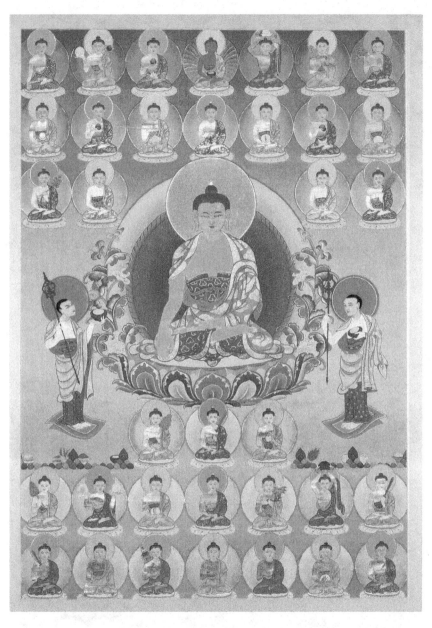

1. Thirty-five Buddhas, thangka painting by
master painter Gega Lama, Nepal

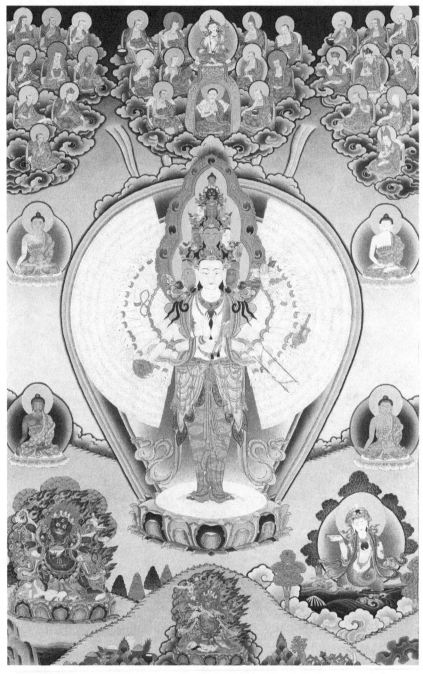

2. Thousand-Armed Chenrezig, thangka painting by disciples
of master painter Gega Lama, Nepal

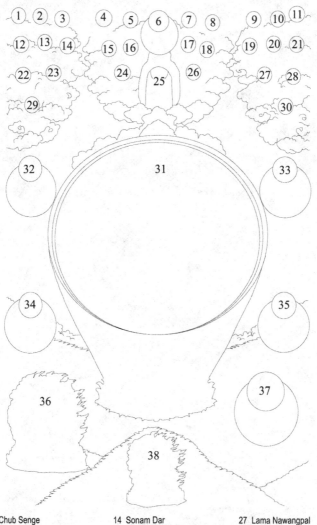

1 Jang Chub Senge	14 Sonam Dar	27 Lama Nawangpal
2 Konchok Zangpo	15 Chogyal Dewanchenpa	28 Karma Nyedun
3 Sherab Bumpo	16 Pandita Penyawa	29 Tenzin Gyurme
4 Shangton Drajig	17 Bodhisattva Dawa Gyeltsen	30 Khenchen Tashi Ozer
5 Dawa Shonnu	18 Khenchen Chuzangwa	31 Thousand-Armed Chenrezig
6 Two-Armed Chenrezig	19 Jangpal Zangpo	32 Buddha Ratnasambhava
7 Yeshe Zangpo	20 Mikyo Dorje	33 Buddha Vairochana
8 Khenchen Tsidulwa	21 Wangchuk Dorje	34 Buddha Akshobhya
9 Bodhisattva Thogme Zangpo	22 Tulku Drubgyu	35 Buddha Amoghasiddhi
10 Lama Nga Wangpa	23 Chokyi Wangchuk	36 Six-Armed Mahakala
11 Khenchen Nyagpukpa	24 Mahasiddha Nyi Phukpa	37 Nyungne Protector Waruna
12 Konchok Yenlak	25 Gelongma Palmo	38 Hayagriva
13 Sangye Nyenpa	26 Supa Dorje Gyalpo	

3. Thousand-Armed Chenrezig, legend

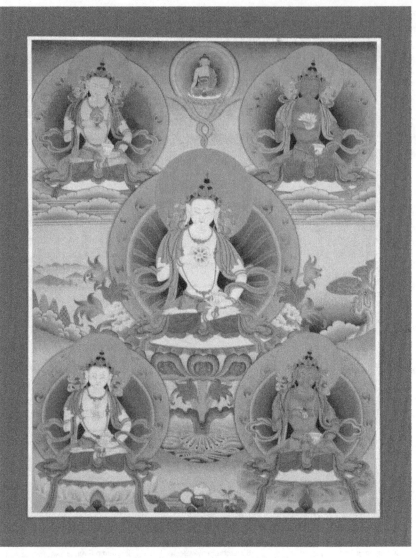

4. Five Dhyani Buddhas, thangka painting by
master painter Gega Lama, Nepal

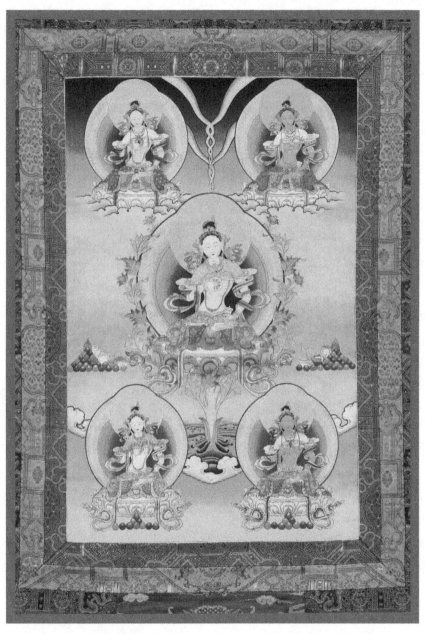

5. Five Female Buddhas, thangka painting by disciples
of master painter Gega Lama, Nepal

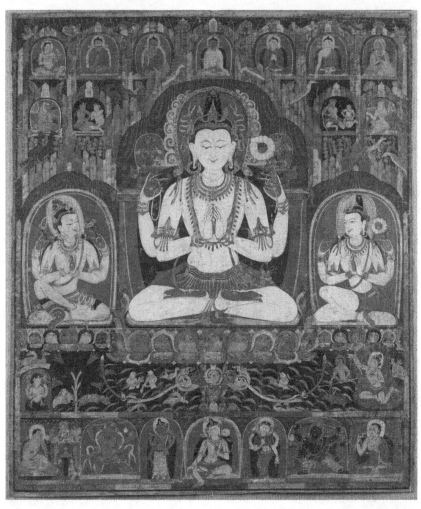

6. Shadakshari Triad and Other Deities (Triple Manifestation of the Six-Syllable Mantra), photograph courtesy of The Walters Art Museum, Baltimore

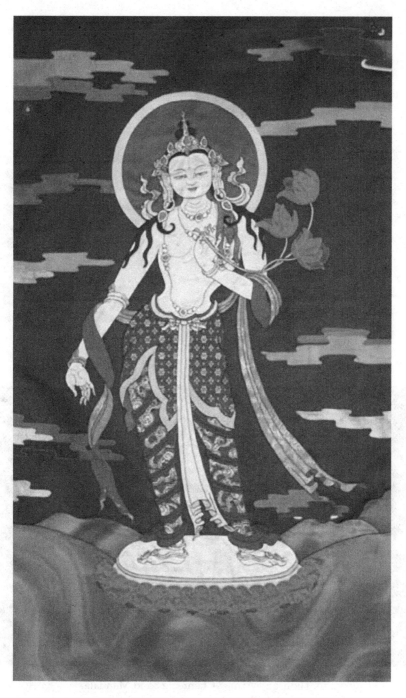

7. Padmapani (Two-Armed Chenrezig): Pieced silk thangka made by
Leslie Rinchen-Wongmo, California, *www.silkthangka.com*

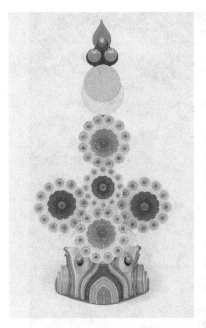

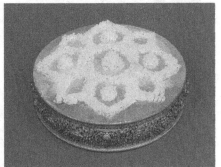

8. Chenrezig Torma

9. Rice Mandala

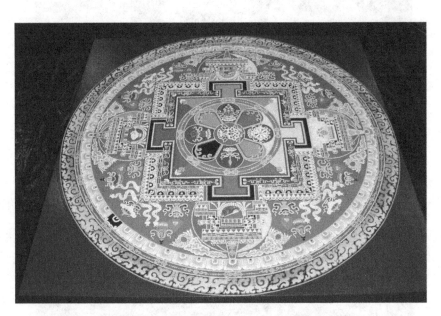

10. Thousand-Armed Chenrezig Sand Mandala,
photograph by Janet Lowry, Austin College, Texas

འཕགས་པ་སྒོ་མཐའ་ཡས་པ་སྒྲུབ་པ་ཞེས་བྱ་བའི་གཟུངས།

Endless Gate Dharani

ཏ་དྱ་ཐཱ།   ཨོཾ་ཨ་ཎེ་མ་ཧཱ་ར་ཎེ་ཨ་ཁེ།

TA YA TA   OM AH NE MA HA RA NE AH KHE

མུ་ཁེ།   མུ་ཁེ།   ས་མན་ཏ་མུ་ཁེ།   སོཾ་མེ་ས།

MU KHE   MU KHE   SA MAN TA MU KHE   SOO ME SA

སོ་རྱ་ར་མེ།   སོ་ཏི་ཡུ་ག་མེ།

SOO RYA RA ME   SOO TI YU GA ME

ནི་རུ་ག་ཏི་ཕ་ཙྲེ་ཧི་ལེ་ཧི་ལེ།   ཀ་ལ་པེ།   ཀེ་ལ་པ།   སི་ས་ལེ།

NI RU GA TI TRA BHE HI LE HI LE   KA LA PE   KE LA PA   SI SA LE

ས་ར་བ་ཏི།   ཧི་ལེ་ཧི་ལེ།   ཧི་ལེ་ཧི་ལེ།   ཧི་ལི་ཧི་ལི་ལི།   མ་ཧཱ་ཧི་ལེ་ལེ།

SA RA WA TI   HI LE HI LE   HI LE HI LE   HI LI HI LI LI   MA HA HI LE LE

ཙན་དེ་ཙ་པ་ནེ།

TSAN DE TSA PA NE

ཙ་ར་ཙ་ར་ཎི།   ཨ་ཙ་ལེ།   མ་ཙྟ་ལེ།   ཨ་ནཾ་ཏེ།   ཨ་ནི་ཏ་མུ་ཁེ།

TSA RA TSA RA NI   AH TSA LE   MA TSA LE   AH NAM TE   AH NI TA MU KHE

ཨ་ནཾ་ཏ་ག་ཏེ་ཨ་ར་ཎེ།

AH NAM TA GA TE AH RA NE

ནིར་མ་ལ་དེ།   ནིར་བ་ལ་ནེ།   ནིར་བ་དྷན་ཏེ།   དྷར་མ་དྷ་རེ།   ནིར་ཧ་རེ།

NIR MA LA DE   NIR BA LA NE   NIR BA DHAN TE   DHAR MA DHA RE   NIR HA RE

གི་མེ་ལེ།

GI ME LE

ཤྲི་མ་པི་ཤོ་ད་ནི།   ཕ་ཀྲི་ཏི་དྷི་པ་ནེ།   བྷ་བ་བེ་བྷ་བ་ནེ།

SHRI MA PI SHO DA NI   TRA KRI TI DHI PA NE   BHA BA BE BHA BA NE

ཨ་སཾ་གེ་ཨ་སཾ་གེ།   བི་ཧ་རེ།

AH SAM GE AH SAM GE   BI HA RE

བི་ད་མེ་ས་མེ།   བི་མ་ལེ།   བི་མ་ལ་པྲ་བྷེ།   སཾ་གར་ཀ་ཎི།

BI DA ME SA ME   BI MA LE   BI MA LA TRA BHE   SAM KAR KA NI

དྷི་རེ་དྷི་དྷི་རེ་ཧ་དྷི་དྷི་རེ།

DHI RE DHI DHI RE HA DHI DHI RE

ཡེ་ཀེ་ཡ་ཀོ་པ་ཏི།   ཙ་ལེ་ཨ་ཙ་ལེ།   མ་ཙ་ལེ།   ས་མ་ཙ་ལེ།

YE KE YA KO PA TI   TSA LE AH TSA LE   MA TSA LE   SA MA TSA LE

ཊ་དྷི་ཏུ་དྲ་སན་དྷི་སྟི་ར།

TRA DHI TRU DHA SAN DHI SA TI RA

ཨ་ས་ག་ཨ་སི་གེ།   བི་ཧ་རེ།   ཨ་སཾ་ག།   ཉིར་ཧ་རེ།   ཉིར་ཧ་ར།   བི་མ་ལེ།

AH SA GA AH SI GE   BI HA RE   AH SAM GA   NIR HA RE   NIR HA RA   BI MA LE

ཉིར་ཧ་ཏ་ཤོ།

NIR HA TRA SHO

ཏ་ནི་ཏ་དྷི་སོ་མེ།   སྟི་རེ་སྟི་མེ།   སྟ་མ་བ་ཏི།   མ་ཧ་པྲ་བྷེ།

TA NI DA DHI SO ME   SA TI RE SA TI ME   SA TA MA WA TI   MA HA TRA BHE

ས་མན་ཏ་པྲ་བྷེ།

SA MAN TA TRA BHE

བི་པུ་ལ་པྲ་བྷེ།   བི་པུ་ལ་རསྨི་སཾ་བྷ་བེ།   ས་མན་ཏ་མུ་ཁེ།   སརྦ་ཏྲ་ཡ་བུ་ག་ཏེ།

BI PU LA TRA BHE BI PU LA RE MI SAM BHA BE   SA MAN TA MU KHE   SAR WA TRA YA BU GA TE

ཚོ་དྱ་ཡན་ཏ་ཚོ་དྱ་ཏི་བྷ་ནི།   དྷ་ར་ཎེ།   ཎི་ནེ་ན།   དྷརྨ་ནི་དྷ་ནཱ་གོ་ཏྲ།

TSE DAYA YAN TA TSE DAYA TRA TI BHA NI   DHA RA NE   NI DE NA   DHAR MA NI DHA NÀ GO TRA

ས་མན་ཏ་བྷ་དྲེ།   སརྦ་ཏ་ཐཱ་ག་ཏ་ཧྲི་ད་ཡ་ཨ་ཛྷིཀ་ཏྲི་ཏེ་སྭཱ་ཧཱ།

SA MAN TA BHA DRE   SAR WA TA THA GA TA HRI DA YA AH DHIK TRI TE SO HA

སྙིང་པོ་ནི།

Essence Mantra

ༀ་པདྨ་ཙིནྟ་མ་ཎི་མ་ཧ་བཛྲ་བྷ་ར་ཧཱུྃ༔

OM PE MA TSIN TA MA NI MA HA BEN DZRA BHA RA HUNG

Sanskrit Vowels

ཨ་ཨཱༀ	ཨི་ཨཱིༀ	ཨུ་ཨཱུༀ	རྀ་རཱྀༀ	ལྀ་ལཱྀༀ	ཨེ་ཨཻༀ	ཨོ་ཨཽༀ	ཨཾ་ཨཿༀ
AH AH	I I	U U	RI RI	LI LI	E EI	O AO	AM AH

Sanskrit Consonants

ཀ་ཁ་ག་གྷ་ང༔	ཙ་ཚ་ཛ་ཛྷ་ཉ༔	ཊ་ཋ་ཌ་ཌྷཎ༔	ཏ་ཐ་ད་དྷ་ན༔
KA K'A GA GHA NGA	TSA TS'A DZA DZHA NY	TA T'A DA DHA NA	TA T'A DA DHA NA

པ་ཕ་བ་བྷ་མ༔	ཡ་ར་ལ་ཝ༔	ཤ་ཁ་ས་ཧ་ཀྵ༔
PA P'A BA BHA MA	YA RA LA WA	SHA KA SA HA KYA

Essence of Dependent-Arising Mantra

ཡེ་དྷརྨ་ཧེ་ཏུ་པྲ་བྷ་ཝ་ཧེ་ཏུནྟེ༔   ཀནྟ་ཐ་ག་ཏོ་ཧྱ་ཝ་དཏྲ༔

YE DHAR MA HE TU PRA BHA WA HE TUN TE   KAN TA THA GA TO HAYA WA DATRA

ཏེ་ཁྱནྩ་ཡོ་ནི་རོ་དྷ་ཨེ་ཝྃ་བ་དི་མ་ཧཱ་ཤྲ་མ་ཎ་ཡེ་སྭ་ཧཱ༔

TE KHYAN TSA YO NI RO DHA E WAM BA DHI MA HA SHRA MA NA YE SO HA

One-Hundred-Syllable Mantra

ༀ་བཛྲ་ས་ཏྭ་ས་མ་ཡ།   མ་ནུ་པ་ལ་ཡ།   བཛྲ་ས་ཏྭ་ཏེ་ནོ་པ་ཏིཥྛ་དྲྀ་ཌྷོ་མེ་བྷ་ཝ།

OM BEN ZRA SA TO SA MA YA   MA NU PA LA YA   BEN ZRA SA TO TE NO PA TI TA
                                                        DRI DO ME BA WA

 སུ་ཏོ་ཙུ་མེ་བྲ་ཝ།　　　　སུ་པོ་ཙུ་མེ་བྲ་ཝ།　　　ཨ་ནུ་ར་ཏྲོ་མེ་བྲ་ཝ།

SU TO KOY YO ME BA WA   U PO KOY YO ME BA WA   AH NU RA TO ME BA WA

སརྦ་སིདྡྷི་མྱེ་པྲ་ཡ་ཙ

SAR WA SID DI ME PRA YA TSA

སརྦ་ཀརྨ་སུ་ཙ་མེ་ཙི་ཏྃ་ཤྲི་ཡཿ　　　　　ཀུ་རུ་ཧཱུྃ་ཧ་ཧ་ཧ་ཧ་ཧོཿ

SAR WA KAR MA SU TSA ME TSI TANG SHI RI YA   KU RU HUNG HA HA HA HA HA HO

བྷ་ག་སྭེན།

BA GA WEN

སརྦ་ཏ་ཐཱ་ག་ཏ།　　　　བཛྲ་མ་མེ་མུཉྩ　　　　བཛྲི་བྷ་ཝ་མ་ཧཱ་ས་མ་ཡ་ས་ཏྭ་ཨཿ

SAR WA TA TA GA TA   EN ZRA MA ME MUN TSA   BEN ZRI BA WA MA HA SA MA
                                            YA SA TO AH

Essence of Amoghapasha Mantra

ཨོཾ་ཧྲཱིཿཏྲེ་ལོ་ཀྱ་བི་ཛ་ཡ་ཨ་མོ་ཁ་པ་ཤ་ཨ་ཏྲ་ཏི་ཧ་ཏ་ཧྲཱིཿཧ་ཧཱུྃ་ཕཊ་སྭཱ་ཧཱ།

OM HRIH TRE LO KYA BI DZA YA AH MO KHA PHA SHA AH TRA TI HA TA HRIH HA
HUNG PHET SO HA

Traditionally this mantra, Essence of Amoghapasha, is recited each morning immediately after we take the mahayana vow of Restoring and Purifying Ordination. First we recite the Mantra for Purifying Morals, which
follows in our text, seven times. Then we recite the Essence of Amoghapasha Mantra the same number of times.

Explanation of the Po Homage Prayer   10

THIS PRAYER is an homage prayer offered by Gelongma Palmo to Arya Avalokiteshvara (Chenrezig) at the time she had a vision of Chenrezig. The original Tibetan text of the "Po Prayer" is a translation from Sanskrit into Tibetan, and it begins with the title in Sanskrit and Tibetan. The title is omitted in our text and the prayer begins:

|ཨོཾ་འཇིག་རྟེན་མགོན་པོ་ལ་ཕྱག་འཚལ་ལོ།

OM   JIG TEN   GON PO   LA   CH'AG TS'AL LO
OM world protector to I bow

OM, I bow to the Protector of the world.

OM is the supreme syllable that refers to the enlightened form. In this case, it represents the essence of Chenrezig's form. It also generates all kinds of auspiciousness, good fortune, glory, supreme benefits, etc.

In the Buddhist view, the deeper understanding of the nature of the world is its transitoriness, where things constantly change and where protection is definitely needed. Bowing is to the Protector of the world, because he is the real protector.

This first line of the prayer is the original Tibetan translator's homage, not that of Gelongma Palmo. He included it when he began translating, and he was bowing with respect from his body, speech, and mind for the purpose of accomplishing a correct (authentic) translation.

།འཇིག་རྟེན་བླ་མ་སྲིད་པ་གསུམ་གྱིས་བསྟོད་པ་པོ།

JIG TEN LAM SIE PA SUM GYI TOE PA PO

world lama three worlds praise and celebrate

Everyone in the three worlds praises and celebrates the Lama.

Again, the Tibetan word JIG TEN refers to the transitory world, in this case a world that eventually disintegrates. The universe, or world, comes into existence, it exists, and it eventually disintegrates. That is why we call it a transitory world.

These are actually two separate words. JIG describes the transitory state of the world, and TEN describes beings who depend on the world for their existence. Another way of understanding is, one will disintegrate by death and dying (JIG), and one comes into existence by birth (TEN). So, the Lama-protector protects sentient beings whose existence is based on transitory circumstances.

SIE PA SUM refers to the three world spheres, the totality of the realm of samsara, which is the world above, beneath, and between.[44] TOE PA means praise or homage and PO refers to the object of the praise, in this case Chenrezig, who is praised and celebrated by everyone in the three world spheres.

།ལྷ་ཡི་གཙོ་བོ་བདུད་དང་ཚངས་པས་བསྟོད་པ་པོ།

LHA YI TSO WO DUE DANG TS'ANG PE TOE PA PO

god realm primary mara & Brahma praise and celebrate

Even the gods and Brahma celebrate and praise Lord Chenrezig.

This primary god of the desire realm, Devil King of the Sixth Heaven of the World of Desire, (Skt. *Mara*),[45] is actually a very sophisticated demon god whose mind is filled with neurotic emotions, and who would like to see everybody stay in samsara with him. Through his clairvoyance, he knows when anyone gives rise to genuine bodhichitta and a renunciation of samsara and is therefore seeking enlightenment. He can read their mind, and he gets jealous that they are trying to get out of this world that he likes to control. It has been said that he shoots them with five arrows, which are called arrows with flowers. He shoots with the five poisons, and this is

44 This is a Buddhist concept. The world above refers to the god realms, beneath refers to the realms beneath us, and between refers to our human realm.

45 He is also named Freely Enjoying Things Conjured by Others, the king who makes free use of the fruits of others' efforts for his own pleasure. Served by innumerable minions, he obstructs Buddhist practice and delights in sapping the life force of others.

actually temptation. The flowers seem very beautiful to weak, ordinary minds, but if you fall for them, you are trapped in samsara again, where you might remain for a long period of time.

Gelongma Palmo is saying that even this sophisticated demon cannot help but praise Chenrezig. And Brahma, who is the primary god of the form realm, praises Chenrezig as well.

|ཐུབ་པའི་རྒྱལ་མཆོག་བསྟོད་པས་གྲུབ་པར་མཛད་པ་པོ།

T'UB PEI   GYAL CH'OG   TOE PE   DRUB PAR   DZE PA PO

the capable one victorious, praise accomplishment who makes it supreme

One who wishes to attain buddhahood praises the Lord who delivers such accomplishment.

T'UB PEI refers to the Capable One, which is part of Shakyamuni Buddha's name. It derives from his ability to overcome, subdue, or get rid of all negativities. Therefore he is "the Capable One." In general arhats, shravakas, and pratyekabuddhas are also capable of overcoming forces of negativities, but buddhas are victorious and supreme (GYAL CH'OG) among all beings.

The Capable One who wished to attain the perfect, supreme, victorious state praised (TOE PEI) Lord Chenrezig, and through his praise accomplished (DRUB PAR) his wishes.

The last word, DZE PA PO, refers to the one who delivered it, the accomplishment of buddhahood.

|འཇིག་རྟེན་གསུམ་གྱི་མགོན་པོ་མཆོག་ལ་ཕྱག་འཚལ་ལོ།

JIG TEN SUM   GYI   GON PO   CH'OG LA   CH'AG TS'AL LO

three worlds of protector supreme bow down

I bow to the supreme protector of the three worlds.

Chenrezig, the Lord of the three world spheres, is the object of the bow, Gelongma Palmo is the subject, and the manner of bowing is with a great deal of respect from her body, speech, and mind. The time of the bow is Saka Dawa, the full moon day, when she actually had the vision of Chenrezig. The place of the bow is the monastery where she was practicing. And the purpose of the bow is for Gelongma Palmo to follow in the footsteps of all the extraordinary beings, and for her prayer to be completely successful.

This is a traditional, scriptural, analytical explanation of the bow, and if you analyze the homage prayer, you will find all of these detailed noble points. But I presume that when Gelongma Palmo had the vision of Chenrezig, she was in a completely pure state of mind, and she wasn't necessarily thinking of all these points. Without a doubt the entire prayer came spontaneously and naturally from her pure mind. Otherwise, it would not have been possible to have such a vision.

PRAISE TO CHENREZIG'S BODY

།བདེ་གཤེགས་དཔག་མེད་སྐུ་སྟེ་སྐུ་བཟང་འཛིན་པ་པོ།

DE SHEK   PAG ME   KU   TE   KU ZANG   DZIN PA PO

| one thus gone | infinite | form, | of | noble body | holder, one |
| | | body | | | who knows |

Holder of a noble form body, filled with infinite tathagatas,

Gelongma Palmo praises Chenrezig's body, speech, and mind, and the praise begins with the body, follows with the mind, and ends with the speech. Gelongma Palmo saw every pore of Chenrezig's body filled with tathagatas (ones thus gone) and buddha realms, infinite numbers of pure realms and buddhas. As Chenrezig's body, which appeared in the form of one thousand arms and eyes, is a truly noble form, she referred to him as the holder of a noble form body.

།བདེ་གཤེགས་སྣང་བ་མཐའ་ཡས་དབུ་རྒྱན་འཛིན་པ་པོ།

DE SHEK   NANG WA T'A YE   U GYEN   DZIN PA PO
one thus gone boundless light crowned holder, one who holds

You are crowned by Buddha Amitabha.

Buddha Amitabha (Tathagata Amitabha) refers to the topmost head, with a face that is peaceful and red in color.

།ཕྱག་གཡས་མཆོག་སྦྱིན་ཡི་དྭགས་བཀྲེས་སྐོམ་སེལ་བ་པོ།

CH'AG YE   CH'OG CHIN   YI DOK   TRE KOM   SEL WA PO
right hand supreme giving hungry ghosts hunger one who dispels it
                or spirits   and thirst
Your supremely bountiful right hand dispels the suffering of the hungry ghosts;

Chenrezig's right hand, which is in the mudra of supreme giving, is the third right hand. From the fingers of this hand, nectar flows and dispels the suffering of hunger and thirst that the hungry ghosts experience, and they are satisfied.

།ཕྱག་གཡོན་གསེར་གྱི་པདྨ་རྣམ་པར་བརྒྱན་པ་པོ།

CH'AG YON   SER GYI   PE ME   NAM PAR GYEN PA PO
left hand   golden   lotus   adorned by it

Your left hand holds a golden lotus.

The left hand holding the golden lotus is Chenrezig's second left hand. The lotus symbolizes Chenrezig's freedom from any samsaric stain, and its golden color symbolizes the abundant quality of complete insight; therefore he is adorned by this precious golden lotus.

།དྲི་ཞིམ་རལ་པའི་ཕྲེང་བ་དམར་སེར་འཁྱུག་པ་པོ།

DRI SH'IM   RAL PEI   TR'ENG WA   MAR SER   K'YUG PA PO

sweet scents   hair   necklaces   yellow and red   sparkling

Your sweetly scented red and yellow hair sparkles like necklaces.

This refers to the hair of the wrathful face, which sparkles with orange color and drapes neatly over the hair of the other faces, yet does not intermingle with it. The common explanation of TR'ENG WA is "necklace" or "mala," but here the understanding is actually more "in orderly rows."

།ཞལ་རས་རྒྱས་པ་ཟླ་བ་ལྟ་བུར་མཛེས་པ་པོ།

SH'AL RE   GYE PA   DA WA TA BUR   DZE PA PO

face   expanse   like a moon   beautiful

The expanse of your face is as lovely as a full moon.

The entire circle of Chenrezig's face is praised by comparing it to the beauty of an autumn full moon.

།སྤྱན་གྱི་པདྨ་མཆོག་ཏུ་བཟང་ཞིང་ཡངས་པ་པོ།

CHEN GYI   PE MA   CH'OG TU   ZANG SH'ING   YANG PA PO

eyes   lotus   supreme   sublime   wide

Like the sublimely supreme lotus, your eyes are beautifully wide.

This refers to the eyes on all the peaceful faces, which are compared to a sublime lotus flower, beautifully extended. "Wide" further refers to Chenrezig's vast vision of the three times: past, present, and future.

ཁ་བ་དུང་ལྟར་རྣམ་དཀར་དྲི་ངད་ལྡན་པ་པོ།

K'A WA   DUNG   TAR   NAM KAR   DRI NGE   DEN PA PO

snow   shell   like white appearance   sweet smell   possessor of

Your sweet-smelling form is like a snow-white conch shell.

Chenrezig's form body is compared to the whiteness of snow and a conch shell, and praised because white is the color of purity. Furthermore, his body emits a sweet scent.

དྲི་མེད་འོད་ཆགས་མུ་ཏིག་ཚོམ་བུ་འཛིན་པ་པོ།

DRI ME   OE CH'AG   MU TIG   TS'OM BU   DZIN PA PO

stainless   radiates   pearl   cluster   holder, one who holds

You hold a mala of stainless, glowing pearls,

Chenrezig holds a stainless cluster of glowing pearls, which is a symbol of his unblemished nature. This is actually a mala (rosary).

མཛེས་པའི་འོད་ཟེར་སྐྱ་རེངས་དམར་པོས་བརྒྱན་པ་པོ།

DZE PEI   OE ZER   KYA RENG   MAR PO   GYEN PA PO

beautiful   light radiation   dawn   red   ornamented by

And radiate stunning beams of light, red as dawn.

Chenrezig's body is adorned by beautiful red light rays that radiate from his white body, a sight so beautiful to behold it takes one's breath away, like seeing the first red rays of the morning sun.

པདྨའི་མཚོ་ལྟར་ཕྱག་ནི་མཛར་བར་བྱས་པ་པོ།

PE MEI TS'O   TAR   CH'AG   NI NGAR WAR   JE PA PO

lotus lake   like   hand   properly arranged   beautiful one

Your body is like a lake; from it hands, like lotuses, are perfectly arranged.

Just as in a lotus-filled lake, many beautiful lotus flowers appear perfectly arranged.

ཿསྟོན་ཀའི་སྤྲིན་གྱི་མདོག་དང་ལྡན་ཞིང་གཞོན་པ་པོ།

TON KEI   TRIN GYI   DOG   DANG   DEN SH'ING   SH'ON PA PO

autumn   clouds   colored   and   having youthful

They are youthful and like autumn clouds, white and bright and clear.

The color of Chenrezig's youthful-looking hands is compared to autumn clouds, which are white, free from dust and stains, smoothly shining, and fresh.

ཿརིན་ཆེན་མང་པོས་དཔུང་པ་གཉིས་ནི་བརྒྱན་པ་པོ།

RIN CH'EN   MANG PO   PUNG PA   NYI NI   GYEN PA PO

precious jewels   many   shoulder   two ornamented

Both shoulders are adorned with many precious jewels.

Chenrezig's two shoulders are ornamented with lapis lazuli and many other precious jewels.

ཿལོ་མའི་མཆོག་ལྟར་ཕྱག་མཐིལ་གཞོན་ཞིང་འཇམ་པ་པོ།

LO MEI   CH'OG TA   CH'AG T'IL   SH'ON SH'ING   JAM PA PO

leaves   supremelike   palm of the hand   youthful   soft one

Your youthful palms are soft like the most supreme leaves.

The palms of Chenrezig's hands are so beautiful and youthful looking; they are compared to supreme leaves, which are leaves from a wish-ful-filling tree.

ཿརི་དྭགས་པགས་པས་ནུ་མ་གཡོན་པ་བཀབ་པ་པོ།

RI DOK   PAK PE   NU MA   YON PA   KAB PA PO

deer   skin   breast   left   one who's covered

Your left breast is covered with a tenasera skin.

Chenrezig wears a deerskin on his left shoulder, which is a special symbol of natural compassion. There is an extraordinary story which relates to a deer with natural compassion, known as a *tenasera* in Sanskrit. This deer is supposed to be very special and extremely rare. Its fur is a golden color, and it is a naturally born bodhisattva deer, a deer with tremendous love and compassion for all. The story goes that even when this deer eats grass, it will not eat from areas with nicely grown grass, because it thinks others might like to eat it. Instead it goes elsewhere and eats grass that's not as good and things like that. Actually, such deer do exist, such unusual, natural phenomena do occur in the ordinary world. Chenrezig wears this deerskin demonstrating that such extraordinary love and compassion also exist.

།སྙན་ཆ་གདུ་བུས་སྒེག་ཅིང་རྒྱན་རྣམས་འཆང་བ་པོ།

NYEN CH'A DU BU   GEG CHING   GYEN NAM   CH'ANG WA PO

earring   graceful ornaments   one holds

Precious earrings and other ornaments gracefully adorn you.

Chenrezig's ears are ornamented with earrings of precious metal with varieties of beautiful jewels on them, and he appears perfectly graceful. It further implies that he is also adorned with various precious jewel necklaces, and so on.

།དྲི་མ་མེད་པའི་པདྨའི་མཚོག་ལ་གནས་པ་པོ།

DRI MA   ME PEI   PE MEI   CH'OG LA   NE PA PO

blemish   no   lotus supreme   to dwell

You dwell upon a supreme and unblemished lotus.

The supreme lotus flower is unblemished by samsaric stains, and so beautifully thrives and expands like all the enlightened qualities; therefore, Chenrezig dwells on top of the supreme lotus demonstrating his perfection.

།ཁྱེ་བའི་དོས་ནི་པདྨའི་འདབས་ལྟར་འཇམ་པ་པོ།

TE WEI   NGO   NI   PE MEI   DAB TAR   JAM PA PO

navel surface of   lotus lotus petal-like   soft one

Your navel's surface is as soft as a lotus petal.

The understanding here is that all birth takes place from the navel. And the birth of all the buddhas' qualities takes place from bodhichitta. The surface of Lord Chenrezig's navel is soft and lotus-petal-like, which symbolizes the bodhichitta from which the qualities of the bodhisattva phenomena arise.

|གསེར་གྱི་སྐ་རགས་མཆོག་ལ་ནོར་བུ་བྲིས་སྤྲས་པ་པོ|

SER   GYI   KA RAK   CH'OG LA   NOR BU   TRE PA PO

golden of   belt   supreme   jewel encrust

Your belt is of the finest jewel-encrusted gold.

This is praise to the extraordinary belt that Chenrezig is wearing, which is made out of precious gold with a wish-fulfilling jewel on it. This belt is referred to as "supreme among all belts."

|སྐུ་རྱུར་དགྱིས་པའི་རས་བཟང་ཤམ་ཐབས་འཛིན་པ་པོ|

TA ZUR   TRI PEI   RE   ZANG   SHAM T'AB   DZIN PA PO

hips   wrap cloth   noble   lower robe   one who holds

Your lower robe wraps your hips in the noblest cloth.

Chenrezig wears his lower robe, which is made of noble cloth, wrapped around his hips. This noble cloth covers both the right and the left hip, and has the symbolic meaning of expressing the qualities of shame and embarrassment. In the Buddhist moral and ethical context, shame as a state of moral value comes from true integrity within, a principle that would prevent one from engaging in any wrongdoing because of one's own true moral character. Embarrassment is moral value coming from the same principle as shame, but it relates to others. It would prevent one from engaging in wrongdoing out of consideration for others.

PRAISE TO THE QUALITIES OF CHENREZIG'S MIND

Praise to the Quality of Chenrezig's Supreme Knowledge

|ཐུབ་པའི་མཁྱེན་མཆོག་མཚོ་ཆེན་ཕ་རོལ་ཕྱིན་པ་པོ|

T'UB PEI   K'YEN   CH'OG   T'SO CH'EN   P'A ROL   CH'IN PA PO

capable   to know   supreme   great ocean   other shore   one who is gone

Gone to the other shore of the great ocean, you have supreme knowledge and capability.

Supreme among all knowledge is the knowledge of the buddhas. It is vast and profound. It is the wisdom of knowing the nature of phenomena as it is, as well as the wisdom that sees the extent of knowables. This is the quality of Chenrezig's wisdom mind, deep and profound like the mighty ocean, and the perfection of having gone to the other shore.

|མཆོག་བརྙེས་བསོད་ནམས་མང་པོས་ཉེ་བར་བསགས་པ་པོ།

CH'OG	NYE	SOE NAM	MANG PO	NYE WAR	SAK PA PO
supreme	receive	virtue	many	appropriate	one who gathered

You, who properly gathered so much virtue, received the supreme state of being.

This is praise for how and why Chenrezig has all this enlightened wisdom. Here the cause for perfect enlightened wisdom is mainly two perfect accumulations, the accumulation of merit and the accumulation of wisdom, for three countless eons.

Praise to the Quality of Chenrezig's Compassion

|རྟག་ཏུ་བདེ་བའི་འབྱུང་གནས་རྒ་ནད་སེལ་བ་པོ།

TAG TU	DE WEI	JUNG NE	GA NE	SEL WA PO
permanent	joy	source, place	old age and illness	one who dispels

Dispeller of the misery of old age and illness, you are the permanent source of joy.

For as long as samsara exists, Lord Chenrezig is *the* permanent source of joy and happiness for others. This further means that while sentient beings are in samsara, Chenrezig dispels the specific pain and suffering of birth, old age, illness, and death; therefore, he is the source of all happiness.

|གསུམ་མཐར་མཛད་ཅིང་མཁའ་སྤྱོད་སྤྱོད་པ་སྟོན་པ་པོ།

SUM T'AR	DZE CHING	K'A CHOE	CHOE PA	TON PA PO
liberation from three	doing or acting	space dweller	performance	one who shows

You act to liberate beings from the three lower realms, and show and perform equally for space dwellers.

The action of liberating beings "from the three" refers specifically to beings of the three lower realms, those who are creating karma to be born in the three lower realms as well as those who are already there. "Show and perform equally for space dwellers" refers to an understanding of the totality of beings and their individual capacities, which is as expansive as space. Chenrezig's performance of showing the enlightened path through a multitude of emanations equals the magnitude of the entire space-dwelling realm.

།ལུས་ཅན་མཆོག་སྟེ་བདུད་དཔུང་འཇོམས་ལས་རྒྱལ་བ་པོ།

LU CHEN   CH'OG TE   DUE PUNG   TR'UK LE   GYAL WA PO

beings   supreme among   hosts of maras   from battle   victorious one

Supreme among beings, you are victorious in battle over hosts of demons.

"Supreme among beings" refers to Chenrezig's ability to manifest in a multitude of sublime nirmanakaya forms for the benefit of others, and to subdue all beings skillfully; he is victorious over the hosts of maras who generate all kinds of conflict.

།གསེར་གྱི་ཀང་གདུབ་སྒྲ་ཡིས་ཞབས་ཡིད་འོང་བ་པོ།

SER GYI   KANG DUB   DRA YI   SH'AB   YIE ONG WA PO

golden   anklets   sound   feet   agreeable one

Your feet tinkle with the pleasing sound of golden anklets;

།ཚངས་པའི་གནས་པ་བཞི་ཡིས་དབེན་པར་མཛད་པ་པོ།

TS'ANG PEI   NE PA   SH'I YI   WEN PAR   DZE PA PO

Brahma   place   four   silencing   one who makes

And you create the four silences, which are the cause of Brahmahood.

The meanings of the previous line and this one are connected. The previous line mentions that the sounds of his golden anklets please all beings. This line mentions the specific nature of the sounds that please. The sounds are the sounds of the four immeasurables, which are the cause to be born into Brahmahood. The sounds of the four immeasurables wish beings to have happiness and the cause of happiness, and to not have suffering and the cause of suffering; to have joy, which is free from suffering, and to live in equanimity, which is free from attachment and aversion. In this way, they silence the pain and suffering of attachment and aversion of all beings. Without bodhichitta, the four immeasurables are the cause to be born in the Brahma realm. With bodhichitta, they become the cause for enlightenment.

ཁྱད་པའི་འགྲོས་འདྲ་གླང་ཆེན་དྲེགས་ལྟར་གཤེགས་པ་པོ།

NGANG PEI   DRO DRA   LANG CH'EN   DREK TAR   SHEK PA PO

swan   manner of walking   elephant   proud   one who walks

You walk with the grace of a swan and the dignity of an elephant.

Chenrezig walks with a great deal of dignity and grace, like the king of swans and like a great elephant. It is understood here that swans and elephants are known to look back as they walk. With his unconditional love and compassion, Lord Chenrezig walks in the same manner. He looks back and forth because he does not want to leave any sentient beings behind.

PRAISE TO CHENREZIG'S SPEECH

ཚོགས་ཀུན་ཉེ་བར་བསགས་ཤིང་བསྟན་པ་གཉེར་བ་པོ།

TS'OK KUN   NYE WAR   SAK SHING   TEN PA   NYER WA PO

accumulation   appropriate   gathering   buddhadharma   provider
or doctrine

Provider of the doctrine, who has completely and properly accumulated,

During the initial stages he developed bodhichitta, and during the stages of the path he accumulated the two virtues, merit and wisdom. During the resultant stages of buddhahood, he completely gathered and accumulated. These three stages of enlightenment were not for his own welfare, but for the purpose of liberating all beings from the suffering of samsara. In this sense, Chenrezig is the provider of the precious doctrine.

འོ་མའི་མཚོ་དང་ཆུ་ཡི་མཚོ་ལས་སྒྲོལ་བ་པོ།

O MEI   TS'O   DANG   CH'U YI   TS'O   LE   DROL WA PO

milk   ocean   and   water   ocean   from   one who liberates

You liberate from the ocean of milk and the ocean of water.

The ocean of milk refers to the peaceful state, the general nirvana, and the ocean of water refers to samsara. In this metaphor, just as milk is white in color and sweet in taste, the arhats who achieve this state are free from the stain of conflicting emotions (white color), and they also have the wisdom understanding of egolessness of self (sweet taste). At this stage they are not completely liberated from the veils of obstruction to omniscience, therefore they have not obtained the two benefits, perfect benefit for oneself and perfect benefit for others. Although it is liberation from the ocean (samsara), Chenrezig shows them the doctrine of the Great Vehicle in order for them to go beyond the extremes of nirvana.

The second metaphor is liberation from the ocean of water. Just as there are all kinds of bizarre life forms in the ocean, beings in the ocean of samsara are suffering from all kinds of bizarre conflicting negative emotions. Lord Chenrezig shows them the doctrine of the inherently nonexisting nature of phenomena, thereby liberating them from the extremes of samsara.

Praises to the body, speech, and mind of Chenrezig are inclusive of praises to the qualities and activities as well.

BENEFITS OF THE PRAISE

།གང་ཞིག་རྟག་ཏུ་ཐོ་རངས་ལངས་ནས་གུས་པ་ཡིས།

GANG SH'IG   TAG TU   T'O RANG   LANG NE   GU PA YI

whoever   always   dawn   rise   with respect

Whoever will rise with respect at dawn,

།སྤྱན་རས་གཟིགས་ཀྱི་དབང་པོ་ཡིད་ལ་སེམས་བྱེད་ཅིང་།

CHEN RE ZIG   KYI WANG PO   YIE LA   SEM JE CHING

Chenrezig   one with power   in mind   act of thinking

Thinking in their mind of powerful Chenrezig,

།བསྟོད་པའི་མཆོག་འདིས་དག་ཅིང་གསལ་བར་བསྟོད་བྱེད་ན།

TOE PEI   CH'OG   DI   DAG CHING   SAL WAR   TOE JE NA

praise   supreme   this   purely   clearly   act of praising

To purely and clearly extol this supreme praise,

ཁེ་ནི་སྐྱེས་པ་འམ་ནི་བུད་མེད་ཡིན་ཀྱང་རུང་།

DE NI   KYE PA   AM NI   BUE ME   YIN KYANG RUNG

that is   male   or is female   either or

Whether they are male or female,

འཇིག་རྟེན་འདི་འམ་མ་འོངས་སྐྱེ་བ་ཐམས་ཅད་དུ།

JIG TEN   DI AM   MA ONG   KYE WA   T'AM CHE DU

world   this or   future   birth   in all of them

In this life and all future lives,

འཇིག་རྟེན་འཇིག་རྟེན་ལས་འདས་དགོས་པ་ཀུན་འགྲུབ་ཤོག།

JIG TEN   JIG TEN LE DE   GO PA   KUN   DRUB SHOK

this world   world beyond   purpose   all   become accomplished

In this world and the world beyond, all their purposes will be accomplished.

These concluding six lines express the benefits of the homage prayer. Whoever sincerely rises early in the morning, washes thoroughly and wears clean clothing, physically prostrates to Chenrezig with folded hands, recites the prayer with flawless speech and a full voice, repeating it seven or twenty-one times, and mentally recollects the qualities of Chenrezig's body, speech, mind, qualities, and activities, whoever praises sincerely in this manner, whether they are male or female, will benefit in this world and in all future lives. They will attain a higher birth of the human and god realms in this world, and enjoy longevity, freedom from sickness, wealth, happiness, and so on. In the world beyond, they will achieve all the great realizations of the eleven bhumis, complete buddhahood. In summary, all their relative and ultimate wishes will come true.

Benefits of the Prostrations

We recite the "Po Homage Prayer" seven times while performing prostrations to Thousand-Armed Chenrezig. Prostration is a skillful means which has profound symbolic meaning and benefit. First of all, it is a remedy for pride and ego, which are the source of many shortcomings. Where there is a great deal of pride and ego, there is a lack of many wonderful qualities.

Where there is humility and modesty, all kinds of spiritual qualities will follow. Therefore, the practice of prostration has its true place in spiritual growth.

When one touches the top of the head, throat, and heart with folded hands, it is a demonstration of complete respect and homage to the body, speech, and mind of all the buddhas. Through it we have the opportunity to receive the blessings of the body, speech, and mind of the buddhas, as well as to overcome the negativities of body, speech, and mind, and to purify the three poisons. And then we have the opportunity to overcome the sufferings of the three realms and to perfect the three paths, the paths of seeing, meditating, and no more learning. Ultimately we are able to attain the three kayas of the buddhas.

There is profound symbolic benefit with respect to touching five points to the ground as well. Five points is a symbol of homage to the body, speech, mind, activity, and qualities of all the buddhas, and an opportunity to receive the blessings of all these five. It is also an opportunity to purify our body, speech, mind, and a combination of these three together, and to purify negativities associated with latent conditioning, as well as an opportunity to overcome sufferings of the five migrations.[46] It further establishes the potential to go through the five paths, the paths of accumulation, preparation, seeing, meditation, and no more learning. Finally, it establishes the possibility of attaining the body, speech, mind, qualities, and activities of all the buddhas.

So whether you do a bowing prostration or a full body prostration, in order to receive the maximum benefit of this precious spiritual act you must prostrate with all these understandings clearly in your mind.

---

46 "Five migrations" refers to the six realms, with the demi-god realm included in the god realm.

Ending Prayers and Offerings 11

THE SPECIAL WISH PRAYER AND TORMA OFFERINGS

FOLLOWING THE "Po Prayer," the main wish we are making in the "Special Wish Prayer" is that the buddhadharma will last for a long time, and that the dharma holders, the spiritual teachers, will live for a long time. Additionally, we pray that all beings develop bodhichitta, shamatha and special insight meditation, and that we all realize the omniscient wisdom of the buddhas. After sincerely praying, Gelongma Palmo, who is on top of our head, dissolves into us and once again we become Chenrezig. Then we continue with torma offerings.

In general torma can represent several different things. Here it refers to the actual representation of a visualized substance in the form of torma to be used for an offering. It is a skillful means, and there seems to be a definite need for this. As long as we need some enlightened activity to be provided, torma offerings will skillfully make it possible for us to receive benefit. In light of all phenomena having no substantial existence, ultimately speaking, it might not seem necessary; but as long as we are unenlightened beings, such skillful means have their true place, because they provide a basis for receiving enlightened activity.

To offer torma to Chenrezig, we bless the torma with mantra and then imagine that the torma becomes an incredible offering substance, which we then offer to Chenrezig. We do it with the thought, "Please accept this offering on my behalf." And then we say, "Please help me and all sentient beings to develop bodhichitta." The blessings, mantra, and so on are pretty much the same for the torma offering to the nagas. But when we request their help, we are mainly asking them to protect buddhadharma in general and the Nyungne teaching and we practitioners in particular.

It is also a tradition to do additional torma offering prayers during the last session of the day. The first offering is to Mahakala, which is mainly to protect the lineage and practitioners. After that we make torma offering prayers known as the "Three-Torma Offering Ceremony." The first of the three torma offerings is for the guardians of the ten directions. The second one is for gods, nagas, gandharvas, and so on. The last is for obstructing spirits. If you are doing Nyungne practice by yourself, and you have received all the proper instruction and authority to do so but you do not know how to perform these additional torma offerings, then they can be omitted.

Right after torma offering, there is an offering of bathing water to Chenrezig, which has a similar purpose as the torma offering in the sense that it ultimately becomes the cause for our own purification. As one uses water for cleaning the unclean, so can we skillfully apply the same principle by using water for spiritual purposes, the cleansing of negativities. It works perfectly because the nature of phenomena is dependent-arising, and if and when you sincerely make an offering of bathing water to the buddhas, you benefit by it becoming the cause of your own purification.

Next comes the final offering and homage prayer called the "Conclusion of the Ceremony Offering." This offering is done by offering mudras and mantras, and then a short homage prayer. Right after that we receive blessing water while chanting OM MANI PEME HUNG.

RECEIVING BLESSING WATER AT THE END OF THE CEREMONY: FINAL PURIFYING SYMBOL

The teacher who presides over the ceremony will give the purification water, during which time you should visualize three emanations of Chenrezig coming from frontal-visualization Chenrezig's heart center. They are called the Triad of Shadakshari Deities or, in Tibetan, the Six-Syllable Chenrezig Triple Manifestation (Fig. 6). These manifestations are also referred to as father, mother, and son manifestations. The father manifestation, who appears right in the center, is actually Four-Armed Chenrezig and is called Liberator of Beings. He looks exactly the same as Four-Armed Chenrezig except he holds a pearl rosary. The mother manifestation, called Holder of the Mantra Family, also looks exactly like Four-Armed Chenrezig. She sits on father Chenrezig's left side, (which is our right side as we look toward them), and looks up at him with a smile. Her position is called the queen posture; she is sitting on her side with her legs drawn up. The son manifestation is called Holder of the Jewel, and he sits to the right side of father

Chenrezig (which is our left side). He is yellow in color with two arms, the right hand holds a jewel in the heart area and the left hand holds a lotus. He sits in the bodhisattva posture with his right foot extended.

You visualize the Triple Manifestation of Chenrezig right in front of you, giving you the purification water three times. When you receive the nectar the first time, you should think that your veils and obscurations of conflicting emotions are purified. When you receive the nectar the second time, you should think your veils and obscurations to omniscience are removed. When you receive the nectar for the third time, you should think you achieve the realization of unborn dharmakaya nature. During this time you symbolically wash yourself three times with the water and drink the water three times. This is done by sprinkling your face three times with the ring finger and thumb, then sipping the water cupped in your palm three times. Although you are supposed to symbolically drink the water for the purpose of purification, during the fasting day you just wash three times, you don't drink the water.

After receiving the purification water, you should think that Triple Manifestation has dissolved into you, and your body, speech, and mind become vajra body, speech, and mind. In that state, one should meditate on the transcendent wisdom nature of the mind.

If this entire visualization of Triple Manifestation is too complicated, then you can simply visualize Two-Armed Chenrezig standing with his right hand in the mudra of supreme giving and his left hand holding a lotus flower. From Chenrezig's right hand nectar flows three times and you are purified on three levels.

ENDING THE FAST

On the morning of the third day of practice, the fast is broken with the acceptance of the blessing water. If you are doing multiple Nyungne practices, in the extensive version of the practice text, just prior to taking the vow, there is a mandala offering during which you are supposed to think that you offer your Nyungne vow back to the Supreme Deity. Then your fast is over. Since the "Mandala Offering Prayer" does not exist in our brief text, if you can, right after the "Thirty-five Buddhas Confession Prayer," imagine that you are offering the Nyungne vow back to the Supreme Deity and break the fast with a special drink, which is referred to as "feeding our body's bacteria." On the last day of the last practice, the fast is broken by accepting the blessing water.

CONCLUDING THE PRACTICE

Final Confession

This confession prayer is for any shortcomings committed during the practice such as not being able to concentrate, recite, and maintain our visualizations properly. We purify our shortcomings with the recitation of the One-Hundred-Syllable Mantra three times.

Completion Phase

We conclude the ceremony by dissolving the frontal and self-visualized deity into emptiness. First we make a request to the wisdom deity, jnanasattva, to remain in the mandala of the shrine. This is accomplished by saying the following prayer: "Please remain in this very place, within the mandala. Grant us longevity and power, spare us from illness, and grant us the sublime accomplishment in the most excellent way." Then we recite the mantra OM SUTRA TIKTA BENZRAYE SOHA (ༀ་སུ་ཏྲ་ཏིཀྟ་བཛྲ་ཡེ་སྭ་ཧཱ).[47]

If we have a sand mandala, our request to the wisdom deity, jnanasattva, is to remain in the mandala until the end of the final practice. In this case we say a prayer in place of the above mantra as follows: "You perform activity for the benefit of sentient beings, please bestow siddhis accordingly upon us. You may depart for the pure land, but please return to us here. BENZRA MU (བཛྲ་མུ༔)."

The Actual Self-Dissolution

Here are the complete steps of the dissolution, or completion, and the postmeditation phases. The commitment deity of the frontal visualization (samayasattva), along with his palace and retinue of buddhas, dissolves into one's self-visualization of Chenrezig. The self-visualization dissolves into a visualization of Two-Armed Chenrezig. Two-Armed Chenrezig dissolves into the thumb-sized Chenrezig at the heart center, and the thumb-sized Chenrezig dissolves into the seed syllable HRIH (ཧྲཱིཿ) at his own heart center. The letter HRIH (ཧྲཱིཿ) becomes a small sphere of light, which in turn becomes smaller and smaller until it dissolves into emptiness. One should

---

47 Wisdom deity, or jnanasattva, refers to the real Chenrezig. Commitment deity, or samayasattva, is the image which we create by means of our visualization. In this case, the commitment deity is the Thousand-Armed Chenrezig visualized in front of us.

remain in this pure state of mind, a nonconceptual mind free of fabrications and elaborations.

When one arises from meditation, one enters into the next stage, the postmeditative state. In the postmeditative state one instantaneously imagines that one is in the form of Two-Armed Chenrezig. This image of Chenrezig is in the standing position, with the right hand in the gesture of supreme giving and the left hand holding a golden lotus (Fig. 7).

Section Four

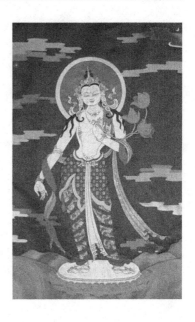

Preparation for the Actual Ceremony 12

PREPARING ONESELF

AS I MENTIONED in the introduction, if one is a Buddhist and on the path of the Great Vehicle in general and the vajrayana path in particular, the basic requirements for preparation are already met. If not, one must be prepared to take the refuge and bodhisattva vows, and the empowerment to do the practice, and be willing to abide by the Nyungne commitments. Actually, the most important factor is faith and confidence in the practice itself. This is more important than being completely familiar with the teaching and text, because complete devotion is the source of true benefit.

If you are going to do a two-day Nyungne practice, it might be necessary to take time off from work. To do eight sets of Nyungne, preparations might have to begin up to a year in advance. Depending on your responsibilities and the nature of your work, you may need to find out the exact dates far in advance and prepare accordingly, so that you really do have the time for this important practice.

A traditionally recommended preparation for eight-session Nyungne practice is to maintain a vegetarian diet for at least one week in advance. This preparation is for the purpose of cleansing, and takes one spiritually in the right direction. Additionally, according to kriya tantra, a substance made out of a newly delivered cow's dung mixed with purified water is put in the bath water, and it is said to have the power to cleanse. One drinks this water for purification as well.

Nyungne practice accomplishes the activity of pacification,[48] and the

---

48 Nyungne is primarily a practice of first-level tantra, or pacification activity. One can achieve that activity the most, and that should be the main focus.

color of pacification is white. Therefore, one's clothing, or at least one article of clothing, should be white. Clothing should not be too fancy, nor should it be too degrading. Here "too fancy" is from the point of view of attachment and ego. "Too degrading" is from the point of view of being disrespectful to this precious practice.

To do the practice you will need the Nyungne practice text, a small bowl of rice which is used as a symbol of flower offering, or actual flower petals for the same purpose, a cushion and table, a bell and dorje, and a mala. In the tradition of the kriya tantra Lotus Family, it is best to use a mala made of lotus seeds; if not lotus seeds, then a mala made of bodhi seeds, crystal, or sandalwood. The mala should not be made out of bone. Tradition specifies that these beads should be strung by a virgin girl who has also spun the thread.

A teacher should bless the mala by mantra, unless one is a good practitioner. If blessing the mala oneself, the mantra is:

ན་མོ་རཏྣ་ཏྲ་ཡ་ཡ།   ན་མོ་ཨཱརྱ་ཨ་ཝ་ལོ་ཀི་ཏེ་ཤྭ་ར་ཡ།

NAMO RATNA TRA YAYA   NAMO ARYA AWALO KITE SHWA RA YA

བོ་དྷི་སཏྭ་ཡ།   ཨོཾ་ཨ་མི་ཏེ་ག་མེ།   ཤྲི་ཡེ་ཤྲི་ཡ་ནི་ལི་སྭ་ཧཱ།

BODHI SATO YA   OM AMI TE GA ME   SHRI YE SHRI YA NI LI SO HA

One recites this mantra seven times, holding the mala between folded hands, and then blows on it. Traditionally the mala is placed in a little white mala pouch, and one recites the mantra secretly while putting one's hand into the pouch to make sure nobody sees it. This is done as a way to protect the blessing power of the mantra recitation. One then keeps the mala hidden in that pouch for the remainder of the practice. In addition, after finishing the recitation of each of the mantras during Nyungne practice, one can continuously bless one's mala by blowing on it, and then imagine that the blessings from the mala are continuously dissolving into you.

Although these practices are in the tradition of kriya tantra, in Tibet they are not generally done. The reason they are not done is because the influence of highest yoga tantra is so strong that they are not considered very important. Also the people who do Nyungne are not necessarily well informed about the tradition. If anybody wants to do the practice as close to the tradition as possible, then I think they should try to perform all of these practices as correctly as they can.

EMPOWERMENT AND INSTRUCTION

It is essential to receive the Chenrezig empowerment before doing the practice. If you have not taken refuge, then you should receive the refuge vows as well. The eight vows of the Restoring and Purifying Ordination are given during the Nyungne practice. You should also receive detailed instructions on visualization from the teacher.

PREPARING THE SHRINE

Here again, if we were to strictly follow kriya tantra tradition, there are all kinds of detailed preparations for the shrine. In most cases, people will not be able to carry out all these details.

The basic requirement is, first and foremost, the mandala (Fig. 10). While a sand mandala is highly recommended in kriya tantra, complete ceremonial knowledge is needed to create one. For anyone not well versed in

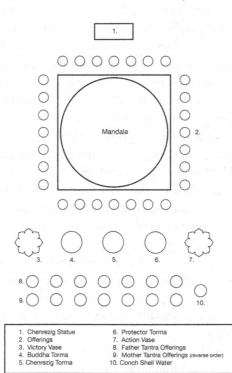

1. Chenrezig Statue
2. Offerings
3. Victory Vase
4. Buddha Torma
5. Chenrezig Torma
6. Protector Torma
7. Action Vase
8. Father Tantra Offerings
9. Mother Tantra Offerings (reverse order)
10. Conch Shell Water

ceremonies, this will probably not be possible; therefore, a painted mandala (Tib. *thangka* [painting]) can also be used. During the practice, the sand or the painted mandala is a symbol upon which the frontal visualization is done. If you cannot produce a sand mandala or a painted mandala, a third possibility is to make a symbolic representation with rice on a mandala offering plate. To do this, make a circle in the center of the plate and eight petals around the circle. Then place small piles of rice in the center of the petals in the four directions and in the center of the circle (Fig. 9).

The other most important preparation, according to the text and commentaries, is a statue of Chenrezig. The best statue is one made out of white sandalwood and filled with relics. The statue is placed on a tripod on top of the mandala, surrounded by offerings in the four directions. If a statue is not possible, then a thangka painting hung right behind the mandala would be the second choice (Fig. 2). If a thangka is also not available, then at minimum you must have a beautiful picture of Chenrezig, which can be placed behind the mandala.

The mandala is surrounded by eight offerings. The offerings are water, flowers, incense, lamps, perfumed water, food, and music, and they should be placed in a clockwise direction. If possible, arrange all eight offerings in each of the four cardinal directions. If not, make as many offerings as you can. In front of these offerings are two different kinds of bumpas. The first is the main bumpa, or victory vase as it is called. The other is the action bumpa. The main bumpa should be tied with a white scarf and placed on the right side of the mandala. The action bumpa should be tied with a red scarf and placed on the left side. (Here, right and left are from the mandala's point of view, which is the opposite of ours.)

In front of the bumpas, a Chenrezig torma is placed in the center, a torma for buddhas and bodhisattvas is placed on the right side, and a torma for the protectors on the left side. The Chenrezig torma is exactly the same as the Green Tara practice torma, which has four lotus flower shapes on the bottom and five ornaments on it. On the top are the sun, moon, and precious gem (Fig. 8).

The Mahakala torma varies, depending on whether it is for Six-Armed or Two-Armed Mahakala, so use the torma for the ceremony to be performed. Only the Chenrezig torma is absolutely necessary. If you do not have the torma for the buddhas and bodhisattvas or the Mahakala torma, these can be omitted.

One complete stacked offering mandala is placed in front of the tormas, and you place an additional set of eight offerings in front of that. The text mentions that one should also put another set of offerings in a counterclockwise direction. Again, this will depend on whatever offerings are available to you. If possible, it is good to add the eight auspicious signs and substances to the shrine as well, and as many offerings as you can in the form of fruit, flowers, etc. White flowers are recommended for the flower offering. On the side, you should have a conch shell with water from the action bumpa. This water is the blessing water one receives during the ceremony, as well as the water used for all of the other purification purposes.

Keep in mind that, in general, a shrine is a representation of Buddha's body, speech, and mind, therefore the basis of the shrine should be any representation of body, speech, and mind. Examples of such representations are statues, texts, and stupas. For Nyungne practice, Thousand-Armed Chenrezig sutras and written mantras should be included in the shrine to represent Chenrezig's speech.

Right in front of all these shrine objects, you should place offering tormas on a lower level. These are offering tormas for the local gods and protectors, and one for the harmful spirits. Most of the time, when participating in Eight Nyungne practices, lamas and monks will prepare these. If you are doing the practice alone, you will need to ask someone to help; or, if you cannot find any help, then cookies and candies can be used for offering. For naga torma, milk should be included because nagas like milk. In addition, you need materials for the bath offering. Bathing water, a pot, a mirror, and a white towel are kept at the side for this purpose.

Offering tormas should not be eaten. They should be taken outside at the end of the practice and put in a high place. They should not be given to four-legged animals such as pigs, which are considered lower forms of animals. Rather they should be given to the birds, which are considered part of the Dakini Family as they are able to fly.

LOCATION OF THE PRACTICE

The text mentions that it is very auspicious to do Nyungne practice in an area where there is a pond with a lotus flower in it, and that this is a sign that your practice will bear fruit. In other words, such a setting provides the cause for one to be successful in the practice. If you do not have a pond with a lotus flower, then you should do the practice in the presence of a stupa with relics. That is also for the purpose of overcoming obstacles and achieving siddhis quickly. In addition to all these preparations, cleaning the shrine and the shrine room is also very important.

AUSPICIOUS DAYS TO DO THE PRACTICE

We follow the Tibetan lunar calendar,[49] according to which the half moon always falls on the eighth day, the full moon always falls on the fifteenth day, and the new moon always falls on the thirtieth day. It has been a Buddhist belief that some days are naturally auspicious in general, such as the full and new moon days, and some are particularly auspicious because they are related to special activities of Lord Buddha.

The first month of the lunar calendar year[50] is called the month of great miracles, because from the first day until the fifteenth day Lord Buddha performed all kinds of extraordinary miracles each day. In addition to it being the month of extraordinary miracles, the fourteenth and fifteenth are especially auspicious for the Kagyu lineage because the fourteenth is the anniversary of Milarepa's parinirvana, and the fifteenth is the anniversary of Marpa's parinirvana.

The fourth month of the lunar calendar is a special month during which three different important events took place. On the eighth day, Lord Buddha was born, and on the fifteenth day he became enlightened under the bodhi tree. Some say Lord Buddha passed away into mahaparinirvana on the eighth day as well. This month is particularly significant for Nyungne practitioners because this is the month when Gelongma Palmo became enlightened, and it is also the month all the lineage holders became enlightened.

On the fourth day of the sixth month, Lord Buddha first turned the wheel of dharma. In the ninth month, on the twenty-second day, Lord Buddha descended from the thirty-three gods realm. These four months, the first, the fourth, the sixth, and the ninth, are called the Four Great Auspicious Times.

On these auspicious days whatever deeds you do, virtuous or nonvirtuous, are multiplied one hundred thousand times, and some say they are multiplied one hundred million times.

The point of mentioning these days is that these are the most auspicious days to do the Nyungne practice. One of our annual Eight Nyungne practices is done during the fourth month because it is the most important month of the year.

---

49 The Tibetan lunar calendar is different from the regular calendar. All the dates and months that we mention here are according to the lunar calendar; therefore, those who want to pay attention to the dates need to use a lunar calendar.

50 The first month usually falls somewhere around February or March of the Western calendar.

It has been further said that the best time to do the practice is when the moon is waxing, from the first to the fifteenth, and it is not auspicious to practice when the moon is waning. However, if you are continually doing the practice for many days, then it doesn't matter as long as you begin in the earlier part of the month. It has also been said that the second, the fourth, the sixth, the ninth, and the twelfth are inauspicious days to start the practice. All of the other ten days are good days, but doing Chenrezig ceremonial practice on the fifth, the seventh, and on full moon days is particularly auspicious.

Inauspicious days derive from a belief that if you do practice on those days, you will be likely to have spiritual obstacles and achieving any siddhis will be difficult. On the other hand, if you do the practice on auspicious days, there will be no obstacles and you will achieve siddhis quickly. This concludes preparation for the actual ceremony.

Actual Practice 13

Three Components of Perfection

To be ultimately correct and pure, every tantric spiritual practice must have three components of perfection: a proper beginning, a proper middle, and a proper end. This means one must begin with proper preparation, and then perform the main body of the practice one-pointedly, and conclude the practice with dedication of merit. So we begin the practice by reaffirming our sincere wish to take refuge in the Three Jewels and Three Roots, since that is the only place one can ultimately take refuge. Then, with correct motivation, we reaffirm our wish to perform the practice by engendering the enlightened attitude, meaning we truly wish to do the practice for the benefit of all sentient beings, not for any selfish reason, since enlightenment is only possible through devotion to the benefit of others, and since there is no example of attaining complete enlightenment by being selfish or self-centered.

To think about everybody else is absolutely the correct and reasonable thing to do, because in reality every single sentient being has been our mother and father in former lives according to Lord Buddha, not just once but countless numbers of times. We know this to be true because Lord Buddha would not falsely make such a statement. Actually, I think this alone is sufficient reason to devote ourselves to doing that which benefits all these beings. This is not just spiritually correct conduct, but it is decent human behavior towards those who have been so kind and generous to us countless numbers of times. If we start the practice with this motivation and a pure mind, it is a perfect beginning.

In the middle, we must engage in the practice with sincerity and with focused attention on the practice by observing the vows correctly, to the best of our ability, and then by saying the prayers, doing the visualizations, reciting the mantras, and meditating, etc. If the visualizations and meditation become a little too difficult, we must do our prayers and prostrations and recitation of mantras correctly and sincerely as much as we can. When we practice in this manner, we perform the middle part of the practice perfectly.

Finally, the conclusion is done by sincerely dedicating the merit and virtue of the practice for the benefit of all beings. The idea of dedication is sometimes explained in terms of sharing the merit with all sentient beings. But actually this is not correct, because the idea of sharing comes from one still wanting to keep some of the merit for oneself, whereas the idea of dedication is to completely give all merit away, with no thought of one's own benefit. One's own benefit is natural and automatic, and an individual spiritual person who wishes to follow in the path of the Great Vehicle is not concerned with himself, because when one does something that is ultimately correct, its result is naturally correct. So, there is no need to think, "What's in it for me?" This dedication not only makes the spiritual practice perfect, but it also makes the merit inexhaustible.

Ordinarily, as much as we would like to, we may not know how to correctly do the dedication. For this reason, the most skillful thing to do is just think and say that we wish to follow in the footsteps of the buddhas of the past, present, and future. The "Dedication Prayer" expresses the correct meaning of dedication perfectly, therefore we need only think that we sincerely wish to dedicate the merit exactly as the prayer states. In this way the end of the practice becomes perfect. These three components of perfection are very important, key points to remember because they are important when doing any spiritual practice, not just Nyungne practice.

NYUNGNE PRACTICE

In the context of the Nyungne practice text, the three components of perfection are as follows. The early morning session starts with praises to Lord Buddha and to Chenrezig, the "Thirty-five Buddhas Confession Prayer," and the taking of the eight-precepts vow. These are all preludes to the actual practice. We then recite the "Lineage Prayer," the "Refuge Prayer," and "Generation of Bodhichitta." Taken together, these constitute a proper beginning.

The main body of the practice begins with accumulation of merit through the recitation of the "Seven-Branch Offering Prayer" and the "Four Immeasurables." This is followed by self-generation of the deity and recitation of the mantra, then frontal generation of the deity and recitation of the mantra.

Next we recite the "Seven-Branch Offering Prayer," the "Mandala Offering Prayer," the "General Confession Prayer," and the "Po Homage Prayer." After that we have a "Specific Request Prayer," then the torma offering, the bathing water offering, the conclusion ceremony offering, and the specific confession of shortcomings in doing the practice. Finally, we perform dissolution of the deity and conclude the main body of the practice.

We end the practice by dedicating the merit, and this dedication is beautifully done by reciting the "Resolve to Practice Excellence,"[51] followed by auspicious omen prayers. In this way we have perfected our practice of Nyungne.

CLEANLINESS

The idea of cleansing plays a central role in Nyungne practice, because this practice derives mainly from the kriya tantra tradition, although charya tantra is also part of it. In kriya tantra, spiritual development is based primarily on physical actions of cleanliness and, while very important, mental visualization and so on are only supporting factors; whereas in charya tantra, physical cleanliness and visualization are both equally important. So this practice of Nyungne is a combination of these two levels of tantra.

According to the kriya tantra tradition, washing and taking showers are very important. One is to engage in the conduct of ritual purification three times a day, which means purification of the physical body by bathing, and then purification of downfalls with confession prayers, and purification of thoughts by being mindful of thoughts and generating bodhichitta.

Next is changing the three types of clothing: outer, inner, and secret. Changing one's outer clothing means to put on clean clothes each day, and changing one's inner clothing means to guard one's vow. Changing one's secret clothing means to visualize the deity. In addition to white clothing, a white shawl might be worn as a dharma robe and as a symbol of purification. The scriptures mention that one should not wear leather of any kind, including on one's mala, one's watch band, leather shoes, etc. They also mention three types of white food one should eat during Nyungne. They are yogurt, milk, and butter.

The strict tradition is to wash one's five limbs, meaning the face, two hands, and two feet, before entering the shrine room. While washing, one is to recite a purification mantra such as the One-Hundred-Syllable Mantra. The most popular One-Hundred-Syllable Mantra is with Vajrasattva,

51 There are other translations of the title such as "Aspiration of Noble Conduct."

but in the tradition of Nyungne the Padmasattva mantra must be used. In addition to this, upon entering the shrine room everyone is given purification water for rinsing the mouth, which one then spits out. This same water is also used for purifying wrong actions done during Nyungne, such as falling asleep, reciting the mantras incorrectly, farting, even yawning, and so on. Traditionally, if one makes any of these mistakes, they are supposed to get up and bow three times, purify themselves by rinsing their mouth and reciting the one-hundred-syllable purification mantra, and then sit down. It is also important to keep everything very clean in the shrine room area.

Although all of these conventions of conduct are in the tradition of Nyungne practice, honestly speaking Tibetan Buddhists are not very good examples of following them. One of the main reasons for this is that truly great, enlightened masters have no need for these cleansing practices. Furthermore, the emphasis in highest yoga tantra is on how to transcend everything, including conceptual notions of what is clean and not clean. As Tibetan Buddhism is predominantly a practicing tradition of highest tantra, the lower tantras are seldom a major focus.

The way my completely enlightened guru, Dorje Chang Kalu Rinpoche, used to teach and behave is a perfect example of this. Since he dwelled in none other than a completely perfect state of mind, in his authentic way of living he neither rejected nor accepted any arising phenomena. Even though he was all for this wonderful tradition if sincere spiritual practitioners were able to carry it out, he himself didn't care one way or the other. And this is the sign of dwelling in a perfectly liberated state of mind, a mind which is free from any kind of bondage. For that reason, it was obvious that he had no attachment to any phenomena whatsoever, including traditions of buddhadharma. At the same time, when asked about certain fine points of traditional practice, he knew them all in precise detail.

POWER OF BREAKING THE VOWS

We take vows to strengthen our spiritual deeds, and the power of the vow is based on our sincere commitment to not engage in specific activities. Therefore, abstention from those activities has great power. It has been said that such power could be compared to an increase in benefit of one hundred thousand times. By the same token, having made a commitment to not engage in wrong deeds and not being able to abide by that commitment, thereby breaking the vow, means wrong deeds increase one hundred thousand times in power as well. Before taking a vow, this point is very important to keep in mind. When and if we cannot keep the vow, the best thing to do is not take it.

To mention something about the power of wrong deeds in general, the karma of killing causes one to be born in the lower realms and, in particular, the hell realm called Reviving Hell (Tib.Yang So, Skt. Samjiva), where people kill each other over and over, thousands of times. Even if one is born as a human, one will have a short life and an ugly body, and one's sanity will be affected. One will experience a great deal of fear, anger, and illness, and suffer a lot. It has been further said that one will have more or less severe negative karma depending on who was killed. One will have to pay with one's own life anywhere from three hundred to 990 times for each killing.

The karma of stealing is cause to be born in the hell realm called Crying and Howling Hell (Tib. Ngu Bo, Skt. Raurava). Even if born as a human, one will experience lack of wealth and prosperity. If one does obtain wealth, it cannot be held on to and it will be very difficult to obtain new wealth. One will be disliked and hated by others.

The karma of sexual misconduct is cause to be born in the hell realm called Loud Crying and Howling Hell (Tib. Ngu Bo Chen Po, Skt. Maharaurava). Even if born as a human, one will be born five hundred times as a woman with a dreadful disease such as leprosy, or as a transsexual, or as the wife of a terrible person. One will experience lots of problems and be hated by others.

The karma of lying is cause to be born in the hell realm of Black Thread Hell (Tib. Thig Nag, Skt. Kalautra). Even if born as a human, one will have speech impediments such as muteness, stuttering, lisping, and so on. One will have very little compassion, be very jealous, and have severe halitosis. In all future lives, one will not comprehend dharma.

The karma of intoxication is cause to be born in the hell realm called Heating Hell (Tib. Tsa Wa, Skt. Tapana). Even if born as a human, one will be very attached to sleeping and will be forgetful and not very bright. One will lack the qualities of shame and humility, and one will be a very jealous and stingy person. One's virtuous spiritual deeds will diminish. One will be born as a harmful spirit, a dog, or mad for five hundred lifetimes.

Whether or not you take a vow, there are severe negative consequences if you engage in these misdeeds. As I mentioned, with a vow the negative karmic consequences multiply one hundred thousand times. On the other hand, the virtuous deed of abstaining from wrong action is truly beneficial and, in particular, the merit of deeds done with a vow and a commitment is multiplied one hundred thousand times. So it is very important to remember the power of taking the vow, as well as the absolute importance of sincerely preserving it.

PURE PHYSICAL ACTION

Since the practice of Nyungne belongs to the category of tantric doctrine known as kriya tantra, or action tantra, completely pure physical action is taught as skillful means. In addition to the fasting and the silence, any food or drink on the nonfasting day must be absolutely pure vegetarian. In this case, the Buddhist idea of pure vegetarianism means completely pure vegetarianism. I stress complete and pure, because people have all kinds of ideas about vegetarianism. Some people consider themselves vegetarian yet still eat fish or certain other types of meat; and there are those who say, "I'm vegetarian," but for health reasons, not for moral reasons. Spiritually speaking it is in the right direction, but this attitude is not completely correct either. If one is willing to be vegetarian, it is better to do it for the right reasons because there is virtue in doing so. Otherwise, there is no benefit beyond the limited health benefits in this life. Here vegetarianism means a completely pure karmic act.

It has been said that during our practice of Nyungne only three white foods should be eaten. Actually this is scriptural terminology referring to pure vegetarianism, although literally the three white foods are dairy products (milk, yogurt, and butter) which are included in the vegetarian diet. Lord Atisha is credited with making a vegetarian diet part of the eight-precepts vow, since it is not formally one of the eight precepts. I presume that in former times people who lived closer to the time of the Buddha automatically adopted correct action; then, possibly they began to fall a little short in this regard. Therefore, Atisha probably felt the need to spell out the correct action clearly by making a vegetarian diet formally part of the eight precepts.

Pure vegetarian action also means that one will not even eat garlic and onions or turnips and mustard seeds. These foods are supposed to contain chemical substances that excite neurosis, and therefore one is not supposed to eat them. There is an ancient story which relates to garlic being an impure substance. The story has to do with the gods and demi-gods (jealous gods). Among the demi-gods, there was one who was always especially jealous of the gods. According to the story, a special vase filled with precious nectar, amrita, was in the gods' palace, and somehow that jealous god managed to break into the palace and grab the vase and run away with it. The gods saw him stealing the vase and they chased after him. The demi-god was unable to outrun the gods, and he knew they were going to get him. But he wasn't going to give back the precious nectar, so instead he drank the whole thing. When the gods finally caught him and realized that he had already drunk the nectar, they got very angry and chopped him into pieces. Pieces of the jealous god's dead body fell down from the sky and eventually hit the earth. From these pieces a very special substance started to grow, and that was garlic.

Today when you eat garlic, modern medicine will tell you that it does very good things for your body. Garlic acts as an antibiotic and as an antioxidant. Large amounts of garlic are supposed to make you look young, as it purifies the blood. Because garlic has so many beneficial properties, you can even purchase garlic pills. All these benefits are due to the amrita. But, spiritually speaking, we also know that garlic is not that good, because it can stir up your emotions. It's good for the body but bad for the mind, and that's because the jealous god's intention was really bad. It's a double-edged sword.

Therefore, substances such as garlic and onions are not to be taken while you do your spiritual practice of Nyungne. Lord Buddha mentions many times that his disciples should not eat meat, garlic, and onions. In addition to stimulating neurosis, it is also understood that those who eat garlic and onions will offend the gods[52] and frighten the poor spirits.

Actually, in strict vegetarianism, one is not supposed to eat anything that grows under the ground. That means excluding potatoes and so forth, but traditionally this is not taken too seriously. Although I have not personally read any reference to such a restriction, I believe the reason for not eating anything that grows underground has to do with the digging and plowing, in the process of which you may kill many insects and other small creatures.

The nineteenth-century teacher Patrul Rinpoche spoke about the karma of people who thought they were very good human beings and didn't do anything wrong. People who live in modern society, with their limited success and education, would very much like to think, egotistically, that they are at the very least "good human beings." Patrul Rinpoche would point out that actually, when you think about it, morally and ethically you are far from being a really good human being when you are eating meat every day.

Patrul Rinpoche went on to talk about the Tibetan diet in which the

52 There is the understanding that godlike beings surround and protect virtuous beings and spiritual practitioners.

main foods are tea and tsampa (roasted barley). He spoke about the bad karma associated with tsampa. He started with what happens when they plow the ground to plant the seeds for the tsampa. All the insects underground are brought to the surface, and those on the surface are forced underground, and many of them die. He also pointed out that the birds are very busy eating these little insects. Then during the harvesting time, all kinds of unfortunate karmic deeds occur. Finally you get to eat the tsampa, and if you think tsampa is a pure substance, well, it's not. That's the point Patrul Rinpoche was trying to make. It's the same thing with the tea, when we consider the hardships the tea growers have to undergo, and so forth. So, in connection with our discussion of diet, anything that's agriculturally grown has a great deal of karma involved with it. Unless one lives a very simple life in caves like Milarepa, and eats only nettles that grow naturally, nothing else other than that, there really is no completely pure way.

Having said all of that, obviously eating vegetables has less severe karmic consequences than eating meat. Therefore, besides the meat, the only vegetables that are prohibited during the practice of Nyungne are garlic and onions, turnips and mustard seeds, etc. However, garlic and onions are strictly prohibited, while the others are traditionally less restricted and therefore I don't restrict them during our practice.

Obviously, the main reason for vegetarianism is to refrain from eating all forms of meat; that includes seafood, red meat, and poultry. In terms of correct and incorrect action, eating meat is incorrect, and it is karmically impure action because of the killing. All these sentient beings are beings with feelings. Just as we like to live, they like to live, and their lives are cut short solely because we want to eat them. From the point of view of action tantra, correct action means absolutely no eating of meat. If you want to be correct, karmically and spiritually, meat eating is not a choice. We only have to think about the animals' pain and suffering to know that this has to be true. The moment they're born, they're only going to die. So many animals are bred under terrible conditions for the purpose of being slaughtered under terrible conditions. People who have seen this are unable to deny the reality that animals are sentient beings, beings with feelings.

ADDITIONAL RULES

Food and Drink

In addition to a strict vegetarian diet, one doesn't eat one's own leftover food, nor should one eat the offering food for the shrine. In Tibet, there was a type of food that enhanced people's ability to travel long distances, climb mountains, and so forth; these specially prepared foods are also not allowed. Peas and the legume family, as well as the salt family, are included in the list of restricted foods; however, these seem less important and less clearly defined.

Although scripture mentions that on the nonfasting day we can drink from morning to evening, Jamgon Kongtrul the Great writes that in Tibet, where tea is customarily drunk, tea drinking is fine, but the tea should be less strong than usual. Similarly, in our time, drinking fruit juice is most probably okay, but like the tea, it should be diluted. In addition, to be completely correct, all the beverages should be blessed with blessing water before being taken.

The correct way of eating the one meal is to begin with a proper offering prayer (page 270). Traditionally Buddhists chant a sutra called *Remembering the Three Jewels*. If you do not know how to do this, then at minimum one should bless the food with the mantra OM AH HUNG and then accept the food while imagining that you are offering it to Lord Chenrezig. We end the meal by blessing and giving away the leftover food to those less fortunate spirit beings who can only receive blessed and dedicated food offerings.

The meal is referred to as a "single sitting," which means one does not get up until the meal is finished. The timing of the meal is also prescribed as noontime. Traditionally, people serve the practitioners so there is no need to get up and sit down again. If possible, we should have this kind of arrangement; however, since this is often difficult to manage, I give my students permission to self-serve even if it means getting up and returning to the table. However, the meal must be taken within the prescribed time frame, which in this case is approximately 12:00-1:00 pm.

Proper eating utensils are also mentioned in the text. Cups and plates should not be made out of precious metals, copper, or brass, nor should they be skull cups or leaves (which were commonly used in India). Bare hands should also not be used.

One should not eat with one's mouth wide open or too much closed, or with noise, and one should not eat while talking or laughing. One should only eat mindfully and with restraint. One should not overeat, nor should one undereat with pretense, meaning putting on the appearance of being able to get along with less food when in fact you are still hungry. In other words, during Nyungne you should eat enough and no more. Of course, these are all among the things that are done during the nonfasting day.

On the fasting day, obviously you do not eat, nor do you drink even a drop of water. There is a tradition of not even swallowing your own saliva; however, in our tradition, Jamgon Kongtrul the Great mentions that either swallowing or not swallowing saliva is fine. People sometimes ask me about brushing their teeth. I think it is okay to brush your teeth because the tradition is, when rules are broken you are supposed to rinse your mouth and purify with purification water along with a confession prayer.[53] Therefore, as long as you don't swallow any water, I think it is okay to brush your teeth as well.

Bending the Rules

The rules are mainly physical and it's not difficult to identify when one is breaking them, such as eating or drinking at times when it's not allowed, talking on a silent day, farting or belching, and falling asleep during practice. Reciting the wrong mantra during practice is also breaking the rules, and one is not supposed to get up even to go to the bathroom. If one does leave the shrine room, one must bow down three times at the door, recite the purification mantra, and cleanse one's mouth with purification water upon returning. This same purification process is necessary for all the other wrongdoings as well.

Perhaps more common is bending the rules. For example, while writing many notes to one another on the silent day is not verbally talking, I think it is bending the rules. The same is true for loud laughter, or grunting at each other as a way of communicating. Some people ask to take medicine. If the medicine is truly necessary, then it can be permitted. But in some cases there is no important health need, for example when someone wants to continue to take vitamins just because they normally take them. This would be bending the rules, because it is not really a life-threatening situation; therefore, it is not permitted.

Another way to bend the rules is to read completely samsaric material like a magazine, whereas reading a dharma book would be okay. Watching TV or listening to the radio is bending the rules. Surfing the internet, sending unnecessary e-mail messages, or making unnecessary phone calls is also bending the rules.

On the other hand, if you simply could not participate in the practice without a means of communication through e-mail or telephones calls, in that case it would still be beneficial to join the practice with the option

---

53 If it's not possible to recite the entire confession prayer, then reciting the One-Hundred-Syllable Mantra and rinsing your mouth will do.

of sending and receiving messages. The important point here is that you must present your situation and receive permission from a teacher for this to be acceptable. In general, the teacher has to make an assessment based on an individual person's needs. Given the situation, what would be the best thing to do? Priority will always be placed on what will make it possible for someone to participate in and benefit from the precious practice.

Samaya Commitments of Nyungne

The samaya commitment (Tib. *dam sig*) consists of the vows made to a teacher and teaching in the vajrayana path. It is the source of all siddhis in the secret mantrayana, or tantric path. Nyungne is part of kriya tantra, and it has been said that in order to receive the ultimate siddhi, the root of the teaching lies in the samaya commitment. Since samaya is the primary factor in spiritual achievement, you must try to keep it to the best of your ability.

The general samaya commitments are:

- Taking refuge in the Three Jewels
- Engendering bodhichitta
- Not discriminating between the deities of the higher tantra and lower tantra, and the male and female deities; rather, with complete sincerity, respecting and honoring them all with delight in your heart.

These three are general commitments and in addition to those there are thirteen specific commitments. They are:

1. Being devoted to the practice deity.
2. Respecting with body, speech, and mind those who have taken tantric vows and entered into the tantric path.
3. Respecting all sangha members, all those who are on the path of buddhadharma, and not finding fault with even the smallest shortcoming.
4. Respecting the guru and absolutely not finding fault with anything they do or say.
5. Not developing any wrong views, even if you practice a lot but don't experience signs of accomplishment through the deity.
6. On auspicious days,[54] making a great deal of offerings to the deity and the Three Jewels.

---

54 The auspicious days are the full moon, new moon, and half moon days, and Saka Dawa.

7. Not worshipping samsaric gods and ordinary spirits.
8. Not refusing food or lodging to someone who comes to you in need.
9. Abandoning even momentary harmful thoughts and actions, and developing beneficial thoughts and actions toward all beings, from humans all the way to tiny insects.
10. Engaging in skillful means to increase the merit by diligently reciting the mantras and keeping the vows.
11. Reciting the mantras properly with correct actions as they have been taught.
12. Not giving up other samaya vows of the secret mantrayana.
13. Keeping the deity and mantra secret from those who did not receive the empowerment and from those who broke the samaya.

If one breaks any of these samaya commitments, the way to purify the broken vow is by confession prayer; and that can be done by reciting the "Thirty-five Buddhas Confession Prayer," the "General Confession," or the One-Hundred-Syllable Mantra. The moment you break the vow and, through mindful awareness, you regret your action, if you don't know the confession prayers, most probably you do know how to recite the One-Hundred-Syllable Mantra and just do that. One very important point to remember is to not let a day go by without purifying your violation.

Furthermore, there is a specific samaya commitment related to Lord Chenrezig. The commitment is: Even if one is not at fault and others, for no reason, do any of the following four things:

• Provoke you,
• Scold you,
• Physically abuse you,
• Proclaim your hidden faults,

even then one still practices patience and does not retaliate. One who practices in this way is considered a true practitioner with the four qualities.

In other words, no matter what others do to you, such as abuse you physically, steal your belongings, speak harsh and ill words, or mentally harbor ill and harmful thoughts towards you, you, as a practitioner, think that these are none other than the blessings of the body, speech, and mind of Lord Chenrezig. These are blessings, because this is how you can overcome defilements and negativities. The bottom line is, no matter what happens, in happiness or in suffering, a practitioner will have nothing but complete faith in Chenrezig.

Further, one will try to develop sacred and pure outlook by thinking that one's dwelling place is the land of Great Bliss, or the Potala Pure Land, and that everyone in it is a manifestation of Chenrezig; that sounds are the supreme Six-Syllable Mantra, and that all thoughts are the vastness of great jnana, the wisdom awareness of the union of compassion and emptiness. One should further develop one's outlook towards others so that you only want to treat them with none other than compassion and kindness in return for all the wrongs that they do to you. Otherwise, it has been said that you will be disappointing Lord Chenrezig. Until you can do these things, your ability to receive true blessing remains a little difficult.

Occasionally, one must try to practice taking and sending and, as a daily prayer, one must recite the long dharani 108 times, or twenty-one times, or a minimum of fifteen times a day. If one recites the supreme Six-Syllable Mantra every day instead of the long dharani, that will be all right too.

If one keeps all of these samaya commitments, the power and benefit of the teaching will infallibly be there. Accordingly, if one does not violate the samaya commitments and engages in this precious practice of Nyungne, one becomes a member of the Vidyadhara Family and has the opportunity to become enlightened in one, three, or a maximum of sixteen lifetimes. Considering the entire situation of samsara, one cannot ask for anything more than what this practice and teaching provide.

Section Five

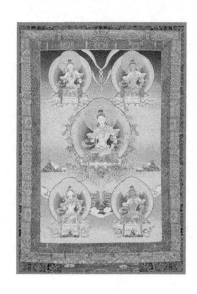

Benefits of Vegetarian Diet and Fasting 14

SINCE FASTING and vegetarianism are a big part of the practice of Nyungne, I think it is important to mention the benefits of fasting as well as the importance of vegetarianism from a Buddhist point of view. There are many benefits to taking the vow of fasting as part of the eight mahayana precepts. The main benefits are that, even if you remain in the samsaric world, in your future lives you will never experience famine, you will never experience wartime, and you will never experience plague: plague, famine, and war. Experiencing war means that you are born in a place where there is war and you are killed by weapons. Experiencing plague means being born in a place where you contract a disease like bubonic plague and die. Experiencing famine means you are born in a place where there are droughts and crops die, and as a result you die of starvation.

Fasting for twenty-four hours may sound a little extreme if you have never done it. This practice is not difficult and fasting has long been recognized as a way to cleanse and heal the body. Now there is growing evidence that fasting every other day contributes to longevity and resistance to serious disease. Recent studies support the health benefits of intermittent fasting in terms of better insulin sensitivity, resistance to a neurotoxin that stimulates Alzheimer's disease, better adaptability to stress, lower heart rates and blood pressure, slowed aging and increased longevity in lab animals and humans. Fasting may make cells less prone to becoming cancerous as well. These benefits are present even when the overall calorie consumption remains the same.

When actually practicing fasting, for those of us who practice regularly, the discomforts of hunger and thirst are quite minor; however it definitely gives us an opportunity to reflect on the sufferings of the lower realms in general and particularly the suffering of the hungry ghost realm. It gives us the opportunity to generate true love and compassion, which is the most important spiritual quality that one can develop. Without a real experience of personal discomfort, it is hard to relate to the suffering of other sentient beings. And if one cannot relate to others' suffering, it is very difficult to generate a genuine compassion. Without a true compassion, becoming a pure enlightened being is out of the question.

VEGETARIAN DIET

While vegetarian diet is an integral part of the Nyungne practice, we generally assume that, as Buddhists, we don't necessarily have to adopt a vegetarian lifestyle. Here I think it is very important to know exactly what Lord Buddha said on the subject.

During the time of Lord Buddha, all his fellow monks and nuns had renounced everything and they lived a simple and pure life of begging for food. Whatever offering they received, they accepted. In the vinaya teaching of the hinayana tradition one can find Lord Buddha giving permission for his fellow monks to eat meat if it is offered, but only if the offering is free from three conditions. The three conditions are: 1) you saw the animal being purposely killed for you; 2) you didn't see it, but you heard about it; and 3) you have a doubt about it, and you think it might have been killed for you. If you know for sure that the meat offering is free from these three conditions, Buddha gave permission to eat it.

The teaching on "free from three conditions" has to do with the degree of karma associated with the eating of meat. Speaking of karma, Lord Buddha's teaching on the various degrees of karma from the butcher to the wholesaler to the retailer and finally to you, as the customer, can all be found in the sutras.

There is a statement by Lord Buddha which says, "Those who eat meat are not my followers." These are seemingly contradictory statements, but in fact Buddhist teachers understand that the former is intended for disciples in the initial stages and the latter is for fully mature followers. So here one has to conclude that the latter is the ultimate statement of the Buddha, while the former is a relative statement. There are other instances when Lord Buddha was trying to correct those who advocated that vegetarianism is the *only* correct spiritual way of life. In order to balance this extreme view, Lord Buddha said, "That's not the only way, there are other ways." Unfortunately some people took liberty to eat meat based on such statements.

As I understand it, in the mahayana tradition, which is based purely on the teaching of bodhichitta, you cannot find one single reference to Lord Buddha giving any permission to eat meat. Not only that but he taught a great deal about mother sentient beings and how one should not eat meat. He elaborated on that a lot: it was like eating your own children's flesh, and so on. There is definitely no permission for meat eating, since the teaching is primarily on true loving-kindness and compassion. As Chinese Buddhists are all followers of the mahayana tradition, they have correctly adopted the vegetarian diet, although my understanding is that it came about through the decree of a Chinese Buddhist emperor. He ordered by decree that they not eat meat, and ever since that time this wonderful tradition has been followed. I am so glad the emperor gave such a tall order.

Tibetan Buddhists are predominantly tantric Buddhists, and they are generally nonvegetarian. If you ask Tibetan Buddhist scholars about meat eating, they will usually quote from the vinaya teaching of Lord Buddha giving permission with the three conditions. Then there are those who, without proper understanding, think that tantric Buddhism is very profound and the highest level of teaching, and since they are the followers of this tradition, everything and anything is okay, including meat eating. This is a complete misunderstanding of the true doctrine. In reality, the greater the understanding of everything there is, the greater the loving-kindness, compassion, and perfect action there should be, and not the other way around. Some will sarcastically quote a popular saying, "He who is truly compassionate should eat meat," meaning that if one is truly compassionate, one will not eat the meat irresponsibly, rather with complete compassion and prayer for the animal, and therefore the animal benefits from it. In my opinion such conditions only apply to a completely enlightened being like my own Lord Guru, Dorje Chang Kalu Rinpoche, and to others like him. Other than that, I think it is an excuse for justifying wrong action.

Having said that, let me explain a little about why everyone eats meat in the country of Tibet, including spiritual beings. I think there are several reasons for this. First of all, Tibet was known as the land of darkness, and people there were almost like the yakshas, flesh-eating beings. I guess even buddhadharma coming to the land of darkness could not stop people from eating meat, which was a habit of the locals for many thousands of years. The other thing is that, being at such a high altitude, vegetables didn't grow in Tibet and people didn't know how to plant them. And then, also, the tantric path being the path of transformation, people took liberty because of that as well. It was all right for truly great practitioners because they really could transform, but for ordinary beings I'm afraid the karma of eating meat is hard to escape.

Although such is the case in Tibetan life, Tibetan people do have some noble habits as well. Most Tibetans would not eat all kinds of little seafood and small animals. They would feel more comfortable sharing one animal that will feed many people than killing many animals to feed a few. I hope I don't sound like I am justifying Tibetans' meat eating. Actually, my point is that if you can be vegetarian, of course that's the best thing to do. But if you cannot, as a Buddhist you must at least try to be responsible. This means eating as little meat as possible and as few sentient beings as possible.

When I was a kid I used to help my enlightened guru collect the bones that were left after a meal. Usually what he did was bless them, and then he crushed them and mixed them with clay and made tsa tsas, miniature clay stupas. From his own point of view, he dwelt in a perfect state of mind that was not affected by any karma, but his actions of collecting bones and saying prayers were to further make sure that the animals that came into contact with him were completely liberated.

In general, Buddhist tantra has four levels and in the first three levels you cannot find any reference to the inclusion of meat. Not only that, meat eating is absolutely forbidden. Perhaps in the highest yoga tantra one will see a reference such as, when engaging in a postmeditative action, one is to neither accept nor reject anything and everything. One simply dwells in the state of mind which is free from attachment and aversion. The only reference point of engaging in meat eating is perhaps during the feast offering ceremony. The feast offerings are a substance representing skillful means and a nectar representing wisdom; meat is supposed to be supreme among substances and the supreme nectar is alcohol. This meat, the supreme substance of skillful means, should be from an animal that died of natural causes. Through ceremonial practices these substances are transformed into a supreme substance that the individual, devoted practitioner in the tradition is to enjoy without hesitation. In other words, if there is such a thing called "okay to eat meat," it has to be in the context of an individual spiritual practitioner's ability to transform and benefit other sentient beings.

Additionally, there are Tibetan lamas who are vegetarian but who will eat the meat of animals that died of natural causes. In a modern society you cannot find such meat, but in Tibet, since a major part of the society is nomadic, there are always animals who have died of natural causes.

Spiritual Benefits

While a vegetarian diet may produce many good results, such as reduced risk of disease and increased longevity, these benefits are only from the point of view of this life. More important are the benefits that affect us in the long term, our endless future lives, and these benefits only come from right action. Avoiding meat eating, which is the result of the killing of animals, and following a vegetarian diet are definitely steps in the right direction as far as ultimate goodness is concerned, which leads to higher birth. In the Buddhist tradition achieving a higher birth means a human birth and birth in the god realms, and so on. Of course if the vegetarianism is practiced for an enlightened reason, then the ultimate result will be enlightenment, freedom from the cycle of rebirth.

The main issue here is what will bring the ultimate benefit? The answer is the practice of Nyungne associated with vegetarian diet and fasting. From this point of view, even if all the research showing the benefits of a vegetarian diet were actually false, it would still be morally and ethically correct to be vegetarian because of the future-life benefits and the ultimate enlightened benefits that follow. In this case it is worth sacrificing a little protein in the body, for example, for the profound benefits that follow. As Buddhists we view wrong action as a complete disregard for one's own future well-being. It's like throwing away your whole life savings in one night on a good party. Doing whatever pleases you in this life, with no regard for your real well-being, is actually disregarding your greater future.

There is a general belief that you won't get enough protein in your diet if you don't eat meat. As I understand it, in the late 1800s doctors conducted research that indicated meat eating was essential to good health. Now, some one hundred years later, scientists and doctors are proving that, in fact, a meatless diet is better for health. There are hundreds of articles based on extensive scientific research demonstrating that the vegetarian diet is not only good, but in fact superior in terms of health benefits and disease prevention. A vegetarian diet is shown to lower the fat/lipids, lower cholesterol levels, slow tumor growth, lower the incidence of cancer, and have many other benefits. In general, a vegetarian diet has fewer calories, increases longevity, is less expensive, and is ecologically sounder and better for the planet and populations of the world at large.[55]

---

55 The American Dietetic Association and the Dietitians of Canada recently published a comprehensive position paper endorsing a vegetarian diet for people of all ages that

My understanding of the scientific explanation of longevity is that it has to do with consuming fewer calories. People who eat more calories tend to age faster and also tend to have higher cholesterol, increased heart disease, and other illnesses. People who eat fewer calories age more slowly and are healthier, so they live longer. According to true dharma and the laws of karma, longevity is primarily a result of your past-life deeds. If you have respected and cherished life in your past lives, then you will enjoy longevity in this one. Even if you didn't have the virtuous deed of cherishing life in your past lives but you do in this one, and instead of taking life you save lives, and if your virtuous deeds in this life are more powerful than those of your past life, then you will have longevity due to these correct actions. A scientific explanation would be that those who eat a vegetarian diet and consume fewer calories will therefore have a longer life, less disease, and so forth. From the point of view of dharma, what is really going on here is correct karmic action. When you are engaging in actions that are all karmically correct, it clicks!

I wish to clarify one point: obviously it will not be correct karmic action if you are a vegetarian for all the wrong reasons. For example, some people look down on animals and reject meat with the unkind attitude that it is dirty and not fit to eat. I have also heard that some extreme vegetarians eat only organic food, and they will not eat anything grown with pesticides and chemical fertilizers. Instead of chemicals, their pesticides and fertilizers are made of dead insects and fish and other animal parts, and that is what they use on their food and consider natural and call "organic." That is completely wrong and not correct action at all. I've heard that some of these people actually kill the insects themselves to make their own pesticides. As a spiritual teacher I'm saddened to hear stories like that, because it's as though these people were almost in the right place and then took a 180 degree turn. I would like to think that cases like this are rare.

Even with all the scientific evidence, you may still not be convinced. You may be skeptical and still think a vegetarian diet might not be good

---

contains 256 references to support their position that such diets are healthy, complete, and beneficial in the prevention and treatment of certain diseases. The paper includes acknowledgment of the "growing appreciation" of the benefits of plant-based diets with minimal if any meat, as evidenced by recommendations by the American Institute for Cancer Research, the World Cancer Research Fund, the American Cancer Society, the American Heart Association, the Heart and Stroke Foundation of Canada, and the Unified Dietary Guidelines developed by the American Cancer Society, the American Heart Association, the National Institutes of Health, and the American Academy of Pediatrics. Such statements from traditional medical organizations were unheard of even twenty years ago.

for you. I thought about some of the things you might worry about, such as low energy, too few calories, or weight loss; you might find it inconvenient to be living among all the meat-eaters, people might ridicule you, you might develop an attitude problem (self-righteousness).[56] Aside from these problems, I don't see that eliminating animal food from your diet would actually jeopardize your longevity, your health, your relationships, or your prosperity. Of course even if you were to suffer them, these are minor concerns when the real issue is the long-term benefit of right action. From the point of view of right and wrong, there can be no question that eating a vegetarian diet is the right thing to do.

56 If you do develop any minor health problems, it's not because you're vegetarian; it may be because you are not following a healthy diet or you may have a condition completely unrelated to your diet.

Animals Are Sentient Beings

Lots of people in the world have no clue that animals really are sentient beings. Instead, many believe that animals are here for us to eat and that they were created by God for that purpose. I remember a story about Catholic missionaries in South America who were experiencing a shortage of food in an area where a particular animal called a capybara lived in the swamp. The capybara is a giant rodent that spends most of its time in the water. The missionaries asked the Vatican to declare that these animals were fish so that they would have permission to eat them. At first I thought that was strange because I knew the missionaries were not vegetarian, and I wondered why they needed to ask that this animal be declared a fish. Later on I found out that Catholics eat only fish during Lent,[57] and the permission must have been for that reason. I understood that they did get written permission from the Vatican; those rodents were declared to be fish and it was okay to eat them as fish.

Another story I remember, again from watching television, concerns an evangelist who was preaching to thousands of people. All of a sudden he said something about India being very poor, where many people were starving, yet they would not eat the cows because the cows were considered holy. He specifically said, "It's stupid for them not to eat them. If they would eat them, people wouldn't have to be so hungry." The Indian belief in the cow being holy may not be ultimately accurate, philosophically speaking; however, morally and ethically they are on the right track, whereas advocating the killing of these cows and the eating of the meat

---

57 In the Catholic tradition, Lent is a period of forty days from Ash Wednesday to Holy Saturday during which time certain restrictions apply for the purpose of purification.

definitely is not. To eat meat is one thing, but to think that it is absolutely the correct thing to do is completely another thing. That is actually putting one wrong action on top of another. I don't mean to attack and disrespect particular beliefs; however, since some of these ideas are so strongly held by so many people, perhaps mentioning them and showing another perspective will shed some light as far as reality is concerned.

Many years ago I went to the University of Southern California to learn something about the philosophical background of most Americans and Europeans. Since I am a Buddhist teacher here in the United States, I wanted to better understand the background of many of my students. One of the classes I went to was comparative religion, and it was taught by an excellent professor in the Philosophy Department. In my opinion, he exhibited all the good, decent American qualities, and I later found out that he was a lay Christian minister as well. On one occasion I talked to him privately about religion and philosophy, and during our conversation I asked what he thought about animals. I asked this question because I was interested in knowing his views as a Christian minister. To my surprise he looked at me, tapped me on the shoulder, and said, "Wangchen, I don't think animals are spirit beings." These were his exact words. I was shocked. That's when I realized that the power of dogma was enormous. Prior to this I believed that Christians who thought that animals were here for us to eat had to be those who lacked education; I really thought that intelligent and educated Christians could not believe that God put animals here for that reason. But you have people like this professor, a reasonably intelligent and highly educated man, who demonstrated very good common sense during his lectures, still ready to deny that animals are sentient beings.

It would be one thing if this were merely an incorrect belief; as long as it is harmless, it doesn't matter. It is entirely another thing to believe in something that is incorrect and also harmful. As much as I like the professor, I am afraid in this case his belief is not only wrong but is harmful as well.

Then there was another professor who told me that those who say animals don't have feelings obviously haven't looked into the eyes of a cat. What she was trying to say is that she had a cat and when she looked into the cat's eyes, she could see there was a mind inside that body. But the interesting thing is that she was ready to deny sentient-beinghood to fleas. She made comments like, "I don't think fleas are sentient beings." I think the point here is that most human opinions are based on this kind of limited judgment. Another example is the person who said to me, "It's absolutely okay to kill bulls in the bullring, because prior to that they have a very good life and receive good care." This is an example of how people jump to conclusions and, without thinking about the moral and ethical implications, are ready to make decisive statements. It is possible that this person was comparing the treatment of bulls to the treatment of other animals prior to being killed, however making such a conclusive statement is wrong.

Another important point to mention with respect to animals being sentient beings is that whenever there is a documentary story about animals, the narrator always describes their behavior in terms of human feelings and perceptions. Naturally this is because they can relate to the animals' behavior with their own feelings, and it is very obvious that the animals have all the same emotions that they have. The only thing that is different is the form. We're bipedal and most animals are quadrupedal. Humans who own pets can readily tell you that animals have feelings and that without a doubt they experience pain and suffering.

There are many people who think that the actions of animals are all based on instinct, not emotion. One story I heard about animals with human emotions is the story of a tiger in a Singapore zoo who lost her cubs after a complicated birth. The tiger became very sick and lethargic. The zookeeper seemed to be an intelligent person. He did research trying to find cubs in another zoo who had no mother. He was unable to find any, and he came up with the solution of dressing little piglets in tiger cloth and the mother tiger adopted them as her own. She also became better. This story definitely shows that animals have similar emotions of loss and grief. If you watch the animal programs on television, you can see the whole range of emotions such as greed, hate, jealousy, and so on as well.

As much as some would like to think that animals are merely food for us humans to eat, one obvious way of understanding that they are not just food but sentient beings is through an interesting tradition that takes place here in the United States. Every year just before Thanksgiving there is the tradition of the president pardoning a turkey. If the traditional Thanksgiving meal were simply sweet potatoes and corn, obviously there would be no such thing as the president pardoning a sweet potato or corn. I remember the year that President George W. Bush pardoned two turkeys rather than just one on Thanksgiving. As I understand it, every year some seventy or eighty million turkeys are slaughtered for that one day. As conscientious human beings we really have to think about these things.

Another story was told to me by one of my students, a wonderful person and a Gnostic priest. Once we were discussing something about animals and how the hyena is a very strange-looking and ferocious beast. My student said he read somewhere that a spiritual mentor of Prince Charles, a highly educated man whose name I don't recall, was in Africa and he described the appearance of a hyena as one who looked like a being condemned by God. I thought, That says it all as far as an animal being sentient is concerned.

There is a Tibetan story as well that concerns a butcher who killed many sheep. One day one of his sheep buried his butcher knife and lay on top of it. When the butcher came back to kill more sheep, he could not find his knife. He looked all around and finally he kicked the sheep who was lying on the ground and he found the knife. Then he realized how much they understood and suffered, and after that he couldn't kill any more.

KARMIC HABITS

Other fascinating stories describe humans and animals behaving exactly the same with regard to their past-life karmic habits. A woman who adopted a boy from North Africa was on the Oprah Winfrey show a few years ago. I think the country was Algeria. A war or famine was going on there, and this boy was in some kind of refugee camp. He was thirteen or fourteen years old and spoke little English. He was interviewed by a journalist and through the journalist's story the adopting mother saw him. She took one look at him and she knew that this was her son and she was determined to go and get him and bring him back. Despite many obstacles, she did. By the time that Oprah told this woman's story the boy had grown up and was graduating from college. When Oprah showed the original piece that was filmed when the boy was young, the mother, who was in the audience, was stunned and cried, "Oh, my son, my son," because he appeared in a very poor condition. Then the son came out in his graduation robe and the mother, in tears, gave him a big hug.

If you look into this whole story from the point of view of karma, it had to have come about from some kind of past-life karmic bond, an unusually powerful one. Even though the lives had changed, and they were born on two different continents, the emotions and feelings were strongly there. The moment one sees the other, they feel related. I don't think there is any other possible explanation.

A similar story is that of a lioness adopting a baby antelope. This didn't take place in a zoo. This was a wild lion filmed by a documentary filmmaker in Africa. Initially the story was on the news all over the world. The lioness and the antelope were together for many days, and they behaved just like a mother and her baby. Both of them had had no food to eat and somehow they stayed together. With each passing day, you weren't sure if the mother lioness was going to eat the little one or not. But it became obvious that no matter how hungry she was, she was not going to eat the baby antelope; this was her child. Then one day, unfortunately, a big male lion came in and killed and ate the baby antelope. The mother lioness looked on helplessly, and afterward she went over to where the killing had taken place. The narrator said she sniffed the blood and the remains as if her own child had been killed.

The human story and the animal story, in my opinion, are identical as far as the emotions and the unique and powerful karma are concerned, even when physical forms have been completely changed in their subsequent lives. This is particularly true with the animals, because ordinarily the lioness would kill the baby antelope.

According to Lord Buddha, all sentient beings are our own mothers and fathers. If you are a Buddhist and you believe in karma and the theory of reincarnation, you must believe in mother sentient beings. This understanding is essential for the development of compassion and devotion to others, and the development of such genuine qualities is the only way one can grow spiritually and achieve enlightenment and understand the truth. One very great Tibetan teacher wrote to encourage every Tibetan to be vegetarian, and he asked them not to cause animals pain and suffering. He said that those animals which are born in the land of Tibet are all our ancestors, they're karmically drawn to us; they couldn't get out of samsara and were born here in Tibet with us. He begged everybody not to treat them badly and then kill them. I believe him when he says they are our ancestors. Maybe all the animals are not the direct ancestors of Tibetans, with their limited history, but the majority of them are karmically tied to that part of the world. And they are certainly all our mothers and fathers. For some of them it's just a matter of how long ago. This is true because we have been living forever, from time without beginning. Therefore we have been living for more than long enough to have circled through all these numerous lives. Our problem is that we humans are so limited in our understanding that we are unable to look beyond this present life to the past or future. Lord Buddha said that sentient beings have been our mother and father not just once or twice, but countless numbers of times.

ANIMAL CRUELTY

There is an abundance of literature documenting animal cruelty for the purpose of human consumption. I wish I could include many of the things that I've been reading about animal cruelty in slaughter houses. They are too painful to read and therefore, at this point, I will only include the following example regarding the treatment of chickens. However, if you wish, one source for information is the Vegetarian Society, the oldest vegetarian organization in England, accessible at http://www.vegsoc.org. Of course, among all forms of cruelty, the worst is animal sacrifice, which still goes on in some areas of the world.

Battery Cages

Approximately three hundred million chickens kept for egg production in the U.S. are confined in "battery cages," where four hens are typically crowded into a wire cage measuring just sixteen inches wide. The cages are stacked in tiers and lined up in rows in huge factory warehouses. The hens are crowded so tightly that they cannot even stretch their wings or legs, and they cannot fulfill normal behavioral patterns or social needs. Constantly rubbing against the wire cages, they suffer from severe feather loss, and their bodies are covered with bruises and abrasions.

Practically all laying hens are "debeaked" in order to reduce injuries resulting from excessive pecking, an aberrant behavior which occurs when the confined birds are bored and frustrated and driven to aggression. Debeaking is a painful procedure which involves cutting through bone, cartilage, and soft tissue to remove part of the beak.

Laying more than 250 eggs per year, laying hens' bodies are severely taxed, and they commonly suffer from diseases like "fatty liver syndrome" and "cage layer fatigue." Calcium deficiency and osteoporosis are rampant among hens in egg factories—caused by intensive egg production and inadequate exercise. The birds lose an exorbitant amount of calcium as one industry journal (*Lancaster Farming*) explains: ". . . a hen will use a quantity of calcium for yearly egg production that is greater than her entire skeleton by thirtyfold or more." Inadequate calcium results in broken bones, paralysis, and even death.

After one year in egg production, the birds are classified as "spent hens," at which time they are either "force molted" or slaughtered. Force molting involves starving the hens for up to eighteen days, keeping them in the dark, and denying them water to shock their bodies into another egg laying cycle. This process causes hens to lose more than 25% of their body weight, and it is common for between 5% and 10% to die. When they are sent to slaughter, spent hens usually end up in soups, pot pies, or similar low grade chicken meat products where their bruised and battered bodies can be shredded and the blemishes hidden from consumers. Spent hens' brittle, calcium-depleted bones typically shatter during handling and/or at the slaughterhouse.[58]

There is no nice way to put it; the bottom line is that meat eating is obviously bad karma no matter how you look at it. It is wrong, it is being careless, it is abusing our power, it is selfish, and it is evil; it makes us like monsters. Slavery in the past is a perfect example of how we humans are capable of abusing power. In those days I'm sure those who were abusing their power justified their behavior. Today nay-sayers of animals being sentient are behaving in the same pattern as those in the past who justified slavery, nothing more than that: no science, no intelligence, no logical reasoning, no common sense. The bottom line is that there is nothing to support this kind of behavior.

A very important point to keep in mind is that most of us humans draw conclusions with respect to everything, including the status of animals, based on what we like to believe. For instance, people will say, "Well I believe in this, and I don't believe in that," regardless of whether something is objectively true or not. Academically speaking, if you are not being objective, it is not considered valid reasoning.

For those who are still not convinced that animals are sentient beings like us, perhaps looking honestly at monkeys and chimpanzees might provide a clue that, as far as fundamental nature is concerned, their existence as beings is the same as ours. My understanding is that chimps have a great deal in common with us such as their DNA, which is over 90% identical to humans. As I recall, from the time the fetus of a chimpanzee first develops until seven months or so you cannot distinguish it from the fetus of a human.

With all the overwhelming evidence of the suffering of animals, if someone still refuses to accept the reality then I would say, with all due respect,

58 *www.freefarmanimals.org*

that there is something really wrong with that individual's common sense. It is a little bit insane to maintain a belief that is so far from reality.

As Buddhists, we have no problem accepting animals as sentient beings. However, practicing completely correct karmic action is another thing altogether. We must try not to be hypocritical, and we must try to practice what we understand as much as we can; first and foremost, that means giving up hurting and harming other sentient beings. Without that, there is no basis for any spiritual growth. In addition, we must practice genuine loving-kindness and compassion for all sentient beings and demonstrate our spiritual sincerity by helping to alleviate the pain and suffering of others as much as we can. This means becoming vegetarian, if possible, and also saving the lives of other animals. Saving lives means buying fish and birds and cattle and chickens and whatever animals would otherwise be put to death for food and releasing them along with saying the mantra OM MANI PEME HUNG, which will plant an enlightened seed as well as give them an opportunity to live. By the way, saying the mantra to all sentient beings, including tiny little ants and other insects, whenever you can is also very beneficial.

Giving life to others is not only a correct action, but such action will result in receiving longevity. Ananda once saw a king in hell undergoing enormous suffering. He asked Lord Buddha for the reason, and Buddha said that it was mainly a karma of eating freshly killed meat all the time. Then Ananda asked Dharmaraja, the Lord of Hell, what could be done to get him out. Dharmaraja said, "There is nothing you can do here. In the human realm, if you give life to others on his behalf, that will make it possible for him to come out of that hell." Ananda did that and the king was able to get out of hell. It has been said that if someone who had only three days to live were to release thirteen animals who are otherwise going to be slaughtered, it would prolong the life of that person for three years. Giving life to thirteen animals equals a virtuous deed that purifies the sinful deeds of ten thousand eons. It has also been said that killing one of those released animals would be equal to killing one hundred times.

According to the karmic laws of nature, giving is receiving, and giving life is receiving life. Who doesn't want longevity? I'm sure everybody would agree that life is more important than fame, fortune, more important than any material possession. Protecting life is obviously one of the greatest virtuous actions, therefore people should make an effort to save lives. In tantric doctrine, within the Five Buddha Family samaya, protecting life is part of the Ratna Family samaya. Nobody needs to doubt or question the correctness of engaging in the action of saving lives. I can give you an example of how anyone and everyone can understand this. When we were doing a fish release a few years ago at Fisherman's Village in Los Angeles, the assistant to the owner of the bait company, a young African-American, was helping us release fish into the water. While doing so, he was talking to himself and saying, "Why doesn't everybody do it?" I distinctly remember that he was very serious. And I thought at the time that he must have had the experience of other human beings not even respecting human life.

Protecting life is naturally engaging in respecting animal rights, human rights, protecting the environment, and so on. If everyone were to respect all lives and were to protect them, there would be no famine, no outbreak of animal plague and bird flu; there would be peace, health, longevity, prosperity, and happiness in the world. These days vegetarianism is gaining in popularity and I'm happy for that. I personally think it is a sign of some kind of positive trend in the world for greater peace, happiness, and spiritual understanding.

I wish that those who cannot give up eating meat and killing animals would consider minimizing the pain and suffering of the animals by any means possible. My own thought is to legislate the manner in which the killing is allowed to take place. Perhaps the method of killing should be putting them to sleep with tranquilizers or anesthetics.

There is a karma for eating meat and it is obviously an unfortunate one. It varies depending on the amount of meat you eat, the number of sentient beings you eat, and how closely you are involved in the killing of the animal. The larger the amount or the greater the number of beings or the closer you are to the killing, the more severe the karmic consequences. Since this is the situation, I encourage everyone to become vegetarian. If you can't become completely vegetarian, at least eat as little meat as possible and as few sentient beings as possible, and avoid eating all small creatures like shrimp and so forth. When eating, one must at the very least say the prayer and mantra OM MANI PEME HUNG for the animals.

One thing to remember is that we human beings really do have a choice. We can choose to eat anything except meat and still have plenty of choices, whereas if we are born as animals, particularly meat-eating animals, then we have no choices. The only choice we would have would be to kill in order to survive. This is really something to think about. At this point we are at a juncture where we can make conscious decisions that will affect our futures.

LUNAR FEAST

It has always been my wish to tell others about the pain and suffering we inflict on animals for our own minute pleasure; however, I was reluctant to do it because I was not a pure vegetarian myself. Although I was a vegetarian as a child, as an adult I was a vegetarian on and off. With the death of my mother I decided to become a complete vegetarian in the name of my kind and compassionate mother and all mother sentient beings. It has given me tremendous joy and happiness to be able to make such a commitment. Now that I am a pure vegetarian I feel privileged to be able to write something about vegetarianism. I hope and wish from the bottom of my heart that those who wish to follow a pure spiritual path will embrace a vegetarian diet. It is my dream to promote vegetarianism with the slogan of "Lunar Feast." Lots of Buddhists eat vegetarian meals on the full moon day and that's where my idea comes from. I am hoping at the very least that all Buddhists will eat vegetarian meals on the full moon, half moon, and new moon days, if they can't give up meat eating altogether.

Those who think that it's very difficult to give up the habit of eating meat should remember what Shantideva said: "With practice, there is nothing that does not grow easier."

CONCLUSION

It is clear that the practice of kriya tantra pure action, the vegetarian diet and fasting with enlightened motivation and intention, will bring endless benefit to all of us. There are those who would like to think and say that Nyungne is a lower tantra practice, and that they are only interested in the highest teaching and practice. To them I say that you cannot make such a statement without being one of those with the highest faculties. In fact, those who really belong to this category would never make such a statement and would take a great deal of joy in seeing others do practices such as Nyungne. Nyungne may not be a highest yoga tantra practice, but one may not have the mental stability to practice a highest tantra either, in which case there is no benefit. With Nyungne you take the vow, observe the precepts, engage in the practice, and there is immediate benefit.

By the blessings of my enlightened guru, it is my wish and prayer that many people will cherish this practice of Nyungne. It is also my hope and dream that some day every Buddhist on planet Earth will, at a minimum, observe the eight precepts on each full moon day and eat vegetarian meals on all full and new moon days. Then, during the auspicious fourth month of the lunar calendar, which is the month of Buddha's birth, enlightenment, and parinirvana, all combined, I hope and pray that all Buddhists will observe the eight precepts and eat a vegetarian meal as well, at least from the first to the fifteenth day, which is from the new moon to the full moon day. May this precious spiritual practice bring happy omens to all beings forever.

Questions and Answers 16

1. *Question*: How does shamatha practice fit in with Nyungne?
   Rinpoche: The idea of shamatha meditation is concentration. Whether you are doing Nyungne or any other practice doesn't matter, as long as you can focus one-pointedly on the practice or on the visualization or on the recitation, whatever; if you can focus your mind without distraction, there you have shamatha meditation.

2. *Question*: Are you saying that tranquility would arise automatically once we have established concentration?
   Rinpoche: Yes, because one-pointed mind is free from neurotic distractions and it is tranquil.

3. *Question*: How does one then cultivate insight or awareness to learn about the nature of one's mind during this practice?
   Rinpoche: During deity visualization, in addition to being able to visualize the deity clearly, knowing that the form is appearing yet empty in its nature is insight meditation. The completion aspect of meditation, which is dissolving everything into emptiness at the end of the practice, is insight meditation as well.

4. *Question*: How does one deal with the realm of extreme experiences (feelings, impulses, ideas) that arise during the Nyungne retreat?
   Rinpoche: One must try to practice according to this tradition, and that is to transform all emotions into Chenrezig's body, speech, and mind. In general, one's state of mind can only function one moment at a time, meaning at the very moment you are experiencing an emotion, at that moment you are unable to experience anything else. The key is

to be mindful of your emotions and to remember to focus your mind on the deity's body, speech, and mind. The moment you can think of that, all other emotions will subside. Basically that is how our mind works. Then there are other forms of remedies, for example practicing compassion if anger is the problem.

For a good meditator there is a much more direct way of dealing with these thoughts and emotions, and that is to see where all those thoughts and emotions come from by looking directly into the nature of mind. By doing so, one will find that they have no real existence.

5. *Question*: Do we cultivate equanimity from learning how to work with these experiences?

Rinpoche: Cultivating equanimity is not the first solution. According to tantra, and Nyungne is a tantric practice, as I already said you have to transform everything into the deity body. The moment you think of the deity body, the emotions are automatically transformed into pure body, speech, and mind. Even on a general level, what you have to cultivate is the remedy for whatever the discursive thought is. Equanimity is only the last resort; if you can't transform, if you can't generate the remedy, then at least practice equanimity.

6. *Question*: What is the benefit of fasting during the Nyungne practice?

Rinpoche: A combination of the vow of fasting with deity visualization, prayer, mantra recitation, etc. has enormous benefit according to Nyungne teaching. Unlike ordinary fasting, Nyungne fasting is done with true enlightened motivation, and therefore the power of pure spiritual intention and action creates correct causes and conditions, which in turn will lead to correct results; that is, purification of negativity and accumulation of merit. The results will be temporary and ultimate benefits. Temporarily the benefits will be freedom from sickness, longevity, and a range of other benefits; ultimately there would be complete freedom from samsara and enlightenment.

7. *Question*: In most spiritual practices, silence is observed to enhance one's internal and external experiences. How would you describe its function in the Nyungne practice?

Rinpoche: The silence is for the purpose of enhancing one's internal and external experiences, and it is a way of minimizing unvirtuous deeds of speech as well as maximizing the power of speech. For example, when one is silent there is natural restraint from negativities of speech. Most of us don't even know how much negativity comes out of our speech. Speech, which is the by-product of our unenlightened mind, generates only expressions of the three poisons. Ordinarily there is no pure speech unless you are reciting prayers and mantras. In addition to that, when one is silent, prayers and mantra recitations have more power, because they are not interrupted by ordinary speech.

8. **Question**: How does the guru interact with the disciple during practice, during silence; what is the nature of the interaction?

Rinpoche: Actually, I think the correct question should be, how does the disciple interact with the guru? Anyway, during Nyungne practice or during any other practice, the guru kindly and compassionately provides teaching and gives guidance and leads others, and the guru sets an example. The disciple's job is to be devoted, follow the instruction, and practice sincerely and diligently, whether being silent or not. If the question is how to interact with the guru when you're observing silence, if you have something important to ask, then you can do it through writing.

9. **Question**: Claim: One has buddha nature, engages in practice in a cave for many years, and can have transformation; in spite of the claim that Nyungne practice is a lower tantra (action meditation), is transformation and ultimately enlightenment possible through the Nyungne practice?

Rinpoche: Nyungne is one of the true spiritual practices and therefore, if one's ambition is to become a buddha in this very lifetime, the practice of Nyungne meditation will definitely deliver the result. The perfect example is the history of the lineage holders of the Nyungne practice.

10. **Question**: How does one cultivate love and compassion for others through the Nyungne practice?

Rinpoche: Generally, the defining characteristics of spiritual development are devotion to the enlightened ones and compassion for those who are unenlightened. Devotion and compassion are principally the same thing. They are two sides of the same coin. Meditating on Lord Chenrezig, who is the embodiment of loving-kindness and compassion, and reciting the mantra OM MANI PEME HUNG are the ways to cultivate love and compassion for others through Nyungne practice.

11. *Question:* Why do we say prayers and mantras out loud during the silent day?

   Rinpoche: Actually, according to the real tradition, practitioners should be completely silent; meditation and recitation of prayers and mantras all should be done mentally. However, since ordinary practitioners are incapable of doing this properly and end up wasting time, it is better for them to recite prayers and mantras out loud. But, it has been said that you should recite them with a soft voice on the silent day.

12. *Question:* If a Nyungne practice presents difficulties physically and mentally, what would be the correct attitude to have?

   Rinpoche: Just think about those who are willing to work so hard in this world for minute benefits. I know a guy who works many hours and three different jobs just for monetary reward and not even a very big reward at that. Then there are those who are willing to make huge physical sacrifices for potential fame and fortune, like the Olympic athletes. The correct attitude during our Nyungne practice should be nothing but gratitude for the opportunity to do this precious practice which has so much benefit. Even just one set of Nyungne practice closes the door forever to the lower realms. Eight sets of Nyungne is the ticket to Dewachen, Amitabha Buddha's pure land of Great Bliss.

13. *Question:* What if you cannot visualize the deity very well?

   Rinpoche: Even if you have difficulty in visualizing the deity, you must continually try your best and not give up. Despite your best effort, if you are unable to visualize the complex body of Thousand-Armed Chenrezig, you can visualize Four-Armed or Two-Armed Chenrezig. If you still have difficulty, you can simply think that you are Chenrezig and recite the mantra, concentrating on the sound. At the very least, if you recite the prayers and mantras very sincerely and observe the vows, you will still receive all the benefits of the practice.

Section Six

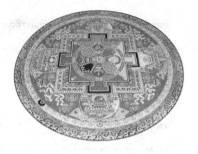

༄༅། །ཐུབ་པའི་དབང་པོ་ལ་མཛད་པ་བཅུ་གཉིས་ཀྱི་སྒོ་ནས་བསྟོད་པ་བཞུགས་སོ།།

Praises to the Buddha, The Twelve Deeds

༄༅། །ཐབས་མཁས་ཐུགས་རྗེ་ཤཱཀྱའི་རིགས་སུ་འཁྲུངས།   །གཞན་གྱིས་མི་ཐུབ་བདུད་ཀྱི་དཔུང་འཇོམས་པ།

T'AB K'E T'UK JE SHA KYEI RIK SU TR'UNG   SH'EN GYI MI T'UB DUE KYI PUNG JOM PA

།གསེར་གྱི་ལྷུན་པོ་ལྟ་བུར་བརྗིད་པའི་སྐུ།   །ཤཱཀྱའི་རྒྱལ་པོའི་ཞབས་ལ་ཕྱག་འཚལ་ལོ།   །གང་གིས་དང་པོ་བྱང་ཆུབ་

SER GYI LHUN PO TA BUR JIE PEI KU   SHA KYEI GYAL POI SH'AB LA CH'AG TS'AL LO   GANG GI DANG PO JANG CH'UB

ཐུགས་བསྐྱེད་ནས།   །བསོད་ནམས་ཡེ་ཤེས་ཚོགས་གཉིས་རྫོགས་མཛད་ཅིང་།   །དུས་འདིར་མཛད་པ་རྒྱ་ཆེན་འགྲོ་བ་ཡི།

T'UK KYE NE   SOE NAM YE SHE TS'OK NYI DZOK DZE CHING   DU DIR DZE PA GYA CH'EN DRO WA YI

།མགོན་གྱུར་ཁྱོད་ལ་བདག་གིས་བསྟོད་པར་བགྱི།   །ལྷ་རྣམས་དོན་མཛད་འདུལ་བའི་དུས་མཁྱེན་ནས།   །ལྷ་ལས་བབས་

GON GYUR K'OE LA DAG GI TOE PAR GYI   LHA NAM DON DZE DUL WEI DU K'YEN NE   LHA LE BAB

ནས་གླང་ཆེན་ལྟར་གཤེགས་ཤིང་།   །རིགས་ལ་གཟིགས་ནས་ལྷ་མོ་སྒྱུ་འཕྲུལ་གྱི།   །ལྷུམས་སུ་ཞུགས་པར་མཛད་ལ།

NE LANG CH'EN TAR SHEK SHING   RIK LA ZIK NE LHA MO GYU TR'UL GYI   LHUM SU SH'UK PAR DZE LA

ཕྱག་འཚལ་ལོ།   །ཟླ་བ་བཅུ་རྫོགས་ཤཱཀྱའི་སྲས་པོ་ནི།   །བཀྲ་ཤིས་ལུམྦིནིའི་ཚལ་དུ་བལྟམས་པའི་ཚེ།   །ཚངས་དང་

CH'AG TS'AL LO   DA WA CHU DZOK SHA KYEI SE PO NI   TRA SHI LUM BI NI TS'AL DU TAM PEI TS'E   TS'ANG DANG

བརྒྱ་བྱིན་གྱིས་བསྟོད་མཚན་མཆོག་ནི།   །བྱང་ཆུབ་རིགས་སུ་ངེས་མཛད་ཕྱག་འཚལ་ལོ།   །གཞོན་ནུ་སྟོབས་ལྡན་མི་ཡི།

GYA JIN GYI TOE TS'EN CH'OG NI   JANG CH'UB RIK SU NGE DZE CH'AG TS'AL LO   SH'ON NU TOB DEN MI YI

སེངྒེ་དེ།   །ཨང་ག་མ་ག་དྷར་ནི་སྒྱུ་རྩལ་བསྟན།   །སྐྱེ་བོ་དྲེགས་པ་ཅན་རྣམས་ཚར་བཅད་ནས།   །འགྲན་ཟླ་མེད་

SENG GE DE   ANG GA MA GA DHAR NI GYU TSAL TEN   KYE WO DREK PA CHEN NAM CH'AR CHEN NE   DREN DA ME

པར་མཛད་ལ་ཕྱག་འཚལ་ལོ།   །འཇིག་རྟེན་ཆོས་དང་མཐུན་པར་བྱ་བ་དང་།   །ཁ་ན་མ་ཐོ་སྤང་ཕྱིར་བཙུན་མོ་ཡི།

PAR DZE LA CH'AG TS'AL LO   JIG TEN CH'O DANG T'UN PAR JA WA DANG   K'A NA MA T'O PANG CH'IR TSUN MO YI

།འཁོར་དང་ལྡན་མཛད་ཐབས་ལ་མཁས་པ་ཡིས།   །རྒྱལ་སྲིད་སྐྱོང་བར་མཛད་ལ་ཕྱག་འཚལ་ལོ།   །འཁོར་བའི་བྱ་བ

K'OR DANG DEN DZE T'AB LA K'E PA YI   GYAL SIE KYONG WAR DZE LA CH'AG TS'AL LO   K'OR WEI JA WA

སྙིང་པོ་མེད་གཟིགས་ནས།   །ཁྱིམ་ནས་བྱུང་སྟེ་མཁའ་ལ་གཤེགས་ནས་ཀྱང་།   །མཆོད་རྟེན་རྣམ་དག་དྲུང་དུ་ཉིད

NYING PO ME JIK NE   K'YIM NE JUNG TE K'A LA SHEK NE KYANG   CH'OE TEN NAM DAG DRUNG DU NYIE

ལ་ཉིད།   །རབ་ཏུ་བྱུང་བར་མཛད་ལ་ཕྱག་འཚལ་ལོ།

LA NYIE   RAB TU JUNG WAR DZE LA CH'AG TS'AL LO

Praises to the Buddha, The Twelve Deeds

He who is skillful, compassionate, born in the lineage of the Shakyas,
Undefeatable by others, destroyer of maras,
And whose body is majestic like golden Mt. Sumeru:
King of the Shakyas, at his feet I prostrate.
He who first developed the mind of enlightenment,
Then perfected the dual accumulations of merit and wisdom,
And in this age performed vast enlightened deeds
And became the protector of beings: to him I offer praise.
Having fulfilled the needs of gods and having known the time
To tame (the human realm), he descended from the god realm,
Came in the form of an elephant, and seeing the lineage of Shakyas,
Entered the womb of Mayadevi: to him I prostrate.
At the completion of ten months, the son of the Shakyas
Was born in the auspicious garden of Lumbini.
At that time, Brahma and Indra praised him and his excellent signs,
Ascertained him to be in the lineage of enlightenment: to him I prostrate.
The powerful youth, the lion of men,
Exhibiting athletic skills at Anga and Magadhar,
Defeated the arrogant competitors
And became unchallengeable: to him I prostrate.
In accordance with the worldly customs and to avoid calumny,
He was accompanied by the retinue of queens.
With skillful means he served the kingdom:
To him I prostrate.
By seeing that mundane activities have no essence,
He left home and, traveling through the sky near Namdag Stupa,
He took the ordination of renunciation from himself:
To him I prostrate.

།བཙོན་པས་བྱང་ཆུབ་བསྒྲུབ་པར་དགོངས་ནས་ནི། ཞེ་རནྱའི་འགྲམ་དུ་ལོ་དྲུག་ཏུ། །དཀའ་བ་སྤྱད་

TSON PE JANG CH'UB DRUB PAR GONG NE NI   NE RANYA DZA NEI DRAM DU LO DRUG TU   KA WA CHE

མཛད་བརྩོན་འགྲུས་མཐར་ཕྱིན་པས། །བསམ་གཏན་མཆོག་བརྙེས་མཛད་ལ་ཕྱག་འཚལ་ལོ། །ཐོག་མ་མེད་ནས་

DZE TSON DRU T'AR CH'IN PE   SAM TEN CH'OG NYE DZE LA CH'AG TS'AL LO   T'OG MA ME NE

འབད་པ་དོན་ཡོད་ཕྱིར། །མ་ག་དྷ་ཡི་བྱང་ཆུབ་ཤིང་དྲུང་དུ། །དཀྱིལ་ཀྲུང་མི་གཡོ་མངོན་པར་སངས་རྒྱས་ནས།

BE PA DON YOE CH'IR   MA GA DHA YI JANG CH'UB SHING DRUNG DU   KYIL TRUNG MI YO NGON PAR SANG GYE NE

།བྱང་ཆུབ་རྫོགས་པར་མཛད་ལ་ཕྱག་འཚལ་ལོ། །ཐུགས་རྗེས་འགྲོ་ལ་མྱུར་དུ་གཟིགས་ནས་ནི། །ཝཱ་ར་ཎཱ་སཱི་ལ་སོགས།

JANG CH'UB DZOK PAR DZE LA CH'AG TS'AL LO   T'UK JE DRO LA NYUR DU ZIK NE NI   WA RA NA SI LA SOK

གནས་མཆོག་ཏུ། །ཆོས་ཀྱི་འཁོར་ལོ་བསྐོར་ནས་གདུལ་བྱ་རྣམས། །ཐེག་པ་གསུམ་ལ་འགོད་མཛད་ཕྱག་འཚལ་ལོ།

NE CH'OG TU   CH'O KYI K'OR LO KOR NE DUL JA NAM   T'EG PA SUM LA GOE DZE CH'AG TS'AL LO

།གཞན་གྱི་རྒོལ་བ་ངན་པ་ཚར་གཅད་ཕྱིར། །མུ་སྟེགས་སྟོན་པ་དྲུག་དང་ལྷས་བྱིན་སོགས། །འཁོར་མོ་འཇིག་གི

SH'EN GYI GOL WA NGEN PA TS'AR CHE CH'IR   MU TEK TON PA DRUG DANG LHE JIN SOK   K'OR MO JIG GI

ཡུལ་དུ་བདུད་རྣམས་བཏུལ། །ཐུབ་པ་གཡུལ་ལས་རྒྱལ་ལ་ཕྱག་འཚལ་ལོ། །སྲིད་པ་གསུམ་ན་དཔེའི་མེད་ཡོན་ཏན་གྱིས།

YUL DU DUE NAM TUL   T'UB PA YUL LE GYAL LA CH'AG TS'AL LO   SIE PA SUM NA PE ME YON TEN GYI

།གཉན་དུ་ཡོད་པར་ཆོ་འཕྲུལ་ཆེན་པོ་བསྟན། །ལྷ་མི་འགྲོ་བ་ཀུན་གྱིས་རབ་མཆོད་པ། །བསྟན་པ་རྒྱས་པར་མཛད་ལ་

NYEN DU YOE PAR CH'O TR'UL CH'EN PO TEN   LHA MI DRO WA KUN GYI RAB CH'OE PA   TEN PA GYE PAR DZE LA

ཕྱག་འཚལ་ལོ། །ལེ་ལོ་ཅན་རྣམས་མྱུར་དུ་བསྐུལ་བའི་ཕྱིར། །རྩ་མཆོག་གྲོང་གི་ས་གཞི་གཙང་མ་རུ

CH'AG TS'AL LO   LE LO CHEN NAM NYUR DU KUL JEI CH'IR   TSA CH'OG DRONG GI SA SH'I TSANG MA RU

།འཆི་མེད་རྡོ་རྗེ་ལྟ་བུའི་སྐུ་གཤེགས་ནས། །མྱ་ངན་འདའ་བར་མཛད་ལ་ཕྱག་འཚལ་ལོ། །ཡང་དག་ཉིད་དུ་འཇིགས

CH'I ME DOR JE TA BUI KU SHEK NE   NYA NGEN DA WAR DZE LA CH'AG TS'AL LO   YANG DAG NYIE DU JIK

པ་མེད་ཕྱིར་དང་། །མ་འོང་སེམས་ཅན་བསོད་ནམས་ཐོབ་བྱའི་ཕྱིར། །དེ་ཉིད་དུ་ནི་རིང་སེལ་མང་སྤྲུལ་ནས།

PA ME CH'IR DANG   MA ONG SEM CHEN SOE NAM T'OB JEI CH'IR   DE NYIE DU NI RING SEL MANG TRUL NE

།སྐུ་གདུང་ཆ་བརྒྱད་མཛད་ལ་ཕྱག་འཚལ་ལོ། །གང་ཚེ་རྐང་གཉིས་གཙོ་བོ་ཁྱོད་བལྟམས་ཚེ། །ས་ཆེན་འདི་ལ་གོམ

KU DUNG CH'A GYE DZE LA CH'AG TS'AL LO   GANG TS'E KANG NYI TSO WO K'YOE TAM TS'E   SA CH'EN DI LA GOM

པ་བདུན་བོར་ནས། །ང་ནི་འཇིག་རྟེན་འདི་ན་མཆོག་ཅེས་གསུངས། །དེ་ཚེ་མཁས་པ་ཁྱོད་ལ་ཕྱག་འཚལ་ལོ།

PA DUN BOR NE   NGA NI JIG TEN DI NA CH'OG CHE SUNG   DE TS'E K'E PA K'YOE LA CH'AG TS'AL LO

Intending to attain enlightenment by efforts,

At the bank of Neranjana for six years he practiced asceticism.

By perfecting perseverance, he attained supreme absorption:

To him I prostrate.

In order to perfect his efforts since beginningless time,

At the foot of the bodhi tree in Magadha

With unmoving cross-legged posture, by attaining the fully enlightened state,

He perfected his enlightenment: to him I prostrate.

Swiftly watching the beings with compassion

In the supreme places such as Varanasi,

By turning the wheel of dharma

He led beings into the three yanas: to him I prostrate.

In order to defeat the others' evil opposition he tamed the six heretical teachers,

Devadatta, and Mara in the country of Khormojig.

To the sage who conquered war I prostrate.

With virtues unequalled in the three worlds he exhibited miracles in Sarasvati,

And was worshipped by all the gods and human beings.

He caused the doctrine to develop: to him I prostrate.

In order to inspire lazy people to practice dharma,

In the clean land of Kushinagar,

His vajralike immortal body passed away and attained nirvana:

To him I prostrate.

Since perfection is indestructible,

And as the object for future beings to accumulate merit,

He manifested his remains with many ringsels

And left them as eight types of reliquaries: to him I prostrate.

When he, the chief of men, was born

He took seven steps on this great earth and proclaimed,

"I am supreme among beings in this world."

To him, the great wise one of that time, I prostrate.

|དང་པོ་དག་ལྡན་ལྷ་ཡི་ཡུལ་ནས་བྱོན། །རྒྱལ་པོའི་ཁབ་ཏུ་ཡུམ་གྱི་ལྷུམས་སུ་ཞུགས། །ལུམྦི་ནི་ཡི་ཚལ་

DANG PO DAG DEN LHA YI YUL NE JON   GYAL POI K'AB TU YUM GYI LHUM SU SH'UK   LUM BI NI YI TS'AL

དུ་ཐུབ་པ་བལྟམས། །བཅོམ་ལྡན་ལྷ་ཡི་ལྷ་ལ་ཕྱག་འཚལ་ལོ། །ཞལ་ཡེ་ཁང་དུ་མ་མ་བརྒྱད་ཀྱིས་མཆོད།

DU T'UB PA TAM   CHOM DEN LHA YI LHA LA CH'AG TS'AL LO   SH'AL YE K'ANG DU MA MA GYE KYI CH'OE

|ཤ་ཀྱའི་དྲུང་དུ་གཞོན་ནུ་རོལ་རྩེད་མཛད། །སེར་སྐྱེའི་གནས་སུ་ས་འཚོ་ཁབ་ཏུ་བཞེས། །སྲིད་གསུམ་

SHA KYAI DRUNG DU SH'ON NU ROL TSE DZE   SER KYEI NE SU SA TS'O K'AB TU SH'E   SIE SUM

མཚུངས་མེད་སྐུ་ལ་ཕྱག་འཚལ་ལོ། །གྲོང་ཁྱེར་སྒོ་བཞིར་སྐྱོ་བའི་ཚུལ་བསྟན་ནས། །མཆོད་རྟེན་རྣམ་དག

TS'UNG ME KU LA CH'AG TS'AL LO   DRONG K'YER GO SH'IR KYO WEI TS'UL TEN NE   CH'OE TEN NAM DAG

དྲུང་དུ་དབུ་སྐྲ་བསིལ། །ནེ་རཉྫ་ནའི་འགྲམ་དུ་དཀའ་ཐུབ་མཛད། །སྒྲིབ་གཉིས་སྐྱོན་དང་བྲལ་ལ་ཕྱག

DRUNG DU U TRA SIL   NE RYAN DZA NEI DRAM DU DAK T'UB DZE   DRIB NYI KYON DANG DRAL LA CH'AG

འཚལ་ལོ། །རྒྱལ་པོའི་ཁབ་ཏུ་གླང་ཆེན་སྨྱོན་པ་བཏུལ། །ཡངས་པ་ཅན་དུ་སྤྲེའུ་ཡིས་སྦྲང་རྩི་འབུལ།

TS'AL LO   GYAL POI K'AB TU LANG CH'EN NYON PA TUL   YANG SA PA CHEN DU TRE-U DRANG TSI BUL

|མ་ག་དྷ་རུ་ཐུབ་པ་མངོན་སངས་རྒྱས། །མཁྱེན་པའི་ཡེ་ཤེས་འབར་ལ་ཕྱག་འཚལ་ལོ། །ཝཱ་ར་ཎཱ་སིར་ཆོས་

MA GA DHA RU T'UB PA NGON SANG GYE   K'YEN PEI YE SHE BAR LA CH'AG TS'AL LO   WA RA NA SIR CH'O

ཀྱི་འཁོར་ལོ་བསྐོར། །རྗེ་དུ་ཚལ་དུ་ཆོ་འཕྲུལ་ཆེན་པོ་བསྟན། །རྩ་མཆོག་གྲོང་དུ་དགོངས་པ་མྱ་

KYI K'OR LO KOR   DZE TEI TS'AL DU CH'O TR'UL CH'EN PO TEN   TSA CH'OG DRONG DU GONG PA NYA

ངན་འདས། །ཐུགས་ནི་ནམ་མཁའ་འདྲ་ལ་ཕྱག་འཚལ་ལོ། །འདི་ལྟར་བསྟན་པའི་བདག་པོ་བཅོམ་ལྡན་གྱི

NGEN DE   T'UK NI NAM K'A DRA LA CH'AG TS'AL LO   DI TAR TEN PEI DAG PO CHOM DEN GYI

|མཛད་པའི་ཚུལ་ལ་མདོ་ཙམ་བསྟོད་པ་ཡི། །དགེ་བས་འགྲོ་བ་ཀུན་གྱི་སྤྱོད་པ་ཡང་། །བདེ་གཤེགས་ཁྱོད་ཀྱི

DZE PEI TS'UL LA DO TSAM TOE PA YI   GE WE DRO WA KUN GYI CHOE PA YANG   DE SHEK K'YOE KYI

མཛད་དང་མཚུངས་པར་ཤོག །དེ་བཞིན་གཤེགས་པ་ཁྱེད་སྐུ་ཅི་འདྲ་དང་། །འཁོར་དང་སྐུ་ཚེའི་ཚེ་དང་

DZE DANG TS'UNG PAR SHOK   DE SH'IN SHEK PA K'YE KU CHI DRA DANG   K'OR DANG KU TS'EI TS'E DANG

ཞིང་ཁམས་དང་། །ཁྱེད་ཀྱི་མཚན་མཆོག་བཟང་པོ་ཅི་འདྲ་བ། །དེ་འདྲ་ཁོ་ནར་བདག་སོགས་འགྱུར་བར

SH'ING K'AM DANG   K'YE KYI TS'EN CH'OG ZANG PO CHI DRA WA   DE DRA K'O NAR DAG SOK GYUR WAR

ཤོག །ཁྱོད་ལ་བསྟོད་ཅིང་གསོལ་བ་བཏབ་པའི་མཐུས། །བདག་སོགས་གང་དུ་གནས་པའི་ས་ཕྱོགས་སུ

SHOK   K'YOE LA TOE CHING SOL WA TAB PEI T'U   DAG SOK GANG DU NE PEI SA CH'OK SU

|ནད་དང་དབུལ་འཕོང་འཐབ་རྩོད་ཞི་བ་དང་། །ཆོས་དང་བཀྲ་ཤིས་འཕེལ་བར་མཛད་དུ་གསོལ།

NE DANG UL P'ONG T'AB TSOE SH'I WA DANG   CH'O DANG TRA SHI P'EL WAR DZE DU SOL

He who first descended from the Tushita Gods' realm,

Entered his mother's womb in the royal state,

And was born as the sage in the Lumbini garden;

The blessed one, god of the gods: to him I prostrate.

In the royal mansion, he who was worshipped by eight nurses

Demonstrated his athletic skill among the Shakya youths,

And in Kapilavastu he accepted Gopa in marriage;

The unequalled body in the three worldly existences: to him I prostrate.

He who showed sadness at the four gates of the city,

Cut off his hair at Namdag Stupa,

And practiced asceticism at the bank of Neranjana,

To him who is free from obscurations I prostrate.

In Rajgrha the sage subdued a mad elephant,

In Vaishali a monkey offered him honey,

And in Magadha he attained enlightenment,

To him who is shining with wisdom I prostrate.

At Varanasi he turned the wheel of dharma,

At the garden of Jeta he exhibited great miracles,

At Kushinagar he passed away into nirvana,

To him whose mind is like space I prostrate.

Thus by the merit of praising the deeds of you,

The Blessed One, the master of the doctrine,

May the activities of all the beings also become equal to your deeds.

May we all become very like the body of the Such Gone Buddha,

And may we have retinues, life extent, buddhafield,

And excellent signs similar to his.

By the power of praying and offering praise to you,

In the area where we are residing,

May the sickness, poverty, and wars be pacified,

And may dharma and auspiciousness increase.

།སྟོན་པ་འཛིག་རྟེན་ཁམས་སུ་བྱོན་པ་དང་།   །བསྟན་པ་ཉི་འོད་བཞིན་དུ་གསལ་བ་དང་།

TON PA JIG TEN K'AM SU JON PA DANG   TEN PA NYI OE SH'IN DU SAL WA DANG

།བསྟན་འཛིན་བུ་སློབ་དར་ཞིང་རྒྱས་པ་ཡི།   །བསྟན་པ་ཡུན་རིང་གནས་པའི་བཀྲ་ཤིས་ཤོག ། ॥

TEN DZIN BU LOB DAR SH'ING GYE PA YI   TEN PA YUN RING NE PEI TRA SHI SHOK

May there be the auspiciousness of the longevity of the doctrine

With buddhas appearing in the world,

The doctrine shining like sunlight, and the development and

Prosperity of the doctrine holders: teachers and disciples.

༄༅། །འཕགས་མཆོག་སྤྱན་རས་གཟིགས་དབང་ཕྱུག་ལ་སྙི་རག་གིས་བསྟོད་པ་རྒྱལ་དབང་མི་སྐྱོད་
ཞབས་ཀྱིས་མཛད་པ་བཞུགས་སོ།།

Heartfelt Praise to Lord Chenrezig

by Glorious Karmapa Mikyo Dorje

༄༅། །ཀྱེ་ལགས་འཕགས་པ་འཇིག་རྟེན་དབང་ཕྱུག་དགོངས། །ཐོག་མེད་དུས་ནས་ངན་སོང་གནས་སུ་བསྡད།

KYE LEK P'AK PA JIG TEN WANG CH'UG GONG T'OG ME DU NE NGEN SONG NE SU DE

།མི་དགེ་བཅུ་ལ་ངོམས་པ་མེད་པར་སྤྱད། །ཡིད་དུ་མི་འོང་འབྲས་བུ་ཁོ་ན་མྱོང་། །བརྩེ་བས་གཟིགས་ཀྱང་བདག་ལ་

MI GE CHU LA NGOM PA ME PAR CHE YI DU MI ONG DRE BU K'O NA NYONG TSI WE ZIK KYANG DAG LA

ཕྲིན་ལས་རྡུགས། །བྱམས་མགོན་བཅོས་མེད་བདག་པས་གཞན་འགའ་མང་། །ཐུགས་རྗེའི་ནུས་པ་སྟོན་ཅིག་སྤྱན་

T'RIN LE NGUK JAM GON CH'O ME DAG PE SH'EN GA MANG T'UK JEI NU PA TON CHIG CHEN

རས་གཟིགས། །ད་ལན་མི་ལུས་ཙམ་པོ་ཐོབ་དུས་འདིར། །རང་བཞིན་ལྷུན་པས་ཚེ་རབས་ཕྱི་མ་ལ། །བདེན་སྙམ་

RE ZIG DA LEN MI LU TSAM PO T'OB DU DIR RANG SH'IN LUN PE TS'E RAB CH'I MA LA DEN NYAM

མི་བགྱིད་གཏི་མུག་འཐུག་པོས་བསྒྲིབས། །ལས་འབྲས་བསླུ་བ་མེད་པའི་དོན་ཅན་ལ། །ཇི་བཞིན་བླང་དོར་མ་ཤེས་

MI GYI TI MUG T'UG PO DRIB LE DRE LU WA ME PEI DON CHEN LA JI SH'IN LANG DOR MA SHE

སྡིག་པ་འཕེལ། །གཏན་དུ་ཐར་དུས་མེད་པའི་ལས་ངན་བསགས། །སྒོ་གསུམ་སྤྱོད་པ་ལེགས་སྤྱད་རློམ་ཀུན་ཀྱང་།

DIG PA P'EL TEN DU T'AR DU ME PEI LE NGEN SAK GO SUM CHOE PA LEK CHE LOM KUN KYANG

།མུན་ནང་མདའ་ལྟར་དགྲ་གཉེན་གང་ལ་ཕོག། །ཆ་མ་འཚལ་བས་ཉེས་པར་སོང་སྲིད་པས། །འཕགས་མཆོག་བརྩེ་

MUN NANG DA TAR DRA NYEN GANG LA P'OG CHA MA TS'AL WE NYE PAR SONG SI PE PA'K CHOG TSE

བས་མི་བཟོད་དྲུང་དུ་བཤགས། །བདག་ནི་ཇི་བྱིས་པའི་རང་བཞིན་གཏོལ་མེད་པས། །ཞིང་མཆོག་གཉེན་པོ་རྣམས་ལ་སྡིག་

WE MI ZOE DRUNG DU SHAK DAG NI JI PEI RANG SH'IN TOL ME PE SH'ING CHOG NYEN PO NAM LA DIG

པའི་ལས། །གང་བསགས་འབྲས་བུ་ཇི་སྙེད་མཆིས་པ་ཀུན། །མཐོང་བའི་ཆོས་ལ་དར་དྲག་རབ་སྨིན་ནས།

PEI LE GANG SAK DRE BU JI NYE CH'I PA KUN T'ONG WEI CH'O LA DAR DRAG RAB MIN NE

།འབྲས་བུ་མྱུར་དུ་ཕྱུང་བར་བྱིན་གྱིས་རློབས། །ལྷག་པར་མཁའ་མཉམ་འགྲོ་བ་ཐམས་ཅད་ཀྱིས། །ངག་གི་སྒོ་ནས་

DRE BU NYUR DU CH'UNG WAR JIN GYI LOB LHEG PAR K'A NYAM DRO WA T'AM CHE KYI NGAG GI GO NE

ཉེས་པ་ཅི་བསགས་པའི། །འབྲས་བུ་ཐམས་ཅད་བདག་ལ་སྨིན་པར་ཤོག། །བདག་གི་ངག་ལ་མི་བཟད་སྡིག་པའི་ལས།

NYE PA CHI SAK PEI DRE BU T'AM CHE DAG LA MIN PAR SHOK DAG GI NGAG LA MI ZE DIG PEI LE

Heartfelt Praise to Lord Chenrezig
by Glorious Karmapa Mikyo Dorje

Oh, noble and exalted Chenrezig, please keep me in mind
From beginningless time until now I have dwelled in the lower realms;
Caught up in the endless entanglement of the ten unvirtuous actions,
I have experienced only the negative results.
Because of this, although you look on me with love,
It doesn't reach me.
Kind Protector, others suffer more than I do.
Chenrezig, please show the power of your compassion.
At this time, having obtained human birth,
Because of our ignorant nature, doubting the truth of future lives,
Clouded by thick obscurations, we do not practice virtue.
Not knowing the infallibility of karmic effect, as it is,
Not knowing right from wrong views,
Our negativities increase,
Trapping us in our accumulation of negative karma.
Even our positive actions are tainted with pride.
Like shooting an arrow in the dark,
Not knowing if it would hit enemy or friend,
Due to not understanding, our actions have been improper.
Great exalted one of limitless love,
In front of you I confess.
As a helpless child, I request to the great field of the remedy
That whatever results from all accumulated negative actions,
However much, you grant your blessings
So they may ripen immediately, in front of my very eyes,
And that I may abandon these actions from this moment onward.
In particular, may all the results of the accumulated negative speech
Of sentient beings as vast as the sky ripen in me.

།འབྲས་བུ་མི་བཟད་སྨྱོང་བས་ཡིད་བྱུང་སྟེ། །མ་རྒན་ངག་གི་སྡུག་བསྔལ་མི་བཟད་པ། །རང་གི་ངག་ལས་འབུམ་འགྱུར་

DRE BU MI ZE NYONG WE YIE JUNG TE MA GEN NGAG GI DUG NGAL MI ZE PA RANG GI NGAG LE BUM GYUR

གཅེས་འཛིན་པའི། །བཅོས་མིན་སེམས་ཅན་ཀུན་གྱི་སེམས་ཁྲལ་ཀུན། །བདག་གི་རྒྱུད་ལ་ལེགས་པར་འཆར་བ་ནས།

CHE DZIN PEI CHO MIN SEM CHEN KUN GYI SEM TR'AL KUN DAG GI GYUE LA LEK PAR CH'AR WA NE

།བདག་གི་ཕན་སེམས་བཟང་པོའི་བདེན་སྟོབས་ཀྱིས། །བདག་གི་ངག་གིས་མཁའ་ཁྱབ་སེམས་ཅན་གྱི། །སྒྲིབ་ཀུན་

DAG GI P'EN SEM ZANG POI DEN TOB KYI DAG GI NGAG GI K'A KY'AB SEM CHEN GYI DRIB KUN

བསལ་བའི་ཆོས་འཁོར་ཐོགས་མེད་དུ། །བསྐོར་ལ་ནུས་པ་ཐོབ་པར་ཐུགས་རྗེས་བཟུང་། །བདག་གི་ངག་ལ་ངག་གི་

SAL WEI CH'O K'OR T'OK ME DU KOR LA NU PA T'OB PAR T'UK JE ZUNG DAG GI NGAG LA NGAG GI

དབང་ཕྱུག་ཤོག། །བདག་གི་ངག་གིས་སྐལ་ལྡན་རེ་སྐོང་ཤོག། །ཅིས་ཀྱང་འཕགས་པའི་ཐུགས་རྗེའི་སྟོབས་ཀྱིས་ཤོག།

WANG CH'UG SHOK DAG GI NGAG GI KAL DEN RE KONG SHOK CHI KYANG P'AK PEI T'UK JEI TOB KYI SHOK

།དཔལ་ལྡན་བླ་མ་དམ་པའི་རྡོ་རྗེའི་གསུང་། །སྒྲིབ་བྲལ་གནས་བརྒྱད་དག་པའི་སྒྲ་དབྱངས་ཅན། །གདུལ་བྱའི་བློ་ལ་

PAL DEN LA MA DAM PEI DOR JEI SUNG DRIB DRAL NE GYE DAG PEI DRA JANG CHEN DUL JEI LO LA

གསལ་པོར་འཆར་བ་ཡིས། །སྨིན་ཅིང་གྲོལ་བའི་རོ་མཆོག་མྱོང་གྱུར་ཅིག།

SAL POR CH'AR WA YI MIN CHING DROL WEI RO CH'OG NYONG GYUR CHIG

With the thought of experiencing the unending results
Of my own countless verbal negativities,
And with the wish for all the worries of all sentient beings,
My mothers whose endless suffering from unvirtuous speech
Is one hundred thousand times more disturbing than my own,
To be taken into my own mind stream, may I,
By the power of the truth of my sincere good intentions,
Obtain the verbal power in my own speech,
Through Chenrezig's compassion,
And continuously turn the wheel of the dharma
Which removes all obscurations of sentient beings pervading space.
Through my speech, may the hopes of the fortunate ones be fulfilled.
With the vajra speech of the glorious holy guru,
Having the eight pure qualities of sound,
Emerging clearly and unobscured in the minds of those to be tamed,
May they experience the sublime taste of full ripening of liberation.

Thirty-five Buddhas Confession Prayer

༄༅། །ཕུང་པོ་གསུམ་པའི་མདོ་བཞུགས་སོ།

Sutra of Three Heaps

༄༅། །སེམས་ཅན་ཐམས་ཅད་རྟག་པར་བླ་མ་ལ་སྐྱབས་སུ་མཆིའོ།
SEM CHEN T'AM CHE TAG PAR LA MA LA KYAB SU CH'I-O

།སངས་རྒྱས་ལ་སྐྱབས་སུ་མཆིའོ།
SANG GYE LA KYAB SU CH'I-O

།ཆོས་ལ་
CH'O LA

སྐྱབས་སུ་མཆིའོ།
KYAB SU CH'I-O

།དགེ་འདུན་ལ་སྐྱབས་སུ་མཆིའོ།
GE DUN LA KYAB SU CH'I-O

།བཅོམ་ལྡན་འདས་དེ་བཞིན་གཤེགས་པ་དགྲ་བཅོམ་པ་ཡང་དག
CHOM DEN DE DE SH'IN SHEK PA DRA CHOM PA YANG DAG

པར་རྫོགས་པའི་སངས་རྒྱས་ཤཱཀྱ་ཐུབ་པ་ལ་ཕྱག་འཚལ་ལོ།
PAR DZOK PEI SANG GYE SHA KYA T'UB PA LA CH'AG TS'AL LO

།རྡོ་རྗེ་སྙིང་པོས་རབ་ཏུ་འཇོམས་པ་ལ་ཕྱག་འཚལ་ལོ།
DOR JE NYING PO RAB TU JOM PA LA CH'AG TS'AL LO

།རིན་ཆེན་འོད་འཕྲོ་ལ་ཕྱག་འཚལ་ལོ།
RIN CH'EN OE TRO LA CH'AG TS'AL LO

།ཀླུ་དབང་གི་རྒྱལ་པོ་ལ་ཕྱག་འཚལ་ལོ།
LU WANG GI GYAL PO LA CH'AG TS'AL LO

།དཔའ་བོའི་སྡེ་ལ་ཕྱག་འཚལ་ལོ།
PA WOI DE LA CH'AG TS'AL LO

།དཔའ་དགྱེས་ལ་ཕྱག་འཚལ་ལོ།
PA GYE LA CH'AG TS'AL LO

།རིན་ཆེན་མེ་ལ་ཕྱག་འཚལ་ལོ།
RIN CH'EN ME LA CH'AG TS'AL LO

།རིན་ཆེན་ཟླ་འོད་ལ་ཕྱག་འཚལ་ལོ།
RIN CH'EN DA OE LA CH'AG TS'AL LO

།མཐོང་བ
T'ONG WA

དོན་ཡོད་ལ་ཕྱག་འཚལ་ལོ།
DON YOE LA CH'AG TS'AL LO

།རིན་ཆེན་ཟླ་བ་ལ་ཕྱག་འཚལ་ལོ།
RIN CH'EN DA WA LA CH'AG TS'AL LO

།དྲི་མ་མེད་པ་ལ་ཕྱག་འཚལ་ལོ།
DRI ME PA LA CH'AG TS'AL LO

།དཔས་བྱིན་ལ་
PE JIN LA

ཕྱག་འཚལ་ལོ།
CH'AG TS'AL LO

།ཚངས་པ་ལ་ཕྱག་འཚལ་ལོ།
TS'ANG PA LA CH'AG TS'AL LO

།ཚངས་པས་བྱིན་ལ་ཕྱག་འཚལ་ལོ།
TS'ANG PE JIN LA CH'AG TS'AL LO

།ཆུ་ལྷ་ལ་ཕྱག་འཚལ་ལོ།
CH'U LHA LA CH'AG TS'AL LO

།ཆུ་ལྷའི་ལྷ་ལ་ཕྱག་འཚལ་ལོ།
CH'U LHEI LHA LA CH'AG TS'AL LO

།དཔལ་བཟང་ལ་ཕྱག་འཚལ་ལོ།
PAL ZANG LA CH'AG TS'AL LO

།ཙན་དན་དཔལ་ལ་ཕྱག་འཚལ་ལོ།
TSEN DEN PAL LA CH'AG TS'AL LO

།གཟི་བརྗིད
ZI JIE

མཐའ་ཡས་ལ་ཕྱག་འཚལ་ལོ།
T'A YE LA CH'AG TS'AL LO

།འོད་དཔལ་ལ་ཕྱག་འཚལ་ལོ།
OE PAL LA CH'AG TS'AL LO

།མྱ་ངན་མེད་པའི་དཔལ་ལ་ཕྱག་འཚལ་ལོ།
NYA NGEN ME PEI PAL LA CH'AG TS'AL LO

།སྲེད་མེད་ཀྱི་བུ་ལ་ཕྱག་འཚལ་ལོ།
SE ME KYI BU LA CH'AG TS'AL LO

།མེ་ཏོག་དཔལ་ལ་ཕྱག་འཚལ་ལོ།
ME TOG PAL LA CH'AG TS'AL LO

།དེ་བཞིན་གཤེགས་པ་ཚངས་པའི་འོད་ཟེར
DE SH'IN SHEK PA TS'ANG PEI OE ZER

རྣམ་པར་རོལ་པས་མངོན་པར་མཁྱེན་པ་ལ་ཕྱག་འཚལ་ལོ།
NAM PAR ROL PE NGON PAR K'YEN PA LA CH'AG TS'AL LO

།དེ་བཞིན་གཤེགས་པ་པདྨའི་འོད་ཟེར་རྣམ་པར་རོལ་པས
DE SH'IN SHEK PA PE MEI OE ZER NAM PAR ROL PE

མངོན་པར་མཁྱེན་པ་ལ་ཕྱག་འཚལ་ལོ།
NGON PAR K'YEN PA LA CH'AG TS'AL LO

།ནོར་དཔལ་ལ་ཕྱག་འཚལ་ལོ།
NOR PAL LA CH'AG TS'AL LO

།དྲན་པའི་དཔལ་ལ་ཕྱག་འཚལ་ལོ།
DRIN PEI PAL LA CH'AG TS'AL LO

Thirty-five Buddhas Confession Prayer

Sutra of Three Heaps[1]

Throughout all times I take refuge in the Gurus, I take refuge in the Buddhas,
I take refuge in the Dharma, I take refuge in the Sangha.
To the Founder, the Transcendent Destroyer, the One Thus Gone, the Foe Destroyer,
The Fully Enlightened One, the Glorious Conqueror from the Shakyas, I bow down.
To the One Thus Gone, the Great Destroyer, Destroying with Vajra Essence, I bow down.
To the One Thus Gone, the Jewel Radiating Light, I bow down.
To the One Thus Gone, the King with Power over the Nagas, I bow down.
To the One Thus Gone, the Leader of the Warriors, I bow down.
To the One Thus Gone, the Glorious Blissful One, I bow down.
To the One Thus Gone, the Jewel Fire, I bow down.
To the One Thus Gone, the Jewel Moonlight, I bow down.
To the One Thus Gone, Whose Pure Vision Brings Accomplishments, I bow down.
To the One Thus Gone, the Jewel Moon, I bow down.
To the One Thus Gone, the Stainless One, I bow down.
To the One Thus Gone, the Glorious Giver, I bow down.
To the One Thus Gone, the Pure One, I bow down.
To the One Thus Gone, the Bestower of Purity, I bow down.
To the One Thus Gone, the Celestial Waters, I bow down.
To the One Thus Gone, the Deity of the Celestial Waters, I bow down.
To the One Thus Gone, the Glorious Good, I bow down.
To the One Thus Gone, the Glorious Sandalwood, I bow down.
To the One Thus Gone, the One of Unlimited Splendor, I bow down.
To the One Thus Gone, the Glorious Light, I bow down.
To the One Thus Gone, the Glorious One Without Sorrow, I bow down.
To the One Thus Gone, the Son of the Desireless One, I bow down.
To the One Thus Gone, the Glorious Flower, I bow down.
To the One Thus Gone, Who Understands Reality Enjoying the Radiant Light of Purity,

1 English translation reprinted from *Pearl of Wisdom*, Book One, with permission from the editor.

།མཚན་དཔལ་ཤིན་ཏུ་ཡོངས་གྲགས་ལ་ཕྱག་འཚལ་ལོ།

TS'EN PAL SHIN TU YONG DRAK LA CH'AG TS'AL LO

།དབང་པོ་ཏོག་གི་རྒྱལ་མཚན་གྱི་རྒྱལ་པོ་ལ་ཕྱག་འཚལ་ལ ོ།

WANG PO TOG GI GYAL TS'EN GYI GYAL PO LA CH'AG TS'AL L O

།ཤིན་ཏུ་རྣམ་པར་གནོན་པའི་དཔལ་ལ་ཕྱག་འཚལ་ལོ།

SHIN TU NAM PAR NON PEI PAL LA CH'AG TS'AL LO

།ཡུལ་ལས་ཤིན་ཏུ་རྣམ་པར་རྒྱལ་བ་ལ་ཕྱག་འཚལ་ལོ།

YUL LE SHIN TU NAM PAR GYAL WA LA CH'AG TS'AL LO

།རྣམ་པར་གནོན་པ་གཤེགས་པའི་དཔལ་ལ་ཕྱག་འཚལ་ལོ།

NAM PAR NON PE SHEK PEI PAL LA CH'AG TS'AL LO

།ཀུན་ནས་སྣང་བ་བཀོད་པའི་དཔལ་ལ་ཕྱག་འཚལ་ལོ།

KUN NE NANG WA KOE PEI PAL LA CH'AG TS'AL LO

།རིན་ཆེན་པདྨ་རྣམ་པར་གནོན་པ་ལ་ཕྱག་འཚལ་ལོ།

RIN CH'EN PE ME NAM PAR NON PA LA CH'AG TS'AL LO

།དེ་བཞིན་གཤེགས་པ་དགྲ་བཅོམ་པ་ཡང་དག་པར་རྫོགས

DE SH'IN SHEK PA DRA CHOM PA YANG DAG PAR DZOK

པའི་སངས་རྒྱས་རིན་པོ་ཆེའི་པདྨ་ལ་རབ་ཏུ་བཞུགས་པ་རི་དབང་གི་རྒྱལ་པོ་ལ་ཕྱག་འཚལ་ལོ།

PEI SANG GYE RIN PO CH'EI PE MA LA RAB TU SH'UK PA RI WANG GI GYAL PO LA CH'AG TS'AL LO

།དེ་དག་ལ་སོགས

DE DAG LA SOK

པ་ཕྱོགས་བཅུའི་འཇིག་རྟེན་གྱི་ཁམས་ཐམས་ཅད་ན་དེ་བཞིན་གཤེགས་པ་དགྲ་བཅོམ་པ་ཡང་དག་པར་རྫོགས་པའི་སངས

PA CH'OK CHUI JIG TEN GYI K'AM T'AM CHE NA DE SH'IN SHEK PA DRA CHOM PA YANG DAG PAR DZOK PEI SANG

རྒྱས་བཅོམ་ལྡན་འདས་གང་ཇི་སྙེད་ཅིག་བཞུགས་ཏེ་འཚོ་ཞིང་གཞེས་པའི་སངས་རྒྱས་བཅོམ་ལྡན་འདས་དེ་དག་ཐམས་ཅད

GYE CHOM DEN DE GANG JI NYE CHIG SH'UK TE TS'O SH'ING SH'E PEI SANG GYE CHOM DEN DE DE DAG T'AM CHE

བདག་ལ་དགོངས་སུ་གསོལ། །བདག་གི་སྐྱེ་བ་འདི་དང་། །སྐྱེ་བ་ཐོག་མ་དང་། །མཐའ་མ་མ་མཆིས་པ་ནས། །འཁོར

DAG LA GONG SU SOL DAG GI KYE WA DI DANG KYE WA T'OG MA DANG T'A MA MA CH'I PA NE K'OR

བ་ན་འཁོར་བའི་སྐྱེ་གནས་ཐམས་ཅད་དུ་སྡིག་པའི་ལས་བགྱིས་པ་དང་། །བགྱིད་དུ་སྩལ་བ་དང་། །བགྱིད་པ་ལ་རྗེས་སུ

WA NA K'OR WEI KYE NE T'AM CHE DU DIG PEI LE GYI PA DANG GYI DU TSAL WA DANG GYI PA LA JE SU

ཡི་རང་བའམ། །མི་དགེ་བ་བཅུའི་ལས་ཀྱི་ལམ་ཡང་དག་པར་བླངས་པ་ལ་ཞུགས་པ་དང་། །འཇུག་ཏུ་སྩལ་བ་དང་།

YI RANG WA AM MI GE WA CHUI LE KYI LAM YANG DAG PAR LANG PA LA SH'UK PA DANG JUG TU TSAL WA DANG

།འཇུག་པ་ལ་རྗེས་སུ་ཡི་རང་བའམ། །ལས་ཀྱི་སྒྲིབ་པ་གང་གིས་བསྒྲིབས་ནས། །བདག་སེམས་ཅན་དམྱལ་བར་མཆི་བའམ།

JUG PA LA JE SU YI RANG WA AM LE KYI DRIB PA GANG GI DRIB NE DAG SEM CHEN NYAL WAR CH'I WA AM

།དུད་འགྲོའི་སྐྱེ་གནས་སུ་མཆི་བའམ། །ཡི་དགས་ཀྱི་ཡུལ་དུ་མཆི་བའམ། །ཡུལ་ཐའ་ཁོབ་ཏུ་སྐྱེ་བའམ།

DUE DROI KYE NE SU CH'I WA AM YI DOG KYI YUL DU CH'I WA AM YUL T'A K'OB TU KYE WA AM

།ཀླ་ཀློར་སྐྱེ་བའམ། །ལྷ་ཚེ་རིང་པོ་རྣམས་སུ་སྐྱེ་བའམ། །དབང་པོ་མ་ཚང་བར་འགྱུར་བའམ།

LA LOR KYE WA AM LHA TS'E RING PO NAM SU KYE WA AM WANG PO MA TS'ANG WAR GYUR WA AM

I bow down.   To the One Thus Gone, Who Understands Reality

Enjoying the Radiant Light of the Lotus, I bow down.

To the One Thus Gone, the Glorious Gem, I bow down.

To the One Thus Gone, the Glorious One Who Is Mindful, I bow down.

To the One Thus Gone, the Glorious One

Whose Name is Extremely Renowned, I bow down.

To the One Thus Gone, the King Holding the Banner

Of Victory over the Senses, I bow down.

To the One Thus Gone, the Glorious One

Who Subdues Everything Completely, I bow down.

To the One Thus Gone, the Victorious One in All Battles, I bow down.

To the One Thus Gone, the Glorious One Gone to Perfect Self-Control, I bow down.

To the One Thus Gone, the Glorious One Who

Enhances and Illuminates Completely, I bow down.

To the One Thus Gone, the Jewel Lotus Who Subdues All, I bow down.

To the One Thus Gone, the Fully Enlightened One, the King with Power

Over Mount Meru, always remaining in the Jewel and the Lotus, I bow down.

All you thirty-five buddhas, and all the others, those thus gone, foe destroyers,

Fully enlightened ones and transcendent destroyers who are existing,

Sustaining and living throughout the ten directions of sentient beings' worlds—

All you buddhas, please give me your attention.

In this life and throughout beginningless lives in all the realms of samsara,

I have created, caused others to create, and rejoiced at the creation of negative karmas

Such as misusing offerings to holy objects, misusing offerings to the Sangha,

Stealing the possessions of the Sangha of the ten directions;

I have caused others to create these negative actions and rejoiced at their creation.

I have created the five heinous actions, caused others to create them,

And rejoiced at their creation.

I have committed the ten nonvirtuous actions,

Involved others in them, and rejoiced at their involvement.

Being obscured by all this karma, I have created the cause

For myself and other sentient beings to be reborn in the hells

།ལྟ་བ་ལོག་པར་འཛིན་པར་འགྱུར་བ་འམ། །སངས་རྒྱས་འབྱུང་བ་ལ་མཉེས་པར་མི་བགྱིད་པར་འགྱུར་བའི་ལས་ཀྱི

TA WA LOG PAR DZIN PAR GYUR WA AM   SANG GYE JUNG WA LA NYE PAR MI GYI PAR GYUR WEI LE KYI

སྒྲིབ་པ་གང་ལག་པ་དེ་དག་ཐམས་ཅད་སངས་རྒྱས་བཅོམ་ལྡན་འདས་ཡེ་ཤེས་སུ་གྱུར་པ།   །སྤྱན་དུ་གྱུར་པ།

DRIB PA GANG LAG PA DE DAG T'AM CHE SANG GYE CHOM DEN DE YE SHE SU GYUR PA   CHEN DU GYUR PA

།དཔང་དུ་གྱུར་པ།   །ཚད་མར་གྱུར་པ།   །མཁྱེན་པ།   །གཟིགས་པ།   །དེ་དག་གི་སྤྱན་སྔར་མཐོལ་ལོ་འཆགས་སོ།

PANG DU GYUR PA   TS'E MAR GYUR PA   K'YEN PA   ZIK PA   DE DAG GI CHEN NGAR T'OL LO CH'AK SO

།མི་འཆབ་བོ།   །མི་སྦེད་དོ།   །ལྷན་ཆད་ཀྱང་གཅོད་ཅིང་སྡོམ་པར་བགྱིད་ལགས་སོ།   །སངས་རྒྱས་བཅོམ་ལྡན་འདས་དེ

MI CH'AB BO   MI BE DO   LEN CH'E KYANG CHOE CHING DOM PAR GYI LAK SO   SANG GYE CHOM DEN DE DE

དག་ཐམས་ཅད་བདག་ལ་དགོངས་སུ་གསོལ།   །བདག་གིས་སྐྱེ་བ་འདི་དང་།   །སྐྱེ་བ་ཐོག་མ་དང་།   །ཐ་མ

DAG T'AM CHE DAG LA GONG SU SOL   DAG GI KYE WA DI DANG   KYE WA T'OG MA DANG   T'A MA

མ་མཆིས་པ་ནས་འཁོར་བ་ན་འཁོར་བའི་སྐྱེ་བ་གཞན་དག་ཏུ་སྦྱིན་པ་ཏ་ན་དུད་འགྲོའི་སྐྱེ་གནས་སུ་སྐྱེས་པ་ལ་ཟས་ཁམ་

MA CH'I PA NE K'OR WA NA K'OR WEI KYE WA SH'EN DAG TU JIN PA T'A NA DU DROI KYE NE SU KYE PA LA ZE K'AM

གཅིག་ཙམ་བསྩལ་བའི་དགེ་བའི་རྩ་བ་གང་ལགས་པ་དང་།   །བདག་གིས་ཚུལ་ཁྲིམས་བསྲུངས་པའི་དགེ་བའི་རྩ་བ་གང

CHIG TSAM TSAL WEI GE WEI TSA WA GANG LAK PA DANG   DAG GI TS'UL TR'IM SUNG PEI GE WEI TSA WA GANG

ལགས་པ་དང་།   །བདག་གིས་ཚངས་པར་སྤྱོད་པ་ལ་གནས་པའི་དགེ་བའི་རྩ་བ་གང་ལགས་པ་དང་།   །བདག་གིས

LAK PA DANG   DAG GI TS'ANG PAR CHOE PA LA NE PEI GE WEI TSA WA GANG LAK PA DANG   DAG GI

སེམས་ཅན་ཡོངས་སུ་སྨིན་པར་བགྱིས་པའི་དགེ་བའི་རྩ་བ་གང་ལགས་པ་དང་།   །བདག་གིས་བྱང་ཆུབ་མཆོག་ཏུ་སེམས

SEM CHEN YONG SU MIN PAR GYI PEI GE WEI TSA WA GANG LAK PA DANG   DAG GI JANG CH'UB CH'OG TU SEM

བསྐྱེད་པའི་དགེ་བའི་རྩ་བ་གང་ལགས་པ་དང་།   །བདག་གི་བླ་ན་མེད་པའི་ཡེ་ཤེས་ཀྱི་དགེ་བའི་རྩ་བ་གང་ལགས་པ་དེ

KYE PEI GE WEI TSA WA GANG LAK PA DANG   DAG GI LA NA ME PEI YE SHE KYI GE WEI TSA WA GANG LAK PA DE

དག་ཐམས་ཅད་གཅིག་ཏུ་བསྡུས་ཤིང་བསྡམས་ཏེ།   །བསྒོམས་ནས་བླ་མ་མཆིས་པ་དང་།   །གོང་ན་མ་མཆིས་པ་དང་།

DAG T'AM CHE CHIG TU DU SHING DUM TE   DOM NE LA NA MA CH'I PA DANG   GONG NA MA CH'I PA DANG

།གོང་མའི་ཡང་གོང་མ།   །བླ་མའི་ཡང་བླ་མར་ཡོངས་སུ་བསྔོ་བས།   །བླ་ན་མེད་པ་ཡང་དག་པར་རྫོགས་པའི་བྱང

GONG MEI YANG GONG MA   LA MEI YANG LA MAR YONG SU NGO WE   LA NA ME PA YANG DAG PAR DZOK PEI JANG

ཆུབ་ཏུ་ཡོངས་སུ་བསྔོ་བར་བགྱིའོ།   །ཇི་ལྟར་འདས་པའི་སངས་རྒྱས་བཅོམ་ལྡན་འདས་རྣམས་ཀྱིས་ཡོངས་སུ་བསྔོས་པ་དང་།

CH'UB TU YONG SU NGO WAR GYI-O   JI TAR DE PEI SANG GYE CHOM DEN DE NAM KYI YONG SU NGO PA DANG

As animals, as hungry ghosts, in irreligious places,
Amongst barbarians, as long-lived gods, with imperfect senses,
Holding wrong views, and being displeased
With the presence of a buddha.
Now before these buddhas, transcendent destroyers
Who have become transcendental wisdom,
Who have become the compassionate eye,
Who have become witnesses,
Who have become valid and see with their omniscient minds,
I am confessing and accepting all these actions as negative.
I will not conceal or hide them, and from now on
I will refrain from committing these negative actions.
Buddhas and transcendent destroyers,
Please give me your attention:
In this life and throughout beginningless lives
In all the realms of samsara, whatever root of virtue I have created
Through even the smallest acts of charity
Such as giving one mouthful of food to a being born as an animal,
Whatever root of virtue I have created
By abiding in pure conduct,
Whatever root of virtue I have created
By fully ripening sentient beings' minds,
Whatever root of virtue I have created
Of the highest transcendent wisdom,
Bringing together all these merits of both myself and others,
I now dedicate them to the highest of which there is no higher,
To that even above the highest,
To the highest of the high,
To the higher of the high.
Thus I dedicate them completely to the highest,
Fully accomplished enlightenment.
Just as the buddhas and transcendent destroyers
Of the past have dedicated,

།ཇི་ལྟར་མ་བྱོན་པའི་སངས་རྒྱས་བཅོམ་ལྡན་འདས་རྣམས་ཀྱིས་ཡོངས་སུ་བསྔོ་བར་འགྱུར་བ་དང་། །ཇི་ལྟར་ད་ལྟར་བྱུང་
JI TAR MA JON PEI SANG GYE CHOM DEN DE NAM KYI YONG SU NGO WAR GYUR WA DANG JI TAR DA TAR JUNG

བའི་སངས་རྒྱས་བཅོམ་ལྡན་འདས་རྣམས་ཀྱིས་ཡོངས་སུ་བསྔོ་བར་མཛད་པ་དེ་བཞིན་དུ་བདག་གིས་ཀྱང་ཡོངས་སུ་བསྔོ་
WEI SANG GYE CHOM DEN DE NAM KYI YONG SU NGO WAR DZE PA DE SH'IN DU DAG GI KYANG YONG SU NGO

བར་བགྱིའོ། །སྡིག་པ་ཐམས་ཅད་ནི་སོ་སོར་གཤགས་སོ། །བསོད་ནམས་ཐམས་ཅད་ལ་རྗེས་སུ་ཡི་རང་ངོ་། །སངས་
WAR GYI-O DIG PA T'AM CHE NI SO SOR SHAK SO SOE NAM T'AM CHE LA JE SU YI RANG NGO SANG

རྒྱས་ཐམས་ཅད་ལ་བསྐུལ་ཞིང་གསོལ་བ་འདེབས་སོ། །བདག་གིས་བླ་ན་མེད་པ་ཡེ་ཤེས་ཀྱི་མཆོག་དམ་པ་ཐོབ་པར་གྱུར་
GYE T'AM CHE LA KUL SH'ING SOL WA DEP SO DAG GI LA NA ME PA YE SHE KYI CH'OG DAM PA T'OB PAR GYUR

ཅིག། །མི་མཆོག་རྒྱལ་བ་གང་དག་ད་ལྟར་བཞུགས་པ་དང་། །གང་དག་འདས་པ་དག་དང་དེ་བཞིན་གང་མ་བྱོན།
CHIG MI CH'OG GYAL WA GANG DAG DA TAR SH'UK PA DANG GANG DAG DE PA DAG DANG DE SH'IN GANG MA JON

།ཡོན་ཏན་བསྔགས་པ་མཐའ་ཡས་རྒྱ་མཚོ་འདྲ་ཀུན་ལ། །ཐལ་མོ་སྦྱར་བར་བགྱིས་ཏེ་སྐྱབས་སུ་ཉེ་བར་མཆིའོ།
YON TEN NGAG PA T'A YE GYA TS'O DRA KUN LA T'AL MO JAR WAR GYI TE KYAB SU NYE WAR CH'I-O

།ལུས་ཀྱི་ལས་ནི་རྣམ་པ་གསུམ། །ངག་གི་རྣམ་པ་བཞི་དག་དང་། །གང་ཡང་ཡིད་ཀྱི་རྣམ་གསུམ་པོ། །མི་དགེ་
LU KYI LE NI NAM PA SUM NGAG GI NAM PA SH'I DAG DANG GANG YANG YIE KYI NAM SUM PO MI GE

བཅུ་པོ་སོ་སོར་བཤགས། །ཐོག་མ་མེད་ནས་ད་ལྟའི་བར། །མི་དགེ་བཅུ་དང་མཚམས་མེད་ལྔ། །སེམས་ནི་ཉོན་
CHU PO SO SOR SHAK T'OG MA ME NE DA TEI BAR MI GE CHU DANG TS'AM ME NGA SEM NI NYON

མོངས་དབང་གྱུར་པའི། །སྡིག་པ་ཐམས་ཅད་བཤགས་པར་བགྱི། །འདོད་ཆགས་ཞེ་སྡང་གཏི་མུག་དབང་གིས་ནི།
MONG WANG GYUR PEI DIG PA T'AM CHE SHAK PAR GYI DOE CH'AK SH'E DANG TI MUG WANG GI NI

།ལུས་དང་ངག་དང་དེ་བཞིན་ཡིད་ཀྱིས་ཀྱང་། །སྡིག་པ་བདག་གིས་བགྱིས་པ་ཅི་མཆིས་པ། །དེ་དག་ཐམས་ཅད་
LU DANG NGAG DANG DE SH'IN YI KYI KYANG DIG PA DAG GI GYI PA CHI CH'I PA DE DAG T'AM CHE

གིས་སོ་སོར་བཤགས། །མཚམས་མེད་ལྔ་པོ་དག་གི་སྡིག་པ་རྣམས། །གང་གིས་མི་ཤེས་དབང་གིས་བྱས་པ་དག།
GI SO SOR SHAK TS'AM ME NGA PO DAG GI DIG PA NAM GANG GI MI SHE WANG GI JE PA DAG

།དེ་ཡིས་ལྟུང་བ་བཤགས་པ་འདི་བཏོན་པས། །དེ་དག་མ་ལུས་ཡོངས་སུ་བྱང་བར་འགྱུར། །བདག་དང་སེམས་ཅན་
DE YI TUNG WA SHAK PA DI TON PE DE DAG MA LU YONG SU JANG WAR GYUR DAG DANG SEM CHEN

ཀུན་གྱི་སྡིག་པའི་ལས། །ཉེས་པར་གྱུར་གང་མཐོལ་ཞིང་བཤགས་པར་བགྱི། །སླན་ཆད་ནམ་ཡང་བགྱིད་པར་མ་གྱུར་ཅིག།
KUN GYI DIG PEI LE NYE PAR GYUR GANG T'OL SH'ING SHAK PAR GYI LEN CH'E NAM YANG GYI PAR MA GYUR CHIG

།ལས་ཀྱི་སྒྲིབ་པའང་གཏན་དུ་ཟད་བྱེད་ཤོག། །ཕྱག་འཚལ་བ་དང་མཆོད་ཅིང་བཤགས་པ་དང་། །རྗེས་སུ་ཡི་རང་
LE KYI DRIB PANG TEN DU ZE JE SHOG CH'AG TS'AL WA DANG CH'E CHING SHAK PA DANG JE SU YI RANG

བསྐུལ་ཞིང་གསོལ་བ་ཡི། །དགེ་བ་ཆུང་ཟད་བདག་གིས་ཅི་བསགས་པ། །ཐམས་ཅད་བདག་གིས་བྱང་ཆུབ་ཕྱིར་བསྔོའོ།།
KUL SH'ING SOL WA YI GE WA CHUNG ZE DAG GI CHI SAK PA T'AM CHE DAG GI JANG CHUB CH'IR NGO-O

Just as the buddhas and transcendent destroyers
Of the future will dedicate,
And just as the buddhas and transcendent destroyers
Of the present are dedicating,
In the same way I make this dedication.
I confess all my negative actions separately
And rejoice in all merits.
I implore the buddhas to grant my request that I may realize
The ultimate, sublime, highest transcendental wisdom.
To the sublime kings of the human beings living now,
To those of the past and to those who have yet to appear,
To all those whose knowledge is as vast as the infinite ocean,
With my hands folded in respect, I go for refuge.
I confess each of the ten unskillful actions I have done,
Be they the three physical, four oral, or three mental ones.
I confess the ten unskillful actions
And the five sins of limitless consequence,
And all the sins I have ever committed
While my mind has been overpowered with ignorance
From time without beginning until this moment.
I confess each and every sin I have committed
With my body, speech, and mind while overpowered
With desire, hatred, and mental dullness.
By means of this presentation of the Confession of Faults,
May the five sins of limitless consequence,
And whatever other sins I have done while overpowered with ignorance,
Be completely purified.
All the faults of all we sentient beings from our bad karma
Being repented, may they never be done again.
May all the veils of karma be completely exhausted.
By prostrations, offerings, repentance, rejoicing in good deeds,
By the calling for the turning of the dharma wheel
And praying for the teachers to remain;
Whatever be the portion of positive karma I accumulate thereby,
I dedicate it all to enlightenment.

༄༅། །འཕགས་པ་བཅུ་གཅིག་ཞལ་གྱི་སྨྱུང་ཚོག་བགྲ་ཤིས་ཀུན་ཁྱབ་ཅེས་བྱ་བ་བཞུགས་སོ། །

The Fasting Ritual of the Noble Eleven-Faced Chenrezig,
Called the Omnipresent Happy Omen

༄༅། །ན་མོ་གུ་རུ་ལོ་ཀེ་ཤུ་ར་ཡེ། །རྒྱལ་ཀུན་ཕྲགས་རྗེའི་རྩ་བ་ནི། །གདས་རིའི་ལྷོངས་ཀྱི་དཔལ་འབར་བ། །བླ་མ་སྤྲུན་
རས་གཟིགས་མགོན་ལ། །བཏུད་ནས་དེ་སྤྲུབ་ཤུང་གསལ་ཏི། །དེ་ལ་མཉམ་དུ་བཟང་ཕྲགས་པའི་སྟེང་པཱུ་འདབ་བརྐྱང་
ཕྱོགས་མཚོན་ནས། །འབྲུ་ཚོམ་དགུ་བཀོད་པའི་མཐར་མཚོ་པས་བསྐོར། །གཏོར་མ་
གཅིག་བཀམ། །བུམ་པ་གཟུངས་རིང་གིས་བགེགས་བསྐྲད་པ་བཞག། །བླ་མཚམ་
རྗེན་གྱི་དུང་ནས་གསོ་སྟོང་གི་སྟོལ་པ་ལེན་པ་ལ། ། །ཐུག་གསུམ་འཚལ།

Sojong Vow

|ཕྱོགས་བཅུན་བཞུགས་པའི་སངས་རྒྱས་དང་བྱང་ཆུབ་སེམས་དཔའ་ཐམས་ཅད་བདག་ལ་དགོངས་སུ་གསོལ།
CH'OK CHU NA SH'UK PEI SANG GYE DANG JANG CH'UB SEM PA T'AM CHE DAG LA GONG SU SOL

|ཇི་ལྟར་སྔོན་གྱི་དེ་བཞིན་གཤེགས་པ་དགྲ་བཅོམ་པ་ཡང་དག་པར་རྫོགས་པའི་སངས་རྒྱས་ཏ་ཆང་ཤེས་ལྟ་བུ་
JI TAR NGON GYI DE SH'IN SHEK PA DRA CHOM PA YANG DAG PAR DZOK PEI SANG GYE TA CHANG SHE TA BU

 གླང་པོ་ཆེན་པོ། །བྱ་བ་བྱས་ཤིང་། །བྱེད་པ་བྱས་པ། །ཁུར་བོར་བ། །རང་གི་དོན་རྗེས་སུ་ཐོབ་པ།
LANG PO CH'EN PO   JA WA JE SH'ING   JE PA JE PA   K'UR BOR WA   RANG GI DON JE SU T'OB PA

|སྲིད་པ་ཀུན་ཏུ་སྦྱོར་བ་ཡོངས་སུ་ཟད་པ། །ཡང་དག་པའི་བཀའ། །ལེགས་པར་རྣམ་པར་གྲོལ་བའི་ཐུགས།
SI PA KUN TU JOR WA YONG SU ZE PA   YANG DAG PEI KA   LEK PAR NAM PAR DROL WEI T'UK

|ལེགས་པར་རྣམ་པར་གྲོལ་བའི་ཤེས་རབ་ཅན་དེ་རྣམས་ཀྱིས། །སེམས་ཅན་ཐམས་ཅད་ཀྱི་དོན་གྱི་ཕྱིར་དང་།
LEK PAR NAM PAR DROL WEI SHE RAB CHEN DE NAM KYI   SEM CHEN T'AM CHE KYI DON GYI CH'IR DANG

|ཕན་པར་བྱ་བའི་ཕྱིར་དང་། །གྲོལ་བར་བྱ་བའི་ཕྱིར་དང་། །ནད་མེད་པར་བྱ་བའི་ཕྱིར་དང་། །མུ་གེ
P'EN PAR JA WEI CH'IR DANG   DROL WAR JA WEI CH'IR DANG   NE ME PAR JA WEI CH'IR DANG   MU GE

མེད་པར་བྱ་བའི་ཕྱིར་དང་། །བྱང་ཆུབ་ཀྱི་ཕྱོགས་ཀྱི་ཆོས་རྣམས་ཡོངས་སུ་རྫོགས་པར་བྱ་བའི་ཕྱིར་དང་།
ME PAR JA WEI CH'IR DANG   JANG CH'UB KYI CH'OK KYI CH'O NAM YONG SU DZOK PAR JA WEI CH'IR DANG

|བླ་ན་མེད་པ་ཡང་དག་པར་རྫོགས་པའི་བྱང་ཆུབ་རྟོགས་པར་བྱ་བའི་ཕྱིར། །གསོ་སྦྱོང་ངེས་པར་བླངས་པ
LA NA ME PA YANG DAG PAR DZOK PEI JANG CH'UB TOK PAR JA WEI CH'IR   SO JONG NGE PAR LANG PA

དེ་བཞིན་ཏུ། །བདག་མིང་...འདི་ཞེས་བགྱི་བས་ཀྱང་། །དུས་འདི་ནས་བཟུང་སྟེ།
DE SH'IN TU   DA MING ... DI SH'E GYI WE KYANG   DU DI NE ZUNG TE

The Fasting Ritual of the Noble Eleven-Faced Chenrezig,
Called the Omnipresent Happy Omen

Namo Guru Lokesharaye! Having bowed respectfully in front of Chenrezig, who protects with the compassion of the Victorious Ones like the moon shining in a glorious blaze on the snowy mountain valley, briefly and clearly I have composed this practice. On a mandala sprinkled with perfumed water, draw an eight-petaled lotus or arrange nine piles of grain indicating the eight directions (in the center), place the offerings (in the bowls), hold a torma, and while reciting the long mantra of the vase, push away obstructions. Then to take the Sojong vow, we prostrate three times in front of the lama, altar, or any other such support.

Sojong Vow

Prostrate three times, then kneel on the right knee with the left knee raised and repeat three times:
All the buddhas and bodhisattvas residing in the ten directions,
Please be gracious to me. Just as the previous tathagatas, arhats,
Perfectly pure and accomplished buddhas,
Who are like the Heavenly Steed and the Great Elephant,
Accomplished in the past what had to be done,
Just as they laid down the burden,
Subsequently attained their own welfare,
And completely relinquished all bonds
To the possibilities of existence;
Their speech is completely pure,
Their minds are completely liberated,
Possessing the completely liberated
Transcendental knowledge;
Just as, for the sake of all beings,
To benefit them, to liberate them,
To spare them from illness, to spare them from famine,
To perfect the aspects of the dharma directed towards awakening,
And to realize the unsurpassable, perfect,
And complete enlightenment,
In the same way, I [say your name],

།ཇི་སྲིད་སང་ཉི་མ་མ་ཤར་གྱི་བར་དུ་གསོ་སྦྱོང་ངེས་པར་བླང་བར་བགྱིའོ། །ལན་གསུམ།
JI SI SANG NYI MA MA SHAR GYI BAR DU SO JONG NGE PAR LANG WAR GYI-O

།དེང་ནས་སྲོག་གཅོད་མི་བྱ་ཞིང་། །གཞན་གྱི་ནོར་ཡང་བླང་མི་བྱ། །འཁྲིག་པའི་ཆོས་ཀྱང་མི་སྤྱད་ཅིང་།
DENG NE SOG CHOE MI JA SH'ING SH'EN GYI NOR YANG LANG MI JA TR'IG PEI CH'O KYANG MI CHE CHING

།རྫུན་གྱི་ཚིག་ཀྱང་མི་སྨྲའོ། །སྐྱོན་ནི་མང་པོ་ཉེར་བརྟེན་པའི། །ཆང་ནི་ཡོངས་སུ་སྤང་བར་བྱ།
DZUN GYI TS'IG KYANG MI MA-O KYON NI MANG PO NYER TEN PEI CH'ANG NI YONG SU PANG WAR JA

།ཁྲི་སྟན་ཆེ་མཐོ་མི་བྱ་ཞིང་། །དེ་བཞིན་དུས་མ་ཡིན་པའི་ཟས། །དྲི་དང་ཕྲེང་བ་དང་ནི་རྒྱན།
TR'I TEN CH'E T'O MI JA SH'ING DE SH'IN DU MA YIN PEI ZE DRI DANG TR'ENG WA DANG NI GYEN

།གར་དང་གླུ་སོགས་སྤང་བར་བྱ། །ཇི་ལྟར་དགྲ་བཅོམ་རྟག་ཏུ་ནི། །སྲོག་གཅོད་ལ་སོགས་མི་བྱེད་ལྟར།
GAR DANG LU SOK PANG WAR JA JI TAR DRA CHOM TAG TU NI SOG CHOE LA SOK MI JE TAR

།དེ་ལྟར་སྲོག་གཅོད་ལ་སོགས་སྤང་། །བླ་མེད་བྱང་ཆུབ་མྱུར་ཐོབ་ཤོག། །སྡུག་བསྔལ་མང་དཀྲུགས་འཇིག་
DE TAR SOG CHOE LA SOK PANG LA ME JANG CH'UB NYUR T'OB SHOK DUG NGAL MANG DRUG JIG

རྟེན་འདི། །སྲིད་པའི་མཚོ་ལས་སྒྲོལ་བར་ཤོག། །ཕྱག་གསུམ། །དེ་ནས་ཚུལ་ཁྲིམས་རྣམ་དག་གི་གཟུངས་བཟླ་བ་ནི།
TEN DI SI PEI TS'O LE DROL WAR SHOK

Mantra for Purifying Morals

།དེ་བཞིན་གཤེགས་པ་ཐམས་ཅད་ལ་ཕྱག་འཚལ་ལོ། །བྱང་ཆུབ་སེམས་དཔའ་སེམས་དཔའ་ཆེན་པོ་འཕགས་པ་
DE SH'IN SHEK PA T'AM CHE LA CH'AG TS'AL LO JANG CH'UB SEM PA SEM PA CH'EN PO P'AK PA

སྤྱན་རས་གཟིགས་དབང་ཕྱུག་ལ་ཕྱག་འཚལ་ལོ།
CHEN RE ZIG WANG CH'UG LA CH'AG TS'AL LO

ཨོཾ་ཨ་མོ་གྷ་ཤཱི་ལ། སམྦྷ་ར་སམྦྷ་ར། བྷ་ར་བྷ་ར། མ་ཧཱ་ཤུདྡྷ་ས་ཏྭ།
OM A MO GHA SHI LA SAM BHA RA SAM BHA RA BHA RA BHA RA MA HA SHUD DHA SA TO

པདྨ་བི་བྷཱུ་ཥི་ཏ་བྷུ་ཛ། དྷ་ར་དྷ་ར། ས་མནྟ། ཨ་ཝ་ལོ་ཀི་ཏེ་ཧཱུྃ་ཕཊ་སྭཱ་ཧཱ། །ལན་བདུན།
PE MA BI BHU KI TA BHU DZA DHA RA DHA RA SA MEN TA A WA LO KI TE HUNG PE SO HA

From this moment until sunrise tomorrow,
Shall definitely undertake the Sojong vow.

Repeat three times.

From now on I will not kill,
I will not take the belongings of others,
I will avoid all sexual activities,
 I will not lie,
I will completely abandon intoxicants,
Which quickly lead to numerous shortcomings,
I will not use high and luxurious seats,
I will not eat at wrong times,
I will use neither perfume nor ornaments,
And I will neither sing nor dance.
Just as the foe destroyers constantly abstain from taking life
And from doing these other actions, in the same way,
Having abandoned all these actions,
May I quickly obtain Unsurpassable Awakening.
May we be freed from the ocean of existence,
The world of destruction, shaken by so many sufferings.

Repeat three times. Recite the mantra for purifying morals
which helps one to preserve the vow:

Mantra for Purifying Morals

I bow to all the buddhas,

and I bow to Bodhisattva Mahasattva Noble Avalokiteshvara.

OM A MO GA SHI LA   SAM BHA RA   SAM BHA RA
BHA RA   BHA RA   MA HA SHUD DHA SA TO
PE MA BI BU KI TA BU DZA   DHA RA DHA RA
SA MEN TA   A WA LO KI TE   HUNG PE SO HA

Repeat seven times

།བདག་སོགས་སེམས་ཅན་ཐམས་ཅད་ཀྱི་རྒྱུད་ལ་ཚུལ་ཁྲིམས་ཀྱི་ཕ་རོལ་ཏུ་ཕྱིན་པའི་ཆོས་རྣམས་ཡོངས་སུ་རྫོགས་པར་

DAG SOK SEM CHEN T'AM CHE KYI GYUE LA TS'UL TR'IM KYI P'A ROL TU CH'IN PEI CH'O NAM YONG SU DZOK PAR

གྱུར་ཅིག   །ཉོན་མོངས་པས་ཚུལ་ཁྲིམས་འཆལ་བ་ལས་བྱུང་བའི་སྡིག་པ་དང་སྒྲིབ་པ་ཐམས་ཅད་བྱང་ཞིང་དག་

GYUR CHIG   NYON MONG PE TS'UL TR'IM CH'AL WA LE JUNG WEI DIG PA DANG DRIB PA T'AM CHE JANG SH'ING DAG

པར་གྱུར་ཅིག   །འཕགས་པ་དགྱེས་པའི་ཚུལ་ཁྲིམས་ཀྱི་སྐལ་པ་དང་ལྡན་པར་གྱུར་ཅིག   །ཉོན་མོངས་པས་མི་རྫི

PAR GYUR CHIG   P'AK PA GYE PEI TS'UL TR'IM KYI KAL PA DANG DEN PAR GYUR CHIG   NYON MONG PE MI DZI

བར་རྣམ་པར་གྲོལ་བའི་བདེ་བ་ལ་གནས་པར་གྱུར་ཅིག   །ཁྲིམས་ཀྱི་ཚུལ་ཁྲིམས་སྐྱོན་མེད་ཅིང་།

BAR NAM PAR DROL WEI DE WA LA NE PAR GYUR CHIG   TR'IM KYI TS'UL TR'IM KYON ME CHING

།ཚུལ་ཁྲིམས་རྣམ་པར་དག་དང་ལྡན   །ཿོམ་སེམས་མེད་པའི་ཚུལ་ཁྲིམས་ཀྱིས   །ཚུལ་ཁྲིམས་ཕ་རོལ་ཕྱིན་རྫོགས་ཤོག

TS'UL TR'IM NAM PAR DAG DANG DEN   LOM SEM ME PEI TS'UL TR'IM KYI   TS'UL TR'IM P'A ROL CH'IN DZOK SHOK

།རྒྱལ་བ་ཀུན་གྱི་རྗེས་སུ་སློབ་གྱུར་ཏེ   །བཟང་པོ་སྤྱོད་པ་ཡོངས་སུ་རྫོགས་བྱེད་ཅིང་།   །ཚུལ་ཁྲིམས་སྤྱོད་པ་དྲི་མེད་

GYAL WA KUN GYI JE SU LOB GYUR TE   ZANG PO CHOE PA YONG SU DZOK JE CHING   TS'UL TR'IM CHOE PA TRI ME

ཡོངས་དག་པར   །ཏྡག་ཏུ་མ་ཉམས་སྐྱོན་མེད་སྤྱོད་པར་ཤོག   །ཅེས་སོགས་སྨོན་ལམ་གདབ་པར་བྱའོ།

YONG DAG PAR   TEG TU MA NYAM KYON ME CHOE PAR SHOK

།བརྒྱུད་རིམ་གྱི་གསོལ་འདེབས་བྱ་འདོད་ན།

Prayer to the Transmission Lineage

།སྤྱན་རས་གཟིགས་དབང་དགེ་སློང་དཔལ་མོ་དང་།

CHEN RE ZIG WANG GE LONG PAL MO DANG

།ཡེ་ཤེས་བཟང་པོ་ཟླ་བ་གཞོན་ནུ་དང་།

YE SHE ZANG PO DA WA SH'ON NU DANG

།པེ་ཉ་བ་དང་བྱང་སེམས་ཟླ་རྒྱལ་ཞབས།

PE NYA WA DANG JANG SEM DA GYAL SH'AB

།ཉི་ཕུག་པ་དང་སུ་སྟོན་རྡོ་རྗེ་རྒྱལ།

NYI P'UG PA DANG SU TON DOR JE GYAL

།ཞང་སྟོན་དྲ་འཇིགས་མཁན་པོ་རྩི་འདུལ་བ།

SH'ANG TON DRA JIK K'EN PO TSI DUL WA

།བདེ་བ་ཅན་པ་མཁས་པ་ཆུ་བཟང་པ།

DE WA CHEN PA K'E PA CH'U ZANG PA

།ཤེས་རབ་འབུམ་པ་རྒྱལ་སྲས་རིན་པོ་ཆེ།

SHE RAB BUM PA GYAL SE RIN PO CH'E

།དཀོན་མཆོག་བཟང་པོ་བླ་མ་ངག་དབང་པ།

KON CH'OG ZANG PO LA MA NGAG WANG PA

།བྱང་ཆུབ་སེང་གེ་མཁན་ཆེན་ཉག་ཕུ་པ།

JANG CH'UB SENG GE K'EN CH'EN NYAG P'U PA

།བསོད་ནམས་དར་དང་འཇམ་དཔལ་བཟང་པོ་དང་།

SOE NAM DAR DANG JAM PAL ZANG PO DANG

May I and all sentient beings be able to completely perfect
The perfection of the doctrine of morality.
May all the moral failings, which come from affliction
And cause negativities and obscurations, be completely purified.
May we have the good fortune to have the morality
which pleases all noble beings.
May we enjoy liberation, which is free from all affliction.

With faultless morality, perfectly pure moral conduct,
Behavior free from vanity, may I take this path
To its transcendental perfection.
Emulating the training of all the victors
And completing my practice of excellence,
May I, with purest motivation,
Engage in stainless moral conduct,
Never weakening and free from fault.

This may be followed by additional prayers.

Prayer to the Transmission Lineage

If we wish, we can say the following prayer
to the Transmission Lineage of this practice:

Powerful Chenrezig, Gelongma Palmo
and Yeshe Zangpo, Dawa Shonnu and
Penyawa, and Chang Sem Dagyal Shab,
Nyipukpa and Suton Dorje Gyal,
Shangton Drajik, Kenpo Tsidulwa,
Dewachenpa, Kepa Chuzangpa,
Sherab Bumpa, Gyalse Rinpoche,
Konchok Zangpo, Lama Ngakwangpa,
Changchub Senge, Kenchen Nyakpupa,
Sonam Dar and Jampal Zangpo and

།སངས་རྒྱས་མཉན་པ་མི་བསྐྱོད་རྡོ་རྗེའི་ཞབས།
SANG GYE NYEN PA MI KYOE DOR JEI SH'AB

།དཀོན་མཆོག་ཡན་ལག་དབང་ཕྱུག་རྡོ་རྗེ་དང་
KON CH'OG YEN LAG WANG CH'UG DOR JE DANG

།ཆོས་ཀྱི་དབང་ཕྱུག་ངག་གི་དབང་ཕྱུག་དང་
CH'O KYI WANG CH'UG NGAG GI WANG CH'UG DANG

།སྤྲུལ་སྐུ་སྒྲུབ་བརྒྱུད་བསྟན་པ་རྣམ་རྒྱལ་དང་
TRUL KU DRUB GYUE TEN PA NAM GYAL DANG

།ཀརྨ་ངེས་དོན་བསྟན་པ་རབ་རྒྱས་དང་
KAR MA NGE DON TEN PA RAB GYE DANG

།མཁས་མཆོག་གྲུབ་དབང་བསྟན་འཛིན་འགྱུར་མེད་སོགས།
K'E CH'OG DRUB WANG TEN DZIN GYUR ME SOK

།རྫ་བརྒྱུད་དཔལ་ལྡན་བླ་མ་མཆོག་རྣམས་ལ།
DZA GYU PAL DEN LA MA CH'OG NAM LA

།གསོལ་བ་འདེབས་སོ་བྱིན་གྱིས་བརླབ་ཏུ་གསོལ།
SOL WA DEB SO JIN GYI LAB TU SOL

།ཆོག་དངོས་ལ་དང་པོ་སྐྱབས་སེམས་ནི།
Refuge and the Generation of the Thought of Enlightenment

།སངས་རྒྱས་ཆོས་དང་ཚོགས་ཀྱི་མཆོག་རྣམས་ལ།
SANG GYE CH'O DANG TS'OK KYI CH'OG NAM LA

།བྱང་ཆུབ་བར་དུ་བདག་ནི་སྐྱབས་སུ་མཆི།
JANG CH'UB BAR DU DAG NI KYAB SU CH'I

།བདག་གིས་སྦྱིན་སོགས་བགྱིས་པའི་བསོད་ནམས་ཀྱིས།
DAG GI JIN SOK GYI PEI SOE NAM KYI

།འགྲོ་ལ་ཕན་ཕྱིར་སངས་རྒྱས་འགྲུབ་པར་ཤོག   །ལན་གསུམ།
DRO LA P'EN CH'IR SANG GYE DRUB PAR SHOK

།ཚོགས་བསགས་ནི།
Accumulation of Beneficial Activity

།བདག་ཉིད་སྤྱན་རས་གཟིགས་གསལ་བའི
DAG NYI CHEN RE ZIG SAL WEI

།ཐུགས་ཀའི་ཧྲཱིཿལས་འོད་འཕྲོས་པས།
T'UK KEI HRIH LE OE TRO PE

།བླ་མ་ཐུགས་རྗེ་ཆེན་པོ་ལ།
LA MA T'UK JE CH'EN PO LA

།སངས་རྒྱས་བྱང་སེམས་ཀྱི་བསྐོར་བ།
SANG GYE JANG SEM KYI KOR WA

།མདུན་མཁར་ཆེན་དྲངས་བཞུགས་པར་གྱུར།
DUN K'AR CHEN DRANG SH'UK PAR GYUR

།ཕྱོགས་བཅུ་དུས་གསུམ་བཞུགས་པ་ཡི།
CH'OK CHU DU SUM SH'UK PA YI

།རྒྱལ་བ་སྲས་བཅས་ཐམས་ཅད་ལ།
GYAL WA SE CHE T'AM CHE LA

།ཀུན་ནས་དང་བས་ཕྱག་འཚལ་ལོ།
KUN NE DONG WE CH'AG TS'AL LO

།མེ་ཏོག་བདུག་སྤོས་མར་མེ་དྲི།
ME TOG DUG PO MAR ME DRI

།ཞལ་ཟས་རོལ་མོ་ལ་སོགས་པ།
SH'AL ZE ROL MO LA SOK PA

།དངོས་འབྱོར་ཡིད་ཀྱིས་སྤྲུལ་ནས་འབུལ།
NGO JOR YIE KYI TRUL NE BUL

།འཕགས་པའི་ཚོགས་ཀྱིས་བཞེས་སུ་གསོལ།
P'AK PEI TS'OK KYI SH'E SU SOL

།ཐོག་མ་མེད་ནས་ད་ལྟའི་བར།
T'OG MA ME NE DA TEI BAR

།མི་དགེ་བཅུ་དང་མཚམས་མེད་ལྔ།
MI GE CHU DANG TS'AM ME NGA

Sangye Nyenpa, Mikyo Dorje Shab,
Konchok Yenlak, Wangchuk Dorje,
and Chokyi Wangchuk, Ngakgi Wangchuk
and Tulku Drubgyu, Tenpa Namgyal
and Karma Ngedon, Tenpa Rabgye
and Kechok Drubwang, Tenzin Gyurme and all the others,
Glorious and Sublime Root Lamas and Lamas of the Lineage,
I beseech you, please grant me your grace.

The rite itself starts with:

Refuge and the Generation of the Thought of Enlightenment

In the Buddhas, Dharma, and Supreme Assembly,
I take refuge until enlightenment.
By the merit of generosity and other virtues,
May I accomplish buddhahood for the benefit of all beings.

Repeat three times.

Accumulation of Beneficial Activity
In order to increase the accumulation of beneficial activity, recite:

I appear clearly as Thousand-Armed Chenrezig.
From the HRIH *in my heart light radiates, inviting the Lama,*
The Great Compassionate One, who appears in the sky in front of me,
Surrounded by the buddhas and bodhisattvas.
To all the buddhas and their sons, who reside in the ten directions
And the three times, with complete sincerity I pay homage.
I offer flowers, incense, butter lamps, perfume, food, music,
And other real and imaginary offerings,
And beseech the noble assembly to accept them.
I confess all the unskillful actions caused by
The power of conflicting emotions,
The ten unvirtuous deeds, and the five sins of limitless consequence

།སེམས་ནི་ཉོན་མོངས་དབང་གྱུར་པའི། ｜སྡིག་པ་ཐམས་ཅད་བཤགས་པར་བགྱི། ｜ཉེན་ཐོས་རང་རྒྱལ་བྱང་

SEM NI NYON MONG WANG GYUR PEI   DIG PA T'AM CHE SHAK PAR GYI   NYEN T'O RANG GYAL JANG

ཆུབ་སེམས། ｜སོ་སོ་སྐྱེ་བོ་ལ་སོགས་པ། ｜དུས་གསུམ་དགེ་བ་ཅི་བསགས་པའི། ｜བསོད་ནམས་ལ་ནི་བདག་ཡི་རང་།

CH'UB SEM   SO SO KYE WO LA SOK PA   DU SUM GE WA CHI SAK PEI   SOE NAM LA NI DAG YI RANG

།སེམས་ཅན་རྣམས་ཀྱི་བསམ་པ་དང་། ｜བློ་ཡི་བྱེ་བྲག་ཇི་ལྟ་བར། ｜ཆེ་ཆུང་ཐུན་མོང་ཐེག་པ་ཡི། ｜ཆོས་ཀྱི

SEM CHEN NAM KYI SAM PA DANG   LO YI JE DRAG JI TA WAR   CH'E CH'UNG T'UN MONG T'EG PA YI   CH'O KYI

འཁོར་ལོ་བསྐོར་དུ་གསོལ། ｜འཁོར་བ་ཇི་སྲིད་མ་སྟོང་བར། ｜མྱ་ངན་མི་འདའ་ཐུགས་རྗེ་ཡིས། ｜སྡུག་བསྔལ

K'OR LO KOR DU SOL   K'OR WA JI SI MA TONG BAR   NYA NGEN MI DA T'UK JE YI   DUG NGAL

རྒྱ་མཚོར་བྱིང་བ་ཡི། ｜སེམས་ཅན་རྣམས་ལ་གཟིགས་སུ་གསོལ། ｜བདག་གིས་བསོད་ནམས་ཅི་བསགས་པ།

GYA TS'OR JING WA YI   SEM CHEN NAM LA ZIK SU SOL   DAG GI SOE NAM CHI SAK PA

།ཐམས་ཅད་བྱང་ཆུབ་རྒྱུར་གྱུར་ནས། ｜རིང་པོར་མི་ཐོགས་འགྲོ་བ་ཡི། ｜འདྲེན་པའི་དཔལ་དུ་བདག་གྱུར་ཅིག །

T'AM CHE JANG CHUB GYUR GYUR NE   RING BOR MI T'OK DRO WA YI   DREN PEI PAL DU DAG GYUR CHIG

།སེམས་ཅན་བདེ་ལྡན་སྡུག་བསྔལ་བྲལ། ｜བདེ་ལས་མི་ཉམས་བཏང་སྙོམས་ཤོག །

SEM CHEN DE DEN DUG NGAL DRAL   DE LE MI NYAM TANG NYOM SHOK

Generation of Oneself as the Deity

ཨོཾ་སྭ་བྷཱ་ཝ་ཤུདྡྷཿསརྦ་དྷརྨ ｜ སྭ་བྷཱ་ཝ་ཤུདྡྷོ྅ཧཾ།

OM SVA BHA WA SHUD DHA SAR VA DHAR MA   SVA BHA WA SHUD DHO HAM

།གཟུང་འཛིན་ཆོས་རྣམས་སྟོང་པར་གྱུར། ｜དེ་ཡི་ངང་ལས་པད་ཟླའི་སྟེང་། ｜རང་སེམས་ཧྲཱིཿཡིག་དཀར་པོ་ལས།

ZUNG DZIN CH'O NAM TONG PAR GYUR   DE YI NGANG LE PE DEI TENG   RANG SEM HRIH YIG KAR PO LE

།འོད་འཕྲོས་སེམས་ཅན་དོན་བྱས་ནས། ｜ཚུར་འདུས་ཧྲཱིཿཡིག་པདྨ་ནི། ｜གསེར་མདོག་འབར་བ་ཧྲཱིཿམཚན་གྱུར།

OE TRO SEM CHEN DON JE NE   TS'UR DUE HRIH YIG PE MA NI   SER DOG BAR WA HRIH TS'EN GYUR

།སླར་ཡང་དེ་ལས་ལྕགས་ཀྱུ་དང་། ｜ཞགས་པ་ལྟ་བུའི་འོད་འཕྲོས་པས། ｜ཕྱོགས་བཅུའི་སངས་རྒྱས་བྱང་སེམས

LAR YANG DE LE CHAK KYU DANG   SH'AK PA TA BUI OE TR'O PE   CH'OK CHUI SANG GYE JANG SEM

རྣམས། ｜སྤྱན་དྲངས་དེ་ལ་ཐིམ་པ་ཡིས། ｜སྐད་ཅིག་ཉིད་ལ་པདྨ་ནི། ｜ཧྲཱིཿདང་བཅས་པ་ཡོངས་གྱུར་ལས།

NAM   CHEN DRANG DE LA T'IM PA YI   KE CHIG NYIE LA PE MA NI   HRIH DANG CHE PA YONG GYUR LE

Done from beginningless time until now.

I rejoice in the spiritual merit of whatever virtue

Shravakas, pratyekabuddhas, bodhisattvas,

And ordinary beings gather throughout the three times.

I pray that the dharma wheel of the mahayana,

Hinayana, and teaching common to both

Be turned in accordance with the wishes and aptitudes of beings.

I beseech the buddhas not to pass into nirvana

As long as samsara is not emptied,

But to look with compassion upon sentient beings

Who wallow in the ocean of suffering.

May whatever merit I have accumulated

Be the cause for the enlightenment of beings,

And may I quickly become a splendid leader of beings.

May all beings be endowed with joy; may they be separated from suffering.

May they never be separated from joy; may they remain in equanimity.

Generation of Oneself as the Deity

OM SVA BHA WA SHUD DHA   SAR VA DHAR MA   SVA BHA WA   SHUD DHO HAM

All aspects of dualistic grasping become emptiness.

From this emptiness, standing on a lotus and moon disk,

My own mind appears in the form of the letter HRIH.

It radiates light beneficial to all beings

And is then absorbed back into the HRIH.

The lotus adorned with the letter HRIH *blazes with the color of gold.*

Again from the HRIH *light radiates in the form of lassos and hooks,*

Inviting all the buddhas and bodhisattvas of the ten directions.

They are absorbed into the HRIH *and in an instant,*

From the complete transformation of the HRIH,

|བདག་ཉིད་འཕགས་པ་སྤྱན་རས་གཟིགས། ཀྲུ་མདོག་དཀར་པོ་ལང་ཚོ་ཅན། བཅུ་གཅིག་ཞལ་གྱི་རྩ་ཞལ་དཀར།

DAG NYIE P'AK PA CHEN RE ZIG   KU DOG KAR PO LANG T'SO CHEN   CHU CHIG SH'AL GYI TSA SH'AL KAR

|གཡས་ལྗང་གཡོན་དམར་དེ་ཡི་སྟེང་། |དབུས་ལྗང་གཡས་དམར་གཡོན་དཀར་བ། |དེ་སྟེང་དབུས་དམར་གཡས་དཀར

YE JANG YON MAR DE YI TENG   UE JANG YE MAR YON KAR WA   DE TENG UE MAR YE KAR

ཞིང་། |གཡོན་ལྗང་བ་རྣམས་ཞི་ཉམས་ཅན། |དེ་སྟེང་ཁྲོ་ཞལ་ནག་པོ་ནི། |སྤྱན་གསུམ་མཁེ་གཚིགས་ཁྲོ་གཉེར

SH'ING   YON JANG WA NAM SH'I NYAM CHEN   DE TENG TRO SH'AL NAG PO NI   CHEN SUM CH'E TSIK TRO NYER

ཅན། |དེ་ཡི་སྟེང་ན་ཞི་ཞལ་ནི། |དམར་པོ་གཙུག་ཏོར་ལྡན་པ་ཉིད། |རྒྱན་སྤང་མགུལ་བཅས་རྣམ་པར་གསལ།

CHEN   DE YI TENG NA SH'I SH'AL NI   MAR PO TS'UK TOR DEN PA NYIE   GYEN PANG GUL CHE NAM PAR SAL

|རྩ་བའི་ཕྱག་བརྒྱད་དང་པོ་གཉིས། |ཐུགས་ཀར་ཐལ་སྦྱར་ཡེ་གཉིས་པས། |བདྲང་ཕྲེང་གསུམ་པ་མཆོག་སྦྱིན

TSA WEI CHAG GYE DANG PO NYI   T'UK KAR T'AL JAR YE NYI PEI   DRANG TRENG SUM PA CH'OG JIN

མཛད། |བཞི་པས་འཁོར་ལོ་འཛིན་པ་སྟེ། |གཡོན་གྱི་གཉིས་པས་པདྨ་དང་། |གསུམ་པས་ཕྱི་ལྔགས་བཞི་པ་ཡིས

DZE   SH'I PE K'OR LO DZIN PA TE   YON GYI NYI PE PE MA DANG   SUM PE CHI LUK SH'I PA YI

|མདའ་གཞུ་ཡོངས་སུ་འཛིན་པའོ། |དེ་ལྷག་ཕྱག་ནི་དགུ་བརྒྱ་དང་། |དགུ་བཅུ་རྩ་གཉིས་མཆོག་སྦྱིན་མཛད།

DA SH'U YONG SU DZIN PA-O   DE LHEG CH'AG NI GU GYA DANG   GU CHU TSA NYI CH'OG JIN DZE

|དེ་ལྟར་སྟོང་ཕྲག་ཕྱག་རྣམས་ཀྱི། |མཐིལ་དུ་སྤྱན་རེ་ལྡན་པའོ། |ནོར་བུ་རིན་ཆེན་རྒྱན་འཆང་ཞིང་།

DE TAR TONG TR'AG CH'AG NAM KYI   T'IL DU JEN RE DEN PA-O   NOR BU RIN CH'EN GYEN CH'ANG SH'ING

|ཀྲུ་སྟོད་ནུ་མ་གཡོན་པ་ནི། |རི་དགས་པགས་པས་ཡོལ་བཀབ་པ། |ཀ་ཤིའི་རས་ཀྱི་ཤམ་ཐབས་ཅན།

KU TOE NU MA YON PA NI   RI DOK PAK PE YONG KAB PA   KA SH'II RE KYI SHAM T'AB CHEN

|ཡིད་འོང་དར་གྱི་ཅོད་པན་འཛིན། |འོད་ཟེར་དཀར་པོ་འཕྲོ་བར་གྱུར། |དེ་ཡི་ཐུགས་ཀར་ཟླ་བའི་སྟེང་།

YIE ONG DAR GYI CHOE PEN DZIN   OE ZER KAR PO TR'O WAR GYUR   DE YI T'UK KAR DA WEI TENG

ཧྲཱིཿཡིག་དཀར་པོའི་འོད་ཟེར་གྱིས། པོ་ཏ་ལ་ནས་སྤྱན་རས་གཟིགས། འཁོར་དང་བཅས་པ་སྤྱན་དྲངས་གྱུར།

HRIH YIG KAR POI OE ZER GYI   PO TA LA NE CHEN RE ZIG   K'OR DANG CHE PA CHEN DRANG GYUR

I clearly appear in the aspect of the Noble Chenrezig,
With a white and youthful body and eleven faces.
The main face is white, the right green, and the left red.
Of the three faces immediately above,
The middle face is green, the right red, the left white.
Above these, the central face is red, the right white,
And the left green. These nine faces are peaceful.
Above them is a black and wrathful three-eyed face
Showing teeth and a gnarled brow.
On top is a peaceful red face, which has a protrusion
 Upon the crown and whose neck is unadorned.
Of the eight main hands, the first two are joined at the heart,
The second right hand holds a rosary, the third is in the gesture
Of Supreme Giving, and the fourth holds a wheel.
The second left hand holds a lotus, the third a golden vase,
And the fourth a bow and arrow.
The remaining nine hundred ninety-two hands
Are in the gesture of Supreme Giving with an eye in each palm.
He is adorned with precious jewels,
His left breast is completely covered by a deerskin,
And his robe is made from the cotton of Benares.
He wears a diadem adorned with ribbons.
Rays of white light spring from his body.
In the heart, upon a moon disk, is the white letter HRIH.
From the HRIH, *light radiates to the Potala,*
Inviting the Noble Chenrezig and his following.

ཨོཾ་བཛྲ་ཨཱཪྒྷཾ་ཨཱཿཧཱུྃ།
OM BEN ZRA AR GHAM AH HUNG

ཨོཾ་བཛྲ་པུཌྱ་ཨཱཿཧཱུྃ།
OM BEN ZRA PAD YAM AH HUNG

ཨོཾ་བཛྲ་པུཥྤེ་ཨཱཿཧཱུྃ།
OM BEN ZRA PUPE AH HUNG

ཨོཾ་བཛྲ་དྷུ་པེ་ཨཱཿཧཱུྃ།
OM BEN ZRA DHU PE AH HUNG

ཨོཾ་བཛྲ་ཨཱ་ལོ་ཀེ་ཨཱཿཧཱུྃ།
OM BEN ZRA A LO KE AH HUNG

ཨོཾ་བཛྲ་གནྡྷེ་ཨཱཿཧཱུྃ།
OM BEN ZRA GEN DHE AH HUNG

ཨོཾ་བཛྲ་ནེ་ཝི་དྱ་ཨཱཿཧཱུྃ།
OM BEN ZRA NE WI DYA AH HUNG

ཨོཾ་བཛྲ་ཤཔྟ་ཨཱཿཧཱུྃ།
OM BEN ZRA SHAP TA AH HUNG

།སྐྱོན་གྱིས་མ་གོས་སྐུ་མདོག་དཀར།
KYON GYI MA GO KU DOG KAR

།རྫོགས་སངས་རྒྱས་ཀྱིས་དབུ་ལ་བརྒྱན།
DZOK SANG GYE KYI U LA GYEN

།ཐུགས་རྗེའི་སྤྱན་གྱིས་འགྲོ་ལ་གཟིགས།
T'UK JEI CHEN GYI DRO LA ZIK

།སྤྱན་རས་གཟིགས་ལ་ཕྱག་འཚལ་ལོ།
CHEN RE ZIG LA CH'AG TS'AL LO

།ཛཿཧཱུྃ་བྃ་ཧོཿགཉིས་མེད་གྱུར།
DZA HUNG BAM HO NYI ME GYUR

།གནས་གསུམ་ཨོཾ་ཨཱཿཧཱུྃ་གིས་མཚན།
NE SUM OM AH HUNG GI TS'EN

།ལར་ཡང་ཧྲཱིཿལས་འོད་འཕྲོས་པས།
LAR YANG HRIH LE OE TR'O PE

།དབང་ལྷ་རིགས་ལྔ་འཁོར་བཅས་བྱོན།
WANG LHA RIK NGA K'OR CHE JON

།དེ་དག་རྣམས་ཀྱི་ཐུགས་ཀ་ནས།
DE DAG NAM KYI T'UK KA NE

།ཡེ་ཤེས་བདུད་རྩི་འཛིན་པ་ཡི།
YE SHE DUE TSI DZIN PA YI

།ཡུམ་ལྔ་འཕྲོས་ནས་བདག་ཉིད་ལ།
YUM NGA TR'O NE DAG NYIE LA

།མངོན་པར་དབང་བསྐུར་ཆུ་ཡི་ལྷག
NGON PAR WANG KUR CH'U YI LHAG

།སྤྱིང་དུ་ལུད་པས་སྤྱི་གཙུག་ཏུ།
TENG DU LUE PE CHI TSUG TU

།བླ་མའི་ངོ་བོ་འོད་དཔག་མེད།
LA MEI NGO WO OE PAG ME

།དཔལ་བར་མི་བསྐྱོད་རྣ་གཡས་སུ།
TRAL WAR MI KYOE NA YE SU

།རིན་འབྱུང་རྣ་གཡོན་དོན་གྲུབ་ཉིད།
RIN JUNG NA YON DON DRUB NYIE

།ཐེག་པར་རྣམ་པར་སྣང་མཛད་དེ།
TEG PAR NAM PAR NANG DZE DE

།རིགས་བདག་རྣམས་ཀྱིས་དབུ་བརྒྱན་གྱུར།
RIK DAG NAM KYI U GEN GYUR

།རང་གི་ཐུགས་ཀར་པད་ཟླའི།
RANG GI T'UK KAR PE DEI

སྟེང་། །ཡེ་ཤེས་སེམས་དཔའི་ངོ་བོ་ཉིད།
TENG   YE SHE SEM PEI NGO WO NYIE

།ཐུགས་རྗེ་ཆེན་པོ་ཚོན་གང་བ།
T'UK JE CH'EN PO TS'ON GANG WA

།དེ་ཡི་ཐུགས་ཀར་ཏིང་ངེ་འཛིན།
DE YI T'UK KAR TING NGE DZIN

།སེམས་དཔའ་ཧྲཱིཿཡིག་དཀར་པོ་ལས།
SEM PA HRIH YIG KAR PO LE

།འོད་འཕྲོས་འགྲོ་བའི་སྒྲིབ་སྦྱངས་ནས།
OE TR'O DRO WEI DRIB JANG NE

།ཐུགས་རྗེ་ཆེན་པོའི་སྐུར་གྱུར་པ།
T'UK JE CH'EN POI KUR GYUR PA

།ཚུར་འདུས་ཧྲཱིཿལ་ཐིམ་པར་གྱུར།
TS'UR DU HRIH LA T'IM PAR GYUR

OM BEN ZRA AR GHAM AH HUNG   OM BEN ZRA PAD YAM AH HUNG

OM BEN ZRA PUPE AH HUNG   OM BEN ZRA DHU PE AH HUNG

OM BEN ZRA A LO KE AH HUNG   OM BEN ZRA GEN DHE AH HUNG

OM BEN ZRA NE WI DYA AH HUNG   OM BEN ZRA SHAP TA AH HUNG

Lord with white body, not veiled by fault,

Whose head is adorned by a perfect buddha,

Who looks upon all beings with the eyes of compassion,

To you, Chenrezig, I pay homage.

We become undifferentiated.

At the three places are the syllables OM AH HUNG.

Again light radiates from the HRIH,

Causing the empowerment deities to come,

The Five Victorious Ones and their following.

From their hearts emanate the Five Feminine Aspects

Who possess the supreme nectar of knowledge,

Which they pour forth bestowing their power upon me.

The nectar overflows upon my head

And it becomes Amitabha, the essence of the Lama.

Above my forehead it becomes Akshobhya (blue); above the right ear,

Ratnasambhava (yellow); above the left ear, Amoghasiddhi (green);

And above the back of my head, Vairochana (white).

Thus I am crowned by the masters of the five lineages.

At the heart level, upon a lotus and moon disk,

The very essence of the deities of supreme knowledge appears,

The Great Compassionate One, the size of a thumb.

In his heart is the white letter HRIH,

Which is the entity of the state of absorption of the deity.

From it springs white light which purifies the obscurations of all beings,

And they become the Great Compassionate One.

They melt into light, which is absorbed back into the HRIH.

ན་མོ་རཏྣ་ཏྲ་ཡཱ་ཡ།

NA MO RAT NA TRA YA YA

ན་མ་ཨཱརྱ་ཡ་ཛྙཱན་ས་ག་ར་བེ་རོ་ཙ་ན་བ་ཡུ་ཧ་ར་ཛ་ཡ།

NA MA AR YA JNYA NA SA GA RA BE RO TSA NA BA YU HA RA DZA YA

ཏ་ཐཱ་ག་ཏ་ཡ།

TA THA GA TA YA

ཨརྷ་ཏེ་སམྱཀྶཾ་བུདྡྷ་ཡ།

AR HA TE SAM YAK SAM BUD DHA YA

ན་མ་སཪྦ་ཏ་ཐཱ་ག་ཏེ་བྷྱཿ

NA MA SAR VA TA THA GA TE BHE

ཨརྷ་ཏེ་བྷྱཿ

AR HA TE BHE

སམྱཀྶཾ་བུདྡྷེ་བྷྱཿ

SAM YAK SAM BUD DHE BHE

ན་མཿཨཱརྱ་ཨ་ཝ་ལོ་ཀི་ཏེ་ཤྭ་ར་ཡ།

NA MA AR YA A WA LO KI TE SHVA RA YA

བོ་དྷི་ས་ཏྭ་ཡ།

BO DHI SA TO YA

མ་ཧཱ་ས་ཏྭ་ཡ།

MA HA SA TO YA

མ་ཧཱ་ཀཱ་རུ་ཎི་ཀཱ་ཡ།

MA HA KA RU NI KA YA

ཏདྱཐཱ།

TA YA TA

ཨོཾ་དྷ་ར་དྷ་ར།

OM DHA RA DHA RA

དྷི་རི་དྷི་རི།

DHI RI DHI RI

དྷུ་རུ་དྷུ་རུ།

DHU RU DHU RU

ཨི་ཊེ་ཝི་ཊེ།

IT TE WIT TE

ཙ་ལེ་ཙ་ལེ།

TSA LE TSA LE

ཏྲ་ཙ་ལེ་ཏྲ་ཙ་ལེ།

TRA TSA LE TRA TSA LE

ཀུ་སུ་མེ་ཀུ་སུ་མ་ཝ་རེ།

KU SU ME KU SU MA WA RE

ཨི་ལི་མི་ལི་ཙི་ཏི་ཛྫོ་ལ་མ་པ་ན་ཡ་སྭཱ་ཧཱ།

I LI MI LI TSI TI DZO LA MA PA NA YA SO HA

།གཟུངས་རིང་ཆར་གཅིག་གིས་དུངས་པའི་གཟུངས་ཐུང་བཅུ་རྩ་བཅུད།

ཨོཾ་མ་ཎི་པདྨེ་ཧཱུྂ།

OM MANI PEME HUNG

།ཡིག་དྲུག་ཅི་ནུས་བཟླ། ། དེ་ནས་མདུན་བསྐྱེད་ནི།

Generating the Deity, Frontal Visualization

ཨོཾ་ཧ་ཡ་གྲཱི་ཝ་ཧཱུྂ་ཕཊ།

OM HA YA GRI WA HUNG PE

ཨོཾ་སྭ་བྷཱ་ཝ་ཤུདྡྷཿ

OM SVA BHA WA SHUD DHA

སཪྦ་དྷརྨཿ

SAR VA DHAR MA

སྭ་བྷཱ་ཝ་ཤུདྡྷོ྅ཧཾ།

SVA BHA WA SHUD DHO HAM

།ཆོས་རྣམས་ཐམས་ཅད་སྟོང་པར་གྱུར།

CH'O NAM T'AM CHE TONG PAR GYUR

།དེ་ཡི་ངང་ལས་རང་ཉིད་ཀྱི།

DE YI NGANG LE RANG NYIE KYI

།ཐུགས་ཀའི་ཧྲཱིཿལས་ཀྲུྂ་ཡིག་ནི།

T'UK KEI HRIH LE DRUM YIG NI

།མདུན་དུ་འཕྲོས་ནས་ཤུ་བ་ལས།

DUN DU TR'O NE SH'U WA LE

།རིན་ཆེན་ལས་གྲུབ་གཞལ་ཡས་ཁང་།

RIN CH'EN LE DRUB SH'AL YE K'ANG

།གྲུ་བཞིའི་སྒོ་བཞི་ལྡན་པའི་དབུས།

DRU SH'I GO SH'I DEN PEI UE

།རིན་ཆེན་ཁྲི་དང་ཟླ་བའི་སྟེང་།

RIN CH'EN TR'I DANG DA WEI TENG

།སྣ་ཚོགས་པདྨ་འདབ་བརྒྱད་ཀྱི།

NA TS'OK PE MA DAB GYE KYI

།ལྟེ་བར་ཧྲཱིཿལས་རང་འདྲ་བའི།

TE WAR HRIH LE RANG DRA WEI

།ཐུགས་རྗེ་ཆེན་པོའི་རྣམ་པར་གསལ།

T'UK JE CH'EN POI NAM PAR SAL

།ཤར་དུ་ཧཱུྂ་ལས་མི་བསྐྱོད་པ།

SHAR DU HUNG LE MI KYO PA

།སྔོན་པོ་ས་གནོན་ཕྱག་རྒྱ་ཅན།

NGON PO SA NON CH'AG GYA CHEN

I bow to the Three Jewels.
I bow to the ocean of the Arya's exalted wisdom,
the king of marvelous manifestations of Vairochana,
the thus gone, foe destroyer, perfectly completed Buddha.
I bow to all the thus gone, foe destroyer, perfectly completed buddhas.
I bow to Arya Avalokiteshvara, the bodhisattva,
the great heroic being endowed with great perfection.
It is thus: OM, *(you) will hold, will hold; do hold, do hold; hold, hold!*
(I) request power; move, move! Thoroughly move, thoroughly move!
(You) hold a flower, hold an offering flower; method and wisdom, supreme guru;
Burned with mind, may it be removed; arrange it![2]

Recite the entire long mantra once, then from TAYATA 108 times.
(Should be recited in Sanskrit.)
Recite the six-syllable mantra as many times as you can: OM MANI PEME HUNG

Generating the Deity, Frontal Visualization

OM HA YA GRI WA HUNG PE   OM SVA BHA WA SHUD DHA

SAR VA DHAR MA   SVA BHA WA SHUD DHO HAM

All appearance becomes emptiness.
Within that state, from the HRIH *in one's heart*
The letter DRUM *emanates and melts into light*
And becomes a superb jeweled palace in front of us.
It is square and has four doors. In the center stands a jeweled throne
With a multicolored, eight-petaled lotus and moon disk upon it.
From the HRIH *in the center of the moon disk*
The Great Compassionate One appears,
Completely bright and clear and resembling oneself.
In the east, from the syllable HUNG *Akshobhya appears,*
Who is blue in color, in the earth-touching gesture.

---

2 Long dharani translated by Lama Zopa Rinpoche, *Nyung Nä,* www.fpmt.org.

|ཀློ་རུ་ཏྲཾ་ལས་རིན་འབྱུང་ནི། |སེར་པོ་མཆོག་སྦྱིན་ཕྱག་རྒྱ་ཅན། |ནུབ་ཏུ་ཨོཾ་ལས་རྣམ་སྣང་མཛད།

LHO RU TRAM LE RIN JUNG NI   SER PO CH'OG JIN CH'AG GYA CHEN   NUB TU OM LE NAM NANG DZE

|དཀར་པོ་བྱང་ཆུབ་མཆོག་གི་ཚུལ། |བྱང་དུ་ཨཱཿལས་དོན་གྲུབ་ནི། |སྐྱང་གུ་སྐྱབས་སྦྱིན་ཕྱག་རྒྱ་ཅན།

KAR PO JANG CH'UB CH'OG GI TS'UL   JANG DU AH LE DON DRUB NI   JANG GU KYAB CHIN CH'AG GYA CHEN

|སངས་རྒྱས་མཆོག་གི་སྤྲུལ་སྐུའི་ཚུལ། |གནས་གསུམ་ཨོཾ་ཨཱཿ་ཧཱུྃ་གཉིས་ལས། |ཡེ་ཤེས་སེམས་དཔའ་སྤྱན་དྲངས་ཐིམ།

SANG GYE CH'OG GI TRUL KUI TS'UL   NE SUM OM AH HUNG NYIE LE   YE SHE SEM PA CHEN DRANG T'IM

|ཛཿཧཱུྃ་བྃ་ཧོཿགཉིས་མེད་གྱུར། |ལར་ཡང་ཧྲཱིཿལས་འོད་འཕྲོས་པས། |དབང་ལྷ་ཆེན་དྲངས་དབང་བསྐུར་ཏེ།

DZA HUNG BAM HO NYI ME GYUR   LAR YANG HRIH LE OE TR'O PE   WANG LHA CHEN DRANG WANG KUR TE

|ཆུ་ཞབས་ཡར་ལུད་གཙོ་བོ་ལ། |འོད་དཔག་མེད་དང་རིགས་བཞི་པོར། |སོ་སོའི་རིགས་ཀྱི་དབུ་རྒྱན་གྱུར།

CH'U SH'AB YAR LUE TSO WO LA   OE PAG ME DANG RIK SH'I POR   SO SOI RIK KYI U GYEN GYUR

|བདག་དང་མདུན་དུ་བཞུགས་པ་ཡི། |ཐུགས་རྗེ་ཆེན་པོའི་ཕྱག་སོར་ལས། |ཡེ་ཤེས་བདུད་རྩིའི་རྒྱུན་བབས་པས།

DAG DANG DUN DU SH'UK PA YI   T'UK JE CH'EN POI CH'AG SOR LE   YE SHE DUE TSII GYUN BAB PE

|བུམ་གང་ཡི་དྭགས་ཀུན་ཚིམ་གྱུར། |ན་མོ་རཏྣ་ཏྲ་ཡ་ཡ།   ན་མ་ཨཱཪྻ་ཛྙཱ་ན

BUM GANG YI DAG KUN TS'IM GYUR   NA MO RAT NA TRA YA YA   NA MA AR YA JNYA NA

ས་ག་ར་བཻ་རོ་ཙན་བྱུ་ཧ་རཱ་ཛ་ཡ།   ཏ་ཐཱ་ག་ཏ་ཡ།   ཨརྷ་ཏེ་སམྱཀྶཾ་བུདྡྷ་ཡ།

SA GA RA BE RO TSA NA BA YU HA RA DZA YA   TA THA GA TA YA   AR HA TE SAM YAK SAM BUD DHA YA

ན་མཿསཪྦ་ཏ་ཐཱ་ག་ཏེ་བྷྱཿ   ཨརྷ་ཏེ་བྷྱཿ   སམྱཀྶཾ་བུདྡྷེ་བྷྱཿ   ན་མ་ཨཱཪྻ་ཨ་ཝ་ལོ་ཀི་ཏེ

NA MA SAR VA TA THA GA TE BHE   AR HA TE BHE   SAM YAK SAM BUD DHE BHE   NA MA AR YA A WA LO KI TE

ཤྭ་ར་ཡ།   བོ་དྷི་ས་ཏོ་ཡ།   མ་ཧཱ་ས་ཏོ་ཡ།   མ་ཧཱ་ཀཱ་རུ་ཎི་ཀཱ་ཡ།   ཏ་དྱ་ཐཱ།   ཨོཾ་དྷ་ར་དྷ་ར།

SHVA RA YA   BOD HI SA TO YA   MA HA SA TO YA   MA HA KA RU NI KA YA   TA YA TA   OM DHA RA DHA RA

དྷི་རི་དྷི་རི།   དྷུ་རུ་དྷུ་རུ།   ཨི་ཊི་ཝི་ཊི།   ཙ་ལེ་ཙ་ལེ།   ཏྲ་ཙ་ལེ་ཏྲ་ཙ་ལེ།   ཀུ་སུ་མེ་ཀུ་སུ་མ་ཝ་རེ།

DHI RI DHI RI   DHU RU DHU RU   IT TI WIT TE   TSA LE TSA LE   TRA TSA LE TRA TSA LE   KU SU ME KU SU MA WA RE

ཨི་ལི་མི་ལི་ཙི་ཏི་ཛྫོ་ལ་མ་པ་ན་ཡ་སྭཱ་ཧཱ། |ཅེས་གཟུངས་རིང་བཀྲུ་བཀྲུ་དང་ཡིག་དྲུག་ཅི་ནུས་བཟླ།   ཨོཾ་མ་ཎི་པདྨེ་ཧཱུྃ།

I LI MI LI TSI TI DZO LA MA PA NA YA SO HA   OM MANI PEME HUNG

|དེ་ནས་བདག་གི་ཡེ་ཤེས་པ། |མདུན་གྱི་གཙོ་བོར་ཐིམ་པར་གྱུར།

DE NE DAG GI YE SHE PA   DUN GYI TSO WOR T'IM PAR GYUR

In the south, from the syllable TRAM *Ratnasambhava appears,*

Who is yellow in color and in the gesture of supreme giving.

In the west, from the syllable OM *Vairochana appears,*

Who is white in color and in the gesture of sublime awakening.

In the north, from the syllable AH *Amoghasiddhi appears,*

Who is green in color and in the gesture of giving refuge.

All of them have the aspect of Buddha's sublime emanation.

From the syllables OM AH HUNG *in their respective places*

The deities of supreme knowledge are invoked. DZA HUNG BAM HO.

Again from the HRIH *light radiates, inviting the deities of empowerment,*

Who bestow their powers with the vase of nectar.

The nectar overflows forming the diadem

Adorning the heads of the main deity, Amitabha Buddha, and

The four other victorious ones, placed according to their lineages.

From my fingers and those of the Great Compassionate One in front of me

The nectar of supreme knowledge flows.

It fills the vase and, by flowing towards the hungry ghosts, it satisfies them

Recite the long mantra 108 times:

NA MO RAT NA TRA YA YA   NA MA AR YA JNYA NA   SA GA RA BE RO TSA NA
BA YU HA RA DZA YA   TA THA GA TA YA   AR HA TE   SAM YAK SAM BUD DHA YA
NA MA SARVA TA THA GA TE BHE   AR HA TE BHE   SAM YAK SAM BUD DHE BHE
NA MA AR YA   A WA LO KI TE SHVA RA YA   BO DHI SA TO YA   MA HA SA TO YA
MA HA KA RU NI KA YA   TA YA TA   OM DHA RA DHA RA   DHI RI DHI RI
DHU RU DHU RU   IT TE WIT TE   TSA LE TSA LE   TRA TSA LE TRA TSA LE
KU SU ME KU SU MA WA RE   I LI MI LI TSI TI DZO LA MA PA NA YA SO HA

Recite the six-syllable mantra as many times as possible: OM MANI PEME HUNG

Then the deity, entity of Supreme Knowledge at the level of my heart,

dissolves into the central Chenrezig in front of me.

Seven-Branch Prayer

།དེ་ནས་ཡན་ལག་བདུན་པ་འབུལ་བ་ནི་ཕྱག་འཚལ་བའི་གནངས་བཅས། ༎དཀོན་མཆོག་གསུམ་ལ་ཕྱག་འཚལ་ལོ།
KON CH'OG SUM LA CH'AG TS'AL LO

ན་མོ་མཉྫུ་ཤྲི་ཡེ། ན་མོ་སུ་ཤྲི་ཡེ། ན་མོ་ཨུཏྟ་མ་ཤྲི་ཡེ་སྭཱ་ཧཱ། །སངས་རྒྱས་ཐམས་ཅད་འདུས་པའི་སྐུ།
NAMO MANJUSHRIYE NAMO SU SHRIYE NAMO UTTAMA SHRIYE SOHA SANG GYE T'AM CHE DU PEI KU

།རྡོ་རྗེ་འཛིན་པའི་ངོ་བོ་ཉིད། །དཀོན་མཆོག་གསུམ་གྱི་རྩ་བ་སྟེ། །བླ་མ་རྣམས་ལ་ཕྱག་འཚལ་ལོ། །དུས་གསུམ
DOR JE DZIN PEI NGO WO NYIE KON CH'OG SUM GYI TSA WA TE LA MA NAM LA CH'AG TS'AL LO DU SUM

བདེ་བར་གཤེགས་པ་ཆོས་ཀྱི་སྐུ། །འགྲོ་དྲུག་སེམས་ཅན་རྣམས་ལ་སྤྱན་རས་གཟིགས། །ནམ་མཁའ་ལྟ་བུར་ཁྱབ
DE WAR SHEK PA CH'O KYI KU DRO DRUG SEM CHEN NAM LA CHEN RE ZIG NAM K'A TA BUR KY'AB

པའི་བཅུ་གཅིག་ཞལ། །གཟི་བརྗིད་འོད་དཔག་མེད་ལ་ཕྱག་འཚལ་ལོ། །ཕྱག་སྟོང་འཁོར་ལོས་སྒྱུར་བའི་རྒྱལ་པོ།
PEI CHU CHIG SH'AL ZI JIE OE PAG ME LA CH'AG TS'AL LO CH'AG TONG K'OR LO GYUR WEI GYAL PO

སྟོང༌། །སྤྱན་སྟོང་བསྐལ་པ་བཟང་པོའི་སངས་རྒྱས་སྟོང༌། །གང་ལ་གང་འདུལ་དེ་ལ་དེར་སྟོན་པའི། །བཙུན་པ
TONG CHEN TONG KAL PA ZANG POI SANG GYE TONG GANG LA GANG DUL DE LA DER TON PEI TSUN PA

སྤྱན་རས་གཟིགས་ལ་ཕྱག་འཚལ་ལོ། །ཆོས་སྐུ་རྣམ་མཁའ་བཞིན་དུ་དབྱེར་མེད་ཀྱང༌། །གཟུགས་སྐུ་ཇ་ཚོན་བཞིན
CHEN RE ZIG LA CH'AG TS'AL LO CH'O KU NAM K'A SH'IN DU JER ME KYANG ZUK KU JA TS'ON SH'IN

དུ་སོ་སོར་གསལ། །ཐབས་དང་ཤེས་རབ་མཆོག་ལ་མངའ་བརྙེས་པ། །རིགས་ལྔ་བདེ་བར་གཤེགས་ལ་ཕྱག་འཚལ་ལོ།
DU SO SOR SAL T'AB DANG SHE RAB CH'OG LA NGA NYE PA RIK NGA DE WAR SHEK LA CH'AG TS'AL LO

།མཁའ་ལྟར་ཁྱབ་པའི་རྒྱལ་བ་སྲས་བཅས་ལ། །བདག་དང་མཁའ་མཉམ་འགྲོ་བ་མ་ལུས་པས། །ལུས་འདི་ཞིང་དུལ
K'A TAR KY'AB PEI GYAL WA SE CHE LA DAG DANG K'A NYAM DRO WA MA LU PE LU DI SH'ING DUL

མཉམ་པར་རབ་སྤྲུལ་ནས། །རྟག་ཏུ་གུས་པའི་ཡིད་ཀྱིས་ཕྱག་འཚལ་ལོ།
NYAM PAR RAB TRUL NE TAG TU GU PEI YIE KYI CH'AG TS'AL LO

།བདག་གི་སྙིང་ཁའི་ས་བོན་ལས། །འཕྲོས་པའི་མེ་ཏོག་བདུག་སྤོས་དང༌། །མར་མེ་དྲི་ཆབ་ཞལ་ཟས་སོགས།
DAG GI NYING K'EI SA BON LE TR'O PEI ME TOG DUG PO DANG MAR ME DRI CH'AB SH'AL ZE SOK

།འཛིན་པའི་ལྷ་མོ་རྣམས་ཀྱིས་མཆོད།
DZIN PEI LHA MO NAM KYI CH'OE

Seven-Branch Prayer

We offer the Seven-Branch Prayer and make prostrations while reciting the mantra, which causes the prostrations to be one hundred times more powerful.

I prostrate in front of the Three Rare and Sublime Ones.

NAMO MANJUSHRIYE   NAMO SU SHRIYE   NAMO UTTAMA SHRIYE SOHA

I prostrate in front of the Lama,

Who is the root of the Three Rare and Sublime Ones,

The essence of Dorje Chang, the united body of all the buddhas.

I prostrate before Amitabha, the Buddha of Infinite Light,

The body of emptiness of all those who have gone to bliss in the three times.

For the benefit of all beings in the three worlds

He appears as the Eleven-Faced Chenrezig, omnipresent as space.

I prostrate in front of the Venerable Chenrezig,

Whose thousand eyes are the thousand buddhas of the virtuous eons,

Whose thousand arms are the thousand great kings, holders of the wheel;

Who shows the appropriate means to tame each and every being.

I prostrate before the victorious ones of the five lineages,

They who have gone to bliss.

I prostrate before the masters of sublime transcendental knowledge

And liberating means, who even though indivisible,

The body of voidness similar to space,

Manifest distinctly in the two formal bodies,

As rainbow colors are differentiated from the sky.

I and all beings whose number is as limitless as space

Give praise to all the buddhas and their sons,

Whose assembly is as vast as space,

By mentally prostrating with a mind continually full of respect,

And with as many emanations as there are particles in all the worlds.

From the syllable in my heart, goddesses emanate carrying flowers,

Incense, light, perfumes, food, and music, and they make offerings.

ༀ་བཛྲ་པུཥྤེ་ཨཱཿཧཱུྃ།

OM BEN ZRA PUPE AH HUNG

ༀ་བཛྲ་དྷུ་པེ་ཨཱཿཧཱུྃ།

OM BEN ZRA DHU PE AH HUNG

ༀ་བཛྲ་ཨཱ་ལོ་ཀེ་ཨཱཿཧཱུྃ།

OM BEN ZRA A LO KE AH HUNG

ༀ་བཛྲ་གནྡྷེ་ཨཱཿཧཱུྃ།

OM BEN ZRA GEN DHE AH HUNG

ༀ་བཛྲ་ནེ་ཝི་དྱ་ཨཱཿཧཱུྃ།

OM BEN ZRA NE WI DYA AH HUNG

ༀ་བཛྲ་ཤཔྟ་ཨཱཿཧཱུྃ།

OM BEN ZRA SHAP TA AH HUNG

ཇི་སྙེད་སུ་དག་ཕྱོགས་བཅུ་འཇིག་རྟེན་ན།

JI NYE SU DAG CH'OK CHU JIG TEN NA

དུས་གསུམ་གཤེགས་པ་མི་ཡི་སེངྒེ་ཀུན།

DU SUM SHEK PA MI YI SENG GE KUN

བདག་གིས་མ་ལུས་དེ།

DAG GIE MA LU DE

དག་ཐམས་ཅད་ལ།

DAG T'AM CHE LA

ལུས་དང་ངག་ཡིད་དང་བས་ཕྱག་བགྱིའོ།

LU DANG NGAG YIE DANG WE CH'AG GYI-O

བཟང་པོ་སྤྱོད་པའི་སྨོན་ལམ་སྟོབས་དག་གིས།

ZANG PO CHOE PEI MON LAM TOB DAG GI

རྒྱལ་བ་ཐམས་ཅད་ཡིད་ཀྱིས་མངོན་སུམ་དུ།

GYAL WA T'AM CHE YIE KYI NGON SUM DU

ཞིང་གི་རྡུལ་སྙེད་ལུས་རབ་བཏུད་པ་ཡིས།

SH'ING GI DUL NYE LU RAB TUE PA YI

རྒྱལ་བ་ཀུན་ལ།

GYAL WA KUN LA

རབ་ཏུ་ཕྱག་འཚལ་ལོ།

RAB TU CH'AG TS'AL LO

རྡུལ་གཅིག་སྟེང་ན་རྡུལ་སྙེད་སངས་རྒྱས་རྣམས།

DUL CHIG TENG NA DUL NYE SANG GYE NAM

སངས་རྒྱས་སྲས་ཀྱི་དབུས་ན།

SANG GYE SE KYI UE NA

བཞུགས་པ་དག

SH'UK PA DAG

དེ་ལྟར་ཆོས་ཀྱི་དབྱིངས་རྣམས་མ་ལུས་པར།

DE TAR CH'O KYI JING NAM MA LU PAR

ཐམས་ཅད་རྒྱལ་བ་དག་གིས་གང་བར་མོས།

T'AM CHE GYAL WA DAG GI GANG WAR MO

དེ་དག་བསྔགས་པ་མི་ཟད་རྒྱ་མཚོ་རྣམས།

DE DAG NGAK PA MI ZE GYA TS'O NAM

དབྱངས་ཀྱི་ཡན་ལག་རྒྱ་མཚོའི་སྒྲ་ཀུན་གྱིས།

JANG KYI YEN LAG GYA TS'OI DRA KUN GYI

རྒྱལ་བ་ཀུན་གྱི་ཡོན།

GYAL WA KUN GYI YON

ཏན་རབ་བརྗོད་ཅིང་།

TEN RAB JOE CHING

བདེ་བར་གཤེགས་པ་ཐམས་ཅད་བདག་གིས་བསྟོད།

DE WAR SHEK PA T'AM CHE DAG GI TOE

མེ་ཏོག་དམ་པ་ཕྲེང་བ་དམ་པ།

ME TOG DAM PA T'RENG WA DAM PA

དང་།

DANG

སིལ་སྙན་རྣམས་དང་བྱུག་པའི་གདུགས་མཆོག་དང་།

SIL NYEN NAM DANG JUG PEI DUK CH'OG DANG

མར་མེ་མཆོག་དང་བདུག་སྤོས་དམ་པ་ཡིས།

MAR ME CH'OG DANG DUG PO DAM PA YI

རྒྱལ་བ་དེ་དག་ལ་ནི་མཆོད་པར་བགྱི།

GYAL WA DE DAG LA NI CH'OE PAR GYI

ན་བཟའ་དམ་པ་རྣམས་དང་དྲི་མཆོག་དང་།

NA ZA DAM PA NAM DANG DRI CH'OG DANG

ཕྱེ་མའི་ཕུར་མ་རི།

CH'E MEI P'UR MA RI

རབ་མཉམ་པ་དང་།

RAB NYAM PA DANG

བཀོད་པ་ཁྱད་པར་འཕགས་པའི་མཆོག་ཀུན་གྱིས།

KOE PA KY'E PAR P'AK PEI CH'OG KUN GYI

རྒྱལ་བ་དེ་དག་ལ་ཡང་མཆོད།

GYAL WA DE DAG LA YANG CH'OE

པར་བགྱི།

PAR GYI

མཆོད་པ་གང་རྣམས་བླ་མེད་རྒྱ་ཆེ་བ།

CH'OE PA GANG NAM LA ME GYA CH'E WA

དེ་དག་རྒྱལ་བ་ཐམས་ཅད་ལ་ཡང་མོས།

DE DAG GYAL WA T'AM CHE LA YANG MO

བཟང་པོ།

ZANG PO

OM BEN ZRA PUPE AH HUNG   OM BEN ZRA DHU PE AH HUNG
OM BEN ZRA A LO KE AH HUNG   OM BEN ZRA GEN DHE AH HUNG
OM BEN ZRA NE WI DYA AH HUNG   OM BEN ZRA SHAP TA AH HUNG

With my voice and body and sincere heart,
I pay homage to all the lions of humanity
Present throughout all time and in all world systems
In every direction with none excepted,
However great their number.
The force of my resolve to practice excellence
Brings all victors clearly to mind;
Emanations of my body,
Numerous as the atoms of all universes,
Bow down in perfect obeisance before them.
All buddhas, numerous as the atoms of all buddha realms,
Stand in a single atom, surrounded by their children.
Similarly, this host of victors stands in every single atom
Throughout the realm of totality.
To them I direct my devotion and faith.
Sounds from an ocean of instruments of melodious speech
Sing of the qualities of all the victors;
The ocean of their qualities is never depleted.
In this way, I praise all the well-gone ones.
To all the victors I present and offer
Perfect flowers and holy garlands, sweet music,
Balms and parasols, oil lamps, and fragrant incense.
Moreover, I offer to all the victors elegant garments
And the finest of scents, powders piled high as Mt. Meru,
All displayed in exceptional splendor.
Vast and unsurpassable offerings
I create and present to all the victors.

སྤྱོད་ལ་དད་པའི་སྟོབས་དག་གིས། །རྒྱལ་བ་ཀུན་ལ་ཕྱག་འཚལ་མཆོད་པར་བགྱི། །འདོད་ཆགས་ཞེ་སྡང་གཏི་མུག་
CHOE LA DAD PEI TOB DAG GI GYAL WA KUN LA CH'AG TS'AL CH'OE PAR GYI DOE CH'AK SH'E DANG TI MUG

དབང་གིས་ནི། །ལུས་དང་ངག་དང་དེ་བཞིན་ཡིད་ཀྱིས་ཀྱང་། །སྡིག་པ་བདག་གིས་བགྱིས་པ་ཅི་མཆིས་པ། །དེ་དག་
WANG GI NI LU DANG NGAG DANG DE SH'IN YIE KYI KYANG DIG PA DAG GI GYI PA CHI CH'I PA DE DAG

ཐམས་ཅད་བདག་གིས་སོ་སོར་བཤགས། །ཕྱོགས་བཅུའི་རྒྱལ་བ་ཀུན་དང་སངས་རྒྱས་སྲས། །རང་རྒྱལ་རྣམས་དང་
T'AM CHE DAG GI SO SOR SHAK CH'OK CHUI GYAL WA KUN DANG SANG GYE SE RANG GYAL NAM DANG

སློབ་དང་མི་སློབ་དང་། །འགྲོ་བ་ཀུན་གྱི་བསོད་ནམས་གང་ལ་ཡང་། །དེ་དག་ཀུན་གྱི་རྗེས་སུ་བདག་ཡི་རང་།
LOB DANG MI LOB DANG DRO WA KUN GYI SOE NAM GANG LA YANG DE DAD KUN GYI JE SU DAG YI RANG

།གང་རྣམས་ཕྱོགས་བཅུའི་འཇིག་རྟེན་སྒྲོན་མ་དག། །བྱང་ཆུབ་རིམ་པར་སངས་རྒྱས་མ་ཆགས་བརྙེས། །མགོན་པོ་དེ་
GANG NAM CH'OK CHUI JIG TEN DRON MA DAG JANG CHUB RIM PAR SANG GYE MA CH'AK NYE GON PO DE

དག་བདག་གི་ཐམས་ཅད་ལ། །འཁོར་ལོ་བླ་ན་མེད་པར་བསྐོར་བར་བསྐུལ། །མྱ་ངན་འདའ་སྟོན་གང་བཞེད་དེ་དག་ལ།
DAG DAG GI T'AM CHE LA K'OR LO LA NA ME PAR KOR WAR KUL NYA NGEN DA TON GANG SH'E DE DAG LA

།འགྲོ་བ་ཀུན་ལ་ཕན་ཞིང་བདེ་བའི་ཕྱིར། །བསྐལ་པ་ཞིང་གི་རྡུལ་སྙེད་བཞུགས་པར་ཡང་། །བདག་གིས་ཐལ་མོ་རབ་
DRO WA KUN LA P'EN SH'ING DE WEI CH'IR KAL PA SH'ING GI DUL NYE SH'UK PAR YANG DAG GI T'AL MO RAB

སྦྱར་གསོལ་བར་བགྱི། །ཕྱག་འཚལ་བ་དང་མཆོད་ཅིང་བཤགས་པ་དང་། །རྗེས་སུ་ཡི་རང་བསྐུལ་ཞིང་གསོལ་བ་ཡི།
JAR SOL WAR GYI CH'AG TS'AL WA DANG CH'OE CHING SHAK PA DANG JE SU YI RANG KUL SH'ING SOL WA YI

།དགེ་བ་ཅུང་ཟད་བདག་གིས་ཅི་བསགས་པ། །ཐམས་ཅད་བདག་གིས་བྱང་ཆུབ་ཕྱིར་བསྔོའོ།
GE WA CHUNG ZE DAG GI CHI SAK PA T'AM CHE DAG GI JANG CH'UB CH'IR NGO-O

།མཎྜལ་ནི།

Mandala Offering

ཨོཾ་བཛྲ་ས་ཏྭ་ས་མ་ཡ། མ་ནུ་པཱ་ལ་ཡ། བཛྲ་ས་ཏྭ་ཏྭེ་ནོ་པ་ཏིཥྛ་དྲི་ཌྷོ་མེ་བྷ་ཝ།
OM BEN ZRA SA TO SA MA YA MA NU PA LA YA BEN ZRA SA TO TE NO PA TI TA DRI DO ME BA WA

སུ་ཏོ་ཥྱོ་མེ་བྷ་ཝ། སུ་པོ་ཥྱོ་མེ་བྷ་ཝ། ཨ་ནུ་རཀྟོ་མེ་བྷ་ཝ། སརྦ་སིདྡྷི་མྨེ་པྲ་ཡཙྪ།
SU TO KOY YO ME BA WA SU PO KOY YO ME BA WA AH NU RAK TO ME BA WA SAR WA SID DHI ME TRA YA TSA

སརྦ་ཀརྨ་སུ་ཙ་མེ་ཙིཏྟཾ་ཤྲི་ཡཿ ཀུ་རུ་ཧཱུྃ་ཧ་ཧ་ཧ་ཧ་ཧོཿ བྷ་ག་ཝཱན།
SAR WA KAR MA SU TSA ME TSI TANG SHIRI YA KU RU HUNG HA HA HA HA HO BAN GA WEN

With a firm appreciation of the practice of excellence,
I render homage and offerings to all the victors.
Overpowered by lust, hatred, and stupidity,
I have perpetrated much evil through my actions, words,
And also in my thoughts; all such evils I confess completely.
With great joy I think of all the merit
Gathered by the victors in all directions, the Buddha's children,
And by the self-realized and partly and thoroughly trained ones.
I rejoice in the merit of all sentient beings.
I urge that the unsurpassable dharma wheel be set in motion
By all the lords, the lights of all worlds in all directions,
Who have traversed the stages of enlightenment
And attained buddhahood,
The state of nonattachment and pure awareness.
With my hands folded in prayer,
I beseech those who have transcended misery,
Whatever be their concern,
To abide for as many eons as there are atoms in all realms,
For the benefit and happiness of beings.
I dedicate to perfect enlightenment all virtue, however slight,
Which I have gathered through homage, offerings,
Confession, rejoicing, entreaty, and supplications.

Mandala Offering

OM BEN ZRA SA TO SA MA YA   MA NU PA LA YA

BEN ZRA SA TO TE NO PA   TI TA DRI DO ME BA WA

SU TO KOY YO ME BA WA   SU PO KOY YO ME BA WA

AH NU RAK TO ME BA WA   SAR WA SID DHI ME TRA YA TSA

SAR WA KAR MA SU TSA ME   TSI TANG SHIRI YA

KU RU HUNG HA HA HA HA HO   BAN GA WEN

སརྦ་ཏ་ཐཱ་ག་ཏ།　　བཛྲ་མུ་མེ་སྨུཉྩ　　བཛྲ་བྷ་བ　　མ་ཧཱ་ས་མ་ཡ་ས་ཏོ་ཨཱཿ

SAR WA TA TA GA TA　　BEN ZRA MA ME MUN TSA　　BEN ZRA BA WA　　MA HA SA MA YA SA TO AH

ༀ་བཛྲ་བྷཱུ་མི་ཨཱཿཧཱུྃ　　　གཞི་རྣམ་པར་དག་པ་དབང་ཆེན་གསེར་གྱི་ས་གཞི།　　　ༀ་བཛྲ་རེ་ཁེ་ཨཱཿཧཱུྃ

OM BEN ZRA BHU MI AH HUNG　　SH'I NAM PAR DAG PA WANG CH'EN SER GYI SA SH'I　　OM BEN ZRA REKE AH HUNG

ཕྱི་ལྕགས་རིའི་འཁོར་ཡུག་གི་ར་བས་ཡོངས་སུ་བསྐོར་བའི་དབུས་སུ་རིའི་རྒྱལ་པོ་རི་བོ་མཆོག་རབ།　　ཤར་ལུས་འཕགས

CH'I CHAK RII K'OR YUG GI RA WE YONG SU KOR WEI UE SU RII GYAL PO RI WO CH'OG RAB　　SHAR LU P'AK

པོ།　ཊློ་ཛཱུ་བུ་གླིང་།　ནུབ་བ་ལང་སྤྱོད།　བྱང་སྒྲ་མི་སྙན།　ལུས་དང་ལུས་འཕགས།　ཇ་ཡབ་དང་

PO　LHO DZAM BU LING　NUB BA LANG CHOE　JANG DRA MI NYEN　LU DANG LU P'AK　NGA YAB DANG

ཇ་ཡབ་གཞན།　ཡོ་ལྡན་དང་ལམ་མཆོག་འགྲོ།　སྒྲ་མི་སྙན་དང་སྒྲ་མི་སྙན་གྱི་ཟླ　　རིན་པོ་ཆེའི་རི་བོ།

NGA YAB SH'EN　YO DEN DANG LAM CH'OG DRO　DRA MI NYEN DANG DRA MI NYEN GYI DA　RIN PO CH'EI RI WO

དཔག་བསམ་གྱི་ཤིང་།　འདོད་འཇོའི་བ།　མ་མོས་པའི་ལོ་ཏོག　འཁོར་ལོ་རིན་པོ་ཆེ　ནོར་བུ་རིན་པོ་ཆེ

PAG SAM GYI SHING　DOE JOI BA　MA MO PEI LO TOG　K'OR LO RIN PO CH'E　NOR BU RIN PO CH'E

བཙུན་མོ་རིན་པོ་ཆེ　བློན་པོ་རིན་པོ་ཆེ　གླང་པོ་རིན་པོ་ཆེ　རྟ་མཆོག་རིན་པོ་ཆེ　དམག་དཔོན་རིན་པོ་ཆེ

TSUN MO RIN PO CH'E　LON PO RIN PO CH'E　LANG PO RIN PO CH'E　TA CH'OG RIN PO CH'E　MAG PON RIN PO CH'E

གཏེར་ཆེན་པོའི་བུམ་པ།　སྒེག་མོ་མ།　ཕྲེང་བ་མ།　གླུ་མ།　གར་མ།　མེ་ཏོག་མ།　བདུག་སྤོས་མ།

TER CH'EN POI BUM PA　GEG MO MA　T'RENG WA MA　LU MA　GAR MA　ME TOG MA　DUG PO MA

སྣང་གསལ་མ།　དྲི་ཆབ་མ།　ཉི་མ།　ཟླ་བ།　རིན་པོ་ཆེའི་གདུགས།　ཕྱོགས་ལས་རྣམ་པར་རྒྱལ་བའི་རྒྱལ་མཚན།

NANG SAL MA　DRI CH'AB MA　NYI MA　DA WA　RIN PO CH'EI DUK　CH'OK LE NAM PAR GYAL WEI GYAL TS'EN

དབུས་སུ་ལྷ་དང་མིའི་དཔལ་འབྱོར་ཕུན་སུམ་ཚོགས་པ་མ་ཚང་བ་མེད་པ　　རབ་འབྱམས་རྒྱ་མཚོའི་དུལ་གྱི་གྲངས་ལས

UE SU LHA DANG MII PAL JOR P'UN SUM TS'OK PA MA TS'ANG WA ME PA　　RAB JAM GYA TS'OI DUL GYI DRANG LE

འདས་པ་མངོན་པར་བཀོད་དེ།　བླ་མ་ཡི་དམ་སངས་རྒྱས་བྱང་ཆུབ་སེམས་དཔའ་དཔའ་བོ་མཁའ་འགྲོ་ཆོས་སྐྱོང་སྲུང་

DE PA NGON PAR KOE DE　LAMA YI DAM SANG GYE JANG CH'UB SEM PA PA WO K'A DRO CH'O KYONG SUNG

མའི་ཚོགས་དང་བཅས་པ་རྣམས་ལ་འབུལ་བར་བགྱིའོ།　　ཐུགས་རྗེས་འགྲོ་བའི་དོན་དུ་བཞེས་སུ་གསོལ།

MEI TS'OK DANG CHE PA NAM LA BUL WAR GYI-O　　T'UK JE DRO WEI DON DU SH'E SU SOL

བཞེས་ནས་བྱིན་གྱིས་བརླབ་ཏུ་གསོལ།

SH'E NE JIN GYI LAB TU SOL

SAR WA TA TA GA TA BEN ZRA MA ME MUN TSA BEN ZRA BA WA MA HA SA MA YA SA TO AH

OM BEN ZRA BHU MI AH HUNG   *The completely pure foundation is the powerful*
golden ground.

OM BEN ZRA REKE AH HUNG   *On the outer rim, completely surrounding it,*
is the circular iron-mountain wall; in the center is
the king of all mountains, Mount Meru.

East Lupakpo.	*South Dzambuling.*
West Balangcho.	*North Draminyen.*
Lu and Lupak.	*Ngayab and Ngayabshen.*
Yoden and Lamchokdro.	*Draminyen and Draminyengida.*
The jewel mountain.	*The wish-fulfilling trees.*
The wish-fulfilling cows.	*The grain that needs no toil.*
The precious wheel.	*The precious gem.*
The precious queen.	*The precious minister.*
The precious elephant.	*The precious horse.*
The precious general.	*The vase of great treasure.*
Goddess of grace.	*Goddess of garlands.*
Goddess of song.	*Goddess of dance.*
Goddess of flowers.	*Goddess of incense.*
Goddess of light.	*Goddess of perfume.*
The Sun. The moon.	*The precious umbrella.*

The royal banner victorious in all directions.

In the center, all the wealth of gods and humans, with nothing lacking.

All this clearly set out and transcending in number

All the atoms in overflowing oceans of galaxies.

To the assembly of lamas, yidams, buddhas, bodhisattvas,

Dakas, dakinis, dharmapalas, and protectors, I offer.

Out of compassion and for the benefit of beings,

Please accept these offerings, we pray.

Having accepted, please grant your blessing.

།ས་གཞི་སྤོས་ཆུས་བྱུགས་ཤིང་མེ་ཏོག་བཀྲམ།

SA SH'I PO CH'UE JUK SHING ME TOG TRAM

།རི་རབ་གླིང་བཞི་ཉི་ཟླ་རྒྱན་པ་འདི།

RI RAB LING SH'I NYI DE GYEN PA DI

།སངས་རྒྱས་ཞིང་དུ་དམིགས་ཏེ་ཕུལ་བ་ཡིས།

SANG GYE SH'ING DU MIK TE P'UL WA YI

།འགྲོ་ཀུན་རྣམ་དག་ཞིང་ལ་སྤྱོད་པར་ཤོག

DRO KUN NAM DAG SH'ING LA CHOE PAR SHOK

།ཞེས་དང་། ༀ་མཎྜལ་པུ་ཛ་མེ་གྷ་ས་མུ་དྲ་ས་ཕ་ར་ཎ་ས་མ་ཡེ་ཨཱཿཧཱུྃ།

OM MAN DAL PU DZA ME GHA SA MU DRA SA PHA RA NA SA MA YE AH HUNG

། སྡིག་པ་བཤགས་པ་ནི།

Confession of Faults

།བླ་མ་རྡོ་རྗེ་འཛིན་པ་ཆེན་པོ་ལ་སོགས་པ་ཕྱོགས་བཅུ་ན་བཞུགས་པའི་སངས་རྒྱས་དང་བྱང་ཆུབ་སེམས་དཔའ་ཐམས་ཅད་

LA MA DOR JE DZIN PA CH'EN PO LA SOK PA CH'OK CHU NA SH'UK PEI SANG GYE DANG JANG CH'UB SEM PA T'AM CHE

དང་། །འཕགས་པ་ཐུགས་རྗེ་ཆེན་པོ་བདག་ལ་དགོངས་སུ་གསོལ། །བདག་མིང་＿＿འདི་ཞེས་བགྱི་བས་ཚེ་འཁོར་བ་

DANG   P'AK PA T'UK JE CH'EN PO DAG LA GONG SU SOL   DAG MING ... DI SH'E GYI WE TS'E K'OR WA

ཐོག་མ་མེད་པ་ནས་ཐ་མ་ད་ཏ་ལ་ལ་ཐུག་གི་བར་དུ་ཉོན་མོངས་པ་འདོད་ཆགས་དང་།   ཞེ་སྡང་དང་   །གཏི་མུག

T'OG MA ME PA NE T'A MA DA TA LA LA T'UG GI BAR DU NYON MONG PA DO CH'AK DANG   SH'E DANG DANG   TI MUG

གི་དབང་གིས་ལུས་དང་ངག་དང་ཡིད་ཀྱི་སྒོ་ནས། །སྡིག་པ་མི་དགེ་བ་བཅུ་བགྱིས་པ་དང་། །མཚམས་མ་མཆིས་པ་ལྔ་

GI WANG GI LU DANG NGAG DANG YI KYI GO NE   DIG PA MI GE WA CHU GYI PA DANG   TS'AM MA CH'I PA NGA

བགྱིས་པ་དང་། །དེ་དང་ཉེ་བ་ལྔ་བགྱིས་པ་དང་། །སོ་སོར་ཐར་པའི་སྡོམ་པ་དང་འགལ་བ་བགྱིས་པ་དང་།

GYI PA DANG   DE DANG NYE WA NGA GYI PA DANG   SO SOR T'AR PEI DOM PA DANG GAL WA GYI PA DANG

།བྱང་ཆུབ་སེམས་དཔའི་བསླབ་པ་དང་འགལ་བ་བགྱིས་པ་དང་། །གསང་སྔགས་ཀྱི་དམ་ཚིག་དང་འགལ་བ་བགྱིས་པ་དང་

JANG CH'UB SEM PEI LAB PA DANG GAL WA GYI PA DANG   SANG NGAK KYI DAM TS'IG DANG GAL WA GYI PA DANG

།དཀོན་མཆོག་གསུམ་ལ་གནོད་པ་བགྱིས་པ་དང་། །དམ་པའི་ཆོས་སྤངས་པ་དང་། །འཕགས་པའི་དགེ་འདུན་ལ་

KON CH'OG SUM LA NOE PA GYI PA DANG   DAM PEI CH'O PANG PA DANG   P'AK PEI GE DUN LA

སྐུར་པ་བཏབ་པ་དང་། །ཕ་དང་མ་ལ་མ་གུས་པ་བགྱིས་ པ་དང་། །མཁན་པོ་དང་སློབ་དཔོན་ལ་མ་གུས་པ་བགྱིས་པ་དང་།

KUR PA TAB PA DANG   P'A DANG MA LA MA GU PA GYI PA DANG   K'EN PO DANG LOB PON LA MA GU PA GYI PA DANG

།གྲོགས་ཚངས་པ་མཆོངས་པར་སྤྱོད་པ་རྣམས་ལ་མ་གུས་པ་བགྱིས་པ་ལ་སོགས་པ་མདོར་ན་མཐོ་རིས་དང་ཐར་པའི་གེགས་

DROK TS'ANG PA TS'UNG PAR CHOE PA NAM LA MA GU PA GYI PA LA SOK PA DOR NA T'O RI DANG T'AR PEI GEK

This golden ground, sprinkled with scented water and strewn with flowers,
Adorned with Mount Meru, the four continents, the sun and the moon,
By visualizing it all as the buddha realm and offering it,
May all beings enjoy the pure realms.

Then:

OM MAN DAL PU DZA ME GHA SA MU DRA SA PHA RA NA SA MA YE AH HUNG

Confession of Faults

Guru, Great Vajra Holder, and other teachers,
All buddhas and bodhisattvas who abide in the ten directions,
And the Great Exalted Compassionate One,
Please consider me. I **[say your name]**,
From time without beginning up to the present moment,
Have committed the ten nonvirtuous actions
In body, speech, and mind,
Because of the power of the defilements—
Passion, aggression, and stupidity.
I have committed the five acts which ripen immediately,
The five which ripen almost immediately,
Violated the vows of individual liberation,
Violated the vows of bodhichitta,
Violated the commitments of the secret mantra,
Injured the Three Jewels,
Abandoned the dharma,
Insulted the sangha,
Been disrespectful to my parents,
Been disrespectful to my teachers and instructors,
And been disrespectful to companions
Who observe pure morals.

ধ্ব্যুম্ডিম্| ।বেনিমি'ম'নম'নেম'নন'শ্লীন'মন'ৰ্জীম'মন'নন'ভ্লীম'নবি'র্ডনিম'উ'মচিম'ম'নি'নন|
SU GYUR CHING   K'OR WA DANG NGEN SONG GI GYUR GYUR PA NYE PA DANG TUNG WEI TS'OK CHI CH'I PA DE DAG

ধমম'ডন| ।শ্ল'ম'ৰ্হি'ৰ্হ'বেই্বিম'ম'ঙৰু'ম্ব'ল'মীনিম'ম'ভ্লীনিম'মন্তুম্ন'মন্তুনিম'মবি'মনিম'ক্কীম'নন| ।শ্লন'ক্কুম্ব'
T'AM CHE   LA MA DOR JE DZIN PA CH'EN PO LA SOK PA CH'OK CHU NA SH'UK PEI SANG GYE DANG   JANG CH'UB

ৰিমম'ন্মন'ধমম'ডন'নন| ।বেধ্মিনিম'ম'ঙ্ক্লীনিম'ৰ্হ'ক্তিন'ম্বি'ৰ্জ্লীন'ম্বিন'ৰ্মনিম'ৰ্লী'নিধ্মিনিম'ৰ্জী| ।মি'বেক্তম'ম্বী|
SEM PA T'AM CHE DANG   P'AK PA T'UK JE CH'EN POI CHEN NGAR T'OL LO SHAK SO   MI CH'AB BO

।মি'ঙ্লীন্ব'ৰ্মী| ।নি'শ্লুম'মঞ্চী্ন'ৰিন'মনিম্ব'ৰ'নন্ম'নবি'ম'ল'মিন'মম'নিৰ্ম'মম'বেৰ্ম্বীন'ক্কীম্ব| ।ম'মঞ্চীম'ম'
MI BE DO   DE TAR T'OL SH'ING SHAK NA DAG DE WA LA REG PAR NE PAR GYUR GYI   MA T'OL MA

নবিমিম্ব'ৰ'নি'শ্লুম'মী'বেক্তীম'ম'ম্মিম্ব'ৰ্জী|
SHAK NA DE TAR MI GYUR WA LAK SO

।মন'ভন'নন্ম'ক্কীম'নুম'ম্বুৰ'ৰ্হু| ধ্লীম'ম'ক্কীম'ম'মন'ক্কীম'ম| ।ক্লীম'মম'ৰ্হি'বেন্লুম'নবিমিম'ম্কীন'ভিন|
GANG YANG DAG GI DUE KUN TU   DIG PA GYI PA GANG GYUR PA   TRAG PE MI DRAR SHAK GYI CHING

।নিন'ৰিম'মন্তুমম'নি'বেছ্ঠীন'মী'নক্কীন| ।নম্বী'ম'ৰ্ক্তমম'ম'ৰ্হি'ৰিম'ল্লী'নন্ম| ।বেনিম'ৰ্লী'নৰ্লীম'ৰিন'মৰ্সীম'ম'বেনীমম|
DENG NE TSAM TE JUNG MI GYIE   GE WA NAM LA JE YI RANG   K'OR LO KOR SH'ING SOL WA DEB

।মনিম'ক্কীম'ম্বন'ক্কুম'ভীন'ক্কীম'মন্তুন| ধমম'ডন'ম্বন'ক্কুম'মৰ্ক্তীম'ৰ্হু'নৰ্লী|
SANG GYE JANG CH'UB YIE KYI ZUNG   T'AM CHE JANG CH'UB CH'OG TU NGO

।নন'ম্বী'ঙ্লী'মৰ'নম্বী'ম্লীন'ম| ।ন্মম'ৰ্লী'নৰিম্বিম'ৰিম'ৰ্হি'ক্তিন'মৰ্হন|
RANG GI CHI WOR GE LONG MA   PAL MO SH'UK NE NGO CH'EN DZE

Po Homage Prayer

ৰ'ৰ্লী'মৰ্ডু'ঝ্লী'ঝি| ৰ'ৰ্লী'মন্তু'ঝ্লী'ঝি| ৰ'ৰ্লী'ভু্ব্ব'ম'ঝ্লী'ঝি'ৰ্জ'ৰ্হ|
NA MO MAN JU SHRI YE   NA MO SU SHRI YE   NA MO UT TA MA SHRI YE SO HA

ৰ্জঁ'বেৰ্ডম'ৰ্হিন'মৰ্মীন'ম্বী'ম'ধ্লুম'বেক্তম'ৰ্লী| ।বেৰ্ডম'ৰ্হিন'শ্ল'ম'ঙ্লীন'ম'নম্বীম'ক্কীম'নর্মীন'ম'ম্বী|
OM JIG TEN GON PO LA CH'AG TS'AL LO   JIG TEN LA MA SIE PA SUM GYI TOE PA PO

।শ্লু'ভি'নার্ডি'ম্বী'নন্ডীন'নন'ক্তনম'মম'নর্মীন'ম'ম্বী| ।শ্লুম'মবি'ক্কুম'মৰ্ক্তীম'নর্মীন'মম'ক্লুম'মম'মৰ্হন'ম'ম্বী|
LHA YI TSO WO DUE DANG TS'ANG PE TOE PA PO   T'UB PEI GYAL CH'OG TOE PE DRUB PAR DZE PA PO

In summary, whatever moral failings or faults I have committed,

Which are obstacles to the higher realms and to freedom,

Or the seeds of samsara and the lower realms,

I acknowledge and confess in the presence of the Guru,

Great Vajra Holder, and other teachers,

All buddhas and bodhisattvas who reside in the ten directions,

And the Great Exalted Compassionate One.

I hide nothing, I conceal nothing, and I vow

To terminate these actions. If I make this sort of confession,

I will remain in the proximity of happiness;

If not, that will not come about.

Whatever errors have been made at any time by me or others,

Looking at them fearfully as if they were a nightmare,

I confess them all. From now on I shall not engage in such actions.

I rejoice in all virtue.

I request the buddhas to turn the wheel of dharma.

Keeping in mind the awakening of the buddhas,

I dedicate all these beneficial actions to Supreme Awakening.

On the top of my head Gelongma Palmo appears,

Who intercedes in my favor.

Po Homage Prayer

NA MO MAN JU SHRI YE   NA MO SU SHRI YE
NA MO UT TA MA SHRI YE SO HA

I bow to the Protector of the world.

Everyone in the three worlds praises and celebrates the Lama.

Even the gods and Brahma celebrate and praise Lord Chenrezig.

One who wishes to attain buddhahood praises the Lord

Who delivers such accomplishment.

།འཇིག་རྟེན་གསུམ་གྱི་མགོན་པོ་མཆོག་ལ་ཕྱག་འཚལ་ལོ། 　　　　།བདེ་གཤེགས་དཔག་མེད་སྐུ་སྟེ་སྐུ་བཟང་འཛིན་པ་པོ།

JIG TEN SUM GYI GON PO CH'OG LA CH'AG TS'AL LO　　　DE SHEK PAG ME KU TE KU ZANG DZIN PA PO

།བདེ་གཤེགས་སྣང་བ་མཐའ་ཡས་དབུ་རྒྱན་འཛིན་པ་པོ།　　　།ཕྱག་གཡས་མཆོག་སྦྱིན་ཡི་དྭགས་བཀྲེས་སྐོམ་སེལ་བ་པོ།

DE SHEK NANG WA T'A YE U GYEN DZIN PA PO　　　CH'AG YE CH'OG JIN YI DOK TRE KOM SEL WA PO

།ཕྱག་གཡོན་གསེར་གྱི་པདྨ་རྣམ་པར་བརྒྱན་པ་པོ།　　　།དྲི་ཞིམ་རལ་པའི་ཕྲེང་བ་དམར་སེར་འཁྱུག་པ་པོ།

CH'AG YON SER GYI PE ME NAM PAR GYEN PA PO　　　DRI SH'IM RAL PEI TR'ENG WA MAR SER K'YUG PA PO

།ཞལ་རས་རྒྱས་པ་ཟླ་བ་ལྟ་བུར་མཛེས་པ་པོ།　　　།སྤྱན་གྱི་པདྨ་མཆོག་ཏུ་བཟང་ཞིང་ཡངས་པ་པོ།

SH'AL RE GYE PA DA WA TA BUR DZE PA PO　　　CHEN GYI PE MA CH'OG TU ZANG SH'ING YANG PA PO

།ཁ་བ་དུང་ལྟར་རྣམ་དཀར་དྲི་ངད་ལྡན་པ་པོ།　　　།དྲི་མེད་འོད་ཆགས་མུ་ཏིག་ཚོམ་བུ་འཛིན་པ་པོ།

K'A WA DUNG TAR NAM KAR DRI NGE DEN PA PO　　　DRI ME OE CH'AG MU TIG TS'OM BU DZIN PA PO

།མཛེས་པའི་འོད་ཟེར་སྐྱ་རེངས་དམར་པོས་བརྒྱན་པ་པོ།　　　།པདྨའི་མཚོ་ལྟར་ཕྱག་ནི་མངར་བར་བྱེད་པ་པོ།

DZE PEI OE ZER KYA RENG MAR PO GYEN PA PO　　　PE MEI TS'O TAR CH'AG NI NGAR WAR JE PA PO

།སྟོན་ཀའི་སྤྲིན་གྱི་མདོག་དང་ལྡན་ཞིང་གཤིན་པ་པོ།　　　།རིན་ཆེན་མང་པོས་དཔུང་པ་གཉིས་ནི་བརྒྱན་པ་པོ།

TON KEI TRIN GYI DOG DANG DEN SH'ING SH'ON PA PO　　　RIN CH'EN MANG PO PUNG PA NYI NI GYEN PA PO

།ལོ་མའི་མཆོག་ལྟར་ཕྱག་མཐིལ་གཤིན་ཞིང་འཇམ་པ་པོ།　　　།རི་དྭགས་པགས་པས་ནུ་མ་གཡོན་པ་བཀབ་པ་པོ།

LO MEI CH'OG TAR CH'AG T'IL SH'ON SH'ING JAM PA PO　　　RI DOK PAK PE NU MA YON PA KAB PA PO

།སྙན་ཆ་དུ་བུས་སྒྲེག་ཅིང་རྒྱན་རྣམས་འཆང་བ་པོ།　　　།དྲི་མ་མེད་པའི་པདྨའི་མཆོག་ལ་གནས་པ་པོ།

NYEN CH'A DU BU GEG CHING GYEN NAM CH'ANG WA PO　　　DRI MA ME PEI PE MEI CH'OG LA NE PA PO

།ལྟེ་བའི་རོ་ནི་པདྨའི་འདབ་བས་ལྟར་འཇམ་པ་པོ།　　　།གསེར་གྱི་སྐ་རགས་མཆོག་ལ་ནོར་བུ་བཀྲེས་པ་པོ།

TE WEI NGO NI PE MEI DAB TAR JAM PA PO　　　SER GYI KA RAK CH'OG LA NOR BU TRE PA PO

།སྐ་རགས་དགྱེས་པའི་རས་བཟང་ཤམ་ཐབས་འཛིན་པ་པོ།　　　།ཐུབ་པའི་མཁྱེན་མཆོག་མཚོ་ཆེན་ཕ་རོལ་ཕྱིན་པ་པོ།

TA ZUR TRI PEI RE ZANG SHAM T'AB DZIN PA PO　　　T'UB PEI K'YEN CH'OG TS'O CH'EN P'A ROL CH'IN PA PO

།མཆོག་བརྙེས་བསོད་ནམས་མང་པོས་ཉེ་བར་བསགས་པ་པོ།　　　།རྟག་ཏུ་བདེ་བའི་འབྱུང་གནས་ཀ་ནད་སེལ་བ་པོ།

CH'OG NYE SOE NAM MANG PO NYE WAR SAK PA PO　　　TAG TU DE WEI JUNG NE GA NE SEL WA PO

།གསུམ་མཐར་མཛད་ཅིང་ཁ་ཆོས་ཆོས་པ་སྟོན་པ་པོ།　　　།ལུས་ཅན་མཆོག་སྟེ་བདུད་དཔུང་འཕྲོགས་ལས་རྒྱལ་བ་པོ།

SUM T'AR DZE CHING K'A CHOE CHOE PA TON PA PO　　　LU CHEN CH'OG TE DUE PUNG TR'UK LE GYAL WA PO

I bow to the supreme protector of the three worlds.

Holder of a noble form body, filled with infinite tathagatas,

You are crowned by Buddha Amitabha.

Your supremely bountiful right hand dispels

The suffering of the hungry ghosts;

Your left hand holds a golden lotus.

Your sweetly scented red and yellow hair sparkles like necklaces.

The expanse of your face is as lovely as a full moon.

Like the sublimely supreme lotus, your eyes are beautifully wide.

Your sweet-smelling form is like a snow-white conch shell.

You hold a mala of stainless, glowing pearls,

And radiate stunning beams of light, red as dawn.

Your body is like a lake; from it hands, like lotuses, are perfectly arranged.

They are youthful and like autumn clouds,

White and bright and clear.

Both shoulders are adorned with many precious jewels.

Your youthful palms are soft like the most supreme leaves.

Your left breast is covered with a tenasera skin.

Precious earrings and other ornaments gracefully adorn you.

You dwell upon a supreme and unblemished lotus.

Your navel's surface is as soft as a lotus petal.

Your belt is of the finest jewel-encrusted gold.

Your lower robe wraps your hips in the noblest cloth.

Gone to the other shore of the great ocean,

You have supreme knowledge and capability.

You, who properly gathered so much virtue,

Received the supreme state of being.

Dispeller of the misery of old age and illness,

You are the permanent source of joy.

You act to liberate beings from the three lower realms,

And show and perform equally for space dwellers.

|གསེར་གྱི་ཀང་གདུབ་སྒྲ་ཡིས་ཞབས་ཡིད་འོང་བ་པོ། ཚངས་པའི་གནས་པ་བཞི་ཡིས་དབེན་པར་མཛད་པ་པོ། །ངང་པའི་

SER GYI KANG DUB DRA YI SH'AB YIE ONG WA PO   TS'ANG PEI NE PA SH'I YI WEN PAR DZE PA PO   NGANG PEI

འགྲོས་འདྲ་གླང་ཆེན་དྲེགས་ལྟར་གཤེགས་པ་པོ། ཚོགས་ཀུན་ཉེ་བར་བསགས་ཤིང་བསྟན་པ་གཉེར་བ་པོ། །ཨོ་མའི་

DRO DRA LANG CH'EN DREK TAR SHEK PA PO   TS'OK KUN NYE WAR SAK SHING TEN PA NYER WA PO   O MEI

མཚོ་དང་ཆུ་ཡི་མཚོ་ལས་སྒྲོལ་བ་པོ། །གང་ཞིག་ཏག་ཏུ་ཐོ་རངས་ལང་ནས་གུས་པ་ཡིས། །སྤྱན་རས་གཟིགས་ཀྱི་

TS'O DANG CH'U YI TS'O LE DROL WA PO   GANG SH'IG TAG TU T'O RANG LANG NE GU PA YI   CHEN RE ZIG KYI

དབང་པོ་ཡིད་ལ་སེམས་བྱེད་ཅིང་། །བསྟོད་པའི་མཆོག་འདི་དག་ཅིང་གསལ་བར་བརྗོད་བྱེད་ན། །དེ་ནི་སྐྱེ་བ་འམ་

WANG PO YIE LA SEM JE CHING   TOE PEI CH'OG DI DAG CHING SAL WAR TOE JE NA   DE NI KYE PA AM

ཉི་བུད་མེད་ཡིན་ཀྱང་རུང་། །འཇིག་རྟེན་འདི་འམ་མ་འོངས་སྐྱེ་བ་ཐམས་ཅད་དུ། །འཇིག་རྟེན་འཇིག་རྟེན་ལས་འདས་

NI BUE ME YIN KYANG RUNG   JIG TEN DI AM MA ONG KYE WA T'AM CHE DU   JIG TEN JIG TEN LE DE

དགོས་པ་ཀུན་འགྲུབ་ཤོག །ཤོགས་ཚར་ཉེར་གཅིག་གསལ་བཏུན་བཟོད།

GO PA KUN DRUB SHOG

Special Wish Prayer

|བསྟན་པ་བསྟན་འཛིན་ཡུན་རིང་གནས་པ་དང་། །བདག་སོགས་འགྲོ་རྣམས་བྱང་ཆུབ་སེམས་འབྱོངས་ཤིང་།

TEN PA TEN DZIN YUN RING NE PA DANG   DAG SOK DRO NAM JANG CH'UB SEM JONG SHING

ཞི་ལྷག་ཟུང་འབྲེལ་ཏིང་འཛིན་རབ་ཐོབ་ནས། །ཀུན་མཁྱེན་ཤེས་རབ་རྟོགས་པར་བྱིན་གྱིས་རློབས།

SH'I LHAG ZUNG DREL TING DZIN RAB T'OB NE   KUN K'YEN SHE RAB TOK PAR JIN GYI LOB

|དེ་ནས་འདས་གཏོར་བསང་སྦྱངས།

Purifying the Torma

ཨོཾ་ཧ་ཡ་གྲི་ས་ཧཱུྃ་ཕཊ། ཨོཾ་སྭ་བྷ་ཝ་ཤུདྡྷ་སརྦ་དྷརྨ་སྭ་བྷ་ཝ་ཤུདྡྷོ྅ཧཾ།

OM HA YA GRI WA HUNG PE   OM SVA BHA WA SHUD DHA SAR VA DHAR MA SVA BHA WA SHUD DHO HAM

ཨོཾ་ཨཱཿཧཱུྃ།   །ལན་གསུམ།   །ཁ་དོག་དྲི་རོ་ནུས་པ་རྣམས། །ཕུན་ཚོགས་ལྡན་པའི་གཏོར་མ་འདི།

OM AH HUNG   K'A DOG DRI RO NU PA NAM   P'UN TS'OK DEN PEI TOR MA DI

|འཕགས་པ་སྤྱན་རས་གཟིགས་དབང་དང་། །རྒྱལ་བ་སྲས་དང་བཅས་ལ་འབུལ། ཨོཾ་མ་ཎི་པདྨེ་ཧཱུྃ།

P'AK PA CHEN RE ZIG WANG DANG   GYAL WA SE DANG CHE LA BUL   OM MANI PEME HUNG

Supreme among beings, you are victorious in battle over hosts of demons.
Your feet tinkle with the pleasing sound of golden anklets;
And you create the four silences, which are the cause of Brahmahood.
You walk with the grace of a swan and the dignity of an elephant.
Provider of the doctrine, who has completely and properly accumulated,
You liberate from the ocean of milk and the ocean of water.
Whoever will rise with respect at dawn,
Thinking in their mind of powerful Chenrezig,
To purely and clearly extol this supreme praise,
Whether they are male or female,
In this life and all future lives,
In this world and the world beyond,
All their purposes will be accomplished.

Recite this prayer seven or twenty-one times.

Special Wish Prayer

Please grant us your grace that the doctrine and its holders remain long,
That I and all beings practice the thought of enlightenment,
And, having obtained the perfect state of absorption,
The inseparability of calm and insight,
That we may realize transcendental knowledge, omniscience.

Purifying the Torma

OM HA YA GRI WA HUNG PE   OM SVA BHA WA SHUD DHA SAR VA
DHAR MA SVA BHA WA SHUD DHO HAM

OM AH HUNG   *Repeat three times.*

This torma, perfect in shape, perfume, and qualities,
I offer to the noble, powerful Chenrezig,
And to the victorious ones and their sons.

OM MANI PEME HUNG   *Recite three times.*

ༀ་ཨ་ཀ་རོ་མུ་ཁཾ་སརྦ་དྷ་ཨུ་ནུ་རྡུ་དུ་ༀ་ཨཱཿཧཱུྃ་པཏ་སྭ་ཧཱ།　　　།ལན་གསུམ།

OM A KA RO MU KAM SAR VA DHAR MA NAM A DYA NUT PAN NA TO TA OM AH HUNG PE SO HA

|བྱང་ཆུབ་སེམས་ནི་རིན་པོ་ཆེ།　　|མ་སྐྱེས་པ་རྣམས་སྐྱེ་གྱུར་ཅིག　|སྐྱེས་པ་ཉམས་པ་མེད་པ་དང་།

JANG CH'UB SEM NI RIN PO CH'E　MA CHE PA NAM KYE GYUR CHIG　KYE PA NYAM PA ME PA DANG

|གོང་ནས་གོང་དུ་འཕེལ་བར་མཛོད།　|ༀ་ཧ་ཡ་གྲི་ཝ་ཧཱུྃ་པཏ།

GONG NE GONG DU P'EL WAR DZOE　OM HA YA GRI WA HUNG PE

ༀ་སྭ་བྷ་ཝ་ཤུཏྡྷ་སརྦ་དྷ་མ་སྭ་བྷ་ཝ་ཤུཏྡྷོ྅ཧཾ།　　　ༀ་ཨཱཿཧཱུྃ།　　　།ལན་གསུམ།

OM SVA BHA VA SHUD DHA SAR VA DHAR MA SVA BHA VA SHUD DHO HAM　OM AH HUNG

ༀ་ད་ཤ་དིག་ལོ་ཀ་པ་ལ་ན་ག་ར་ཛ་ཝ་རུ་ན་བྷུ་མི་པ་ཏི་ས་པ་རི་ཝ་ར་ཨི་དྃ་པ་ལི྅

OM DA SHA DIK LO KA PA LA NA GA RA DZA WA RU NA BHU MI PA TI SA PA RI WA RA I DAM PA LING

ཊ་ཁ་ཁ་ཁཱ་ཧི་ཁཱ་ཧི།　　　།ལན་གསུམ།

TA KHA KHA KHA HI KHA HI

ༀ་བཛྲ་ཨརྒཾ།　　པཱདྱཾ།　　པུཥྤེ།　　དྷུ་པེ།　　ཨ་ལོ་ཀེ།　　གནྡྷེ།　　ནེ་ཝི་དྱ།　　ཤཔྟ་ཨཱཿཧཱུྃ།

OM BEN ZRA AR GAM　PAD YAM　PU PE　DHU PE　A LO KE　GEN DHE　NE WI DYA　SHAP TA AH HUNG

|སངས་རྒྱས་བསྟན་སྲུང་འཇིག་རྟེན་སྐྱོང་།　|འཕགས་པའི་བཀའ་དོ་ལུ་ཡི་རྒྱལ།　|གཞན་ཡང་འབྱུང་པོ་བགེགས།

SANG GYE TEN SUNG JIG TEN KYONG　P'AK PEI KA DOE LU YI GYAL　SH'EN YANG JUNG PO GEK

རིགས་དང་།　|ཡུལ་གཞིའི་གནས་བདག་གྲོང་བདག་རྣམས།　|མཆོད་བསྟོར་གཏོར་མ་འདི་བཞེས་ལ།

RIK DANG　YUL SH'II NE DAG DRONG DAG NAM　CH'OE TOE TOR MA DI SH'E LA

|བྱང་ཆུབ་སེམས་ཀྱི་གཞི་བཟུང་སྟེ།　|བསྟན་འགྲོར་ཕན་བདེའི་ལྷག་བསམ་གྱིས།　|ཡིད་ལ་འདོད་པ་ཀུན་སྒྲུབས་མཛོད།

JANG CH'UB SEM KYI SH'I ZUNG TE　TEN DROR P'EN DEI LHAG SAM GYI　YI LA DOE PA KUN DRUB DZOE

|ལྷ་ཁྲུས་གསོལ་བ།

Prayer of Bath Offering to the Deity

|འགྲོ་བའི་སྒྲོན་མེ་སྤྱན་རས་གཟིགས་མགོན་ལ།　|དྲི་ཞིམ་བདུད་རྩིའི་རྒྱུན་གྱིས་ཁྲུས་གསོལ་བས།

DRO WEI DRON ME CHEN RE ZIG GON LA　DRI SH'IM DUE TSII GYUN GYI TR'U SOL WE

|འགྲོ་བའི་སྒྲིབ་གཉིས་དྲི་མ་ཀུན་བསལ་ནས།　|དྲི་བྲལ་སྐུ་གསུམ་བརྙེས་པའི་བཀྲ་ཤིས་ཤོག

DRO WEI DRIB NYI DRI MA KUN SAL NE　DRI DRAL KU SUM NYE PEI TRA SHI SHOK

OM A KA RO MU KAM SAR VA DHAR MA NAM A DYA NUT PAN NA TO TA

OM AH HUNG PE SO HA   **Repeat three times.**

May the precious thought of enlightenment,

Which has not arisen in us, arise.

Wherever it has arisen, may it not be destroyed,

But increase more and more!

Then, to purify the torma offering to the nagas:

OM HA YA GRI WA HUNG PE OM SVA BHA VA SHUD DHA SAR VA

DHAR MA SVA BHA VA SHUD DHO HAM   OM AH HUNG   *Repeat three times.*

OM DA SHA DIK LO KA PA LA NA GA RA DZA WA RU NA BHU MI PA TI SA PARI WA

RA I DAM PA LING TA KHA KHA KHA HI KHA HI   **Repeat three times.**

OM BEN ZRA AR GAM   PAD YAM   PU PE   DHU PE   A LO KE   GEN DHE

NE WI DYA   SHAP TA AH HUNG

King of the nagas, who observes the rules of the noble Chenrezig,

Please protect the universe and preserve the Buddha's teachings.

Obstructing spirits, genii of the lands and the towns,

Having accepted this torma, these offerings and praises,

Keeping the foundation of the thought of enlightenment,

And with the sublime vow to bring happiness and comfort to all beings,

Grant the realization of all our wishes.

Prayer of Bath Offering to the Deity

I beseech you, Protector Chenrezig, the light for all beings,

To bathe in the continuous flow of perfect nectar.

May this be the happy omen

To the achievement of the three immaculate bodies,

All stains and the two veils having been purified.

།རྫས་མཆོད་པ་བྱིན་རླབས།

Blessing of the Offering

ན་མ་སརྦ་བུད་དྷི་ས་ཏོ་བྷྱཿ

NA MA SAR VA BUD DHA BOD HI SA TO BHE

ༀ་སརྦ་བིད་པུ་ར་པུ་ར་སུ་ར་སུ་ར་ཨ་བཛྲེ་བྷྱུ་སྭཱ་ཧཱ།

OM SAR VA PI PU RA PU RA SU RA SU RA AH WAT TE BHE SO HA

ༀ་བཛྲ་སྥ་ར་ཎ་ཁཾ།

OM BEN ZRA SA PA RA NA KAM

ༀ་ཨྱཱ་ཡ་ལོ་ཀེ་ཤྭ་ར་ས་པ་རི་ལྭ་ར་ཨརྒྷཾ་ཏྲ་ཏི་ཙྪ་སྭཱ་ཧཱ།

OM AR YA LO KE SHVA RA SA PA RI WA RA AR GHAM TRA TI TSA SO HA

ༀ་ཨྱཱ་ཡ་ལོ་ཀེ་ཤྭ་ར་ས་པ་རི་ལྭ་ར་པཱདྱ་པ་ཏི་ཙྪ་སྭཱ་ཧཱ།

OM AR YA LO KE SHVA RA SA PA RI WA RA PAD YAM TRA TI TSA SO HA

ༀ་ཨྱཱ་ཡ་ལོ་ཀེ་ཤྭ་ར་ས་པ་རི་ལྭ་ར་པུཥྤེ་པ་ཏི་ཙྪ་སྭཱ་ཧཱ།

OM AR YA LO KE SHVA RA SA PA RI WA RA PU PE TRA TI TSA SO HA

ༀ་ཨྱཱ་ཡ་ལོ་ཀེ་ཤྭ་ར་ས་པ་རི་ལྭ་ར་དྷུ་པེ་པ་ཏི་ཙྪ་སྭཱ་ཧཱ།

OM AR YA LO KE SHVA RA SA PA RI WA RA DHU PE TRA TI TSA SO HA

ༀ་ཨྱཱ་ཡ་ལོ་ཀེ་ཤྭ་ར་ས་པ་རི་ལྭ་ར་ཨ་ལོ་ཀེ་པ་ཏི་ཙྪ་སྭཱ་ཧཱ།

OM AR YA LO KE SHVA RA SA PA RI WA RA A LO KE TRA TI TSA SO HA

ༀ་ཨྱཱ་ཡ་ལོ་ཀེ་ཤྭ་ར་ས་པ་རི་ལྭ་ར་གནྡྷེ་པ་ཏི་ཙྪ་སྭཱ་ཧཱ།

OM AR YA LO KE SHVA RA SA PA RI WA RA GEN DHE TRA TI TSA SO HA

ༀ་ཨྱཱ་ཡ་ལོ་ཀེ་ཤྭ་ར་ས་པ་རི་ལྭ་ར་ནཻ་བི་དྱ་པ་ཏི་ཙྪ་སྭཱ་ཧཱ།

OM AR YA LO KE SHVA RA SA PA RI WA RA NE WI DYA TRA TI TSA SO HA

ༀ་ཨྱཱ་ཡ་ལོ་ཀེ་ཤྭ་ར་ས་པ་རི་ལྭ་ར་ཤཔྟ་པ་ཏི་ཙྪ་སྭཱ་ཧཱ།

OM AR YA LO KE SHVA RA SA PA RI WA RA SHAP TA TRA TI TSA SO HA

།སྐྱོན་གྱིས་མ་གོས་སྐུ་མདོག་དཀར། KYON GYI MA GO KU DOG KAR

།རྫོགས་སངས་རྒྱས་ཀྱིས་དབུ་ལ་བརྒྱན། DZOK SANG GYE KYI U LA GYEN

།ཐུགས་རྗེའི་སྤྱན་གྱིས་འགྲོ་ལ་གཟིགས། T'UK JEI CHEN GYI DRO LA ZIG

།སྤྱན་རས་གཟིགས་ལ་ཕྱག་འཚལ་ལོ། CHEN RE ZIG LA CH'AG TS'AL LO

Blessing of the Offering

NA MA SAR VA BUD DHA BOD HI SA TO BHE

OM SAR VA PI PU RA PU RA SU RA SU RA AH WAT TE BHE SO HA

OM BEN ZRA SA PA RA NA KAM

OM AR YA LO KE SHVA RA SA PA RI WA RA

AR GHAM TRA TI TSA SO HA

OM AR YA LO KE SHVA RA SA PA RI WA RA

PAD YAM TRA TI TSA SO HA

OM AR YA LO KE SHVA RA SA PA RI WA RA

PU PE TRA TI TSA SO HA

OM AR YA LO KE SHVA RA SA PA RI WA RA

DHU PE TRA TI TSA SO HA

OM AR YA LO KE SHVA RA SA PA RI WA RA

A LO KE TRA TI TSA SO HA

OM AR YA LO KE SHVA RA SA PA RI WA RA

GEN DHE TRA TI TSA SO HA

OM AR YA LO KE SHVA RA SA PA RI WA RA

NE WI DYA TRA TI TSA SO HA

OM AR YA LO KE SHVA RA SA PA RI WA RA

SHAP TA TRA TI TSA SO HA

Lord with white body, not affected by fault,
Whose head is adorned by a perfect buddha,
Who looks upon all beings with the eyes of compassion,
To you, Chenrezig, I pay homage.

།བསྟོད་པར་འོས་པ་ཐམས་ཅད་ལ།   །ཞིང་དུལ་ཀུན་གྱིས་གྲངས་སྙེད་ཀྱིས།   །ལུས་བཏུད་པས་ནི་རྣམ་ཀུན་ཏུ།

TOE PAR OE PA T'AM CHE LA   SH'ING DUL KUN GYI DRANG NYE KYI   LU TUE PE NI NAM KUN TU

།མཆོག་ཏུ་དད་པས་བསྟོད་པར་བགྱི།   ཨོཾ་མ་ཎི་པདྨེ་ཧཱུྃ།

CH'OG TU DE PE TOE PAR GYI   OM MANI PEME HUNG

།མདུན་མཁར་འཕགས་པ་ཡི་གེ་དྲུག །ཕྱོན་པའི་ཕྱག་གཡས་བདུད་རྩི་ཡིས། །ཁྲུས་བྱས་སྒྲིབ་གསུམ་དག་གྱུར་ཏེ།

DUN K'AR P'AK PA YI GE DRUG   JON PEI CH'AG YE DUE TSI YI   T'RU JE DRIB SUM DAG GYUR TE

།ལྷ་ཡང་སྤྱི་བོར་ཐིམ་པར་གྱུར། །བཅོམ་ལྡན་བདག་ལ་དགོངས་སུ་གསོལ། །བདག་ཅག་ཅིང་གོས་དབང་

LHA YANG CHI WOR T'IM PAR GYUR   CHOM DEN DAG LA GONG SU SOL   DAG CHAG JING GOE WANG

གྱུར་པས། །ཏིང་འཛིན་མི་གསལ་སྔགས་མ་དག །གཙང་དྲ་ཆུང་སོགས་བཟོད་པར་གསོལ།

GYUR PE   TING DZIN MI SAL NGAK MA DAG   TSANG DRA CH'UNG SOK ZOE PAR SOL

ཨོཾ་པདྨ་ས་ཏོ་ས་མ་ཡ།   མ་ནུ་པ་ལ་ཡ།   པདྨ་ས་ཏོ   ཏེ་ནོ་པ་ཏི་ཊ་དྲི་དོ་མེ་བྷ་ཝ།

OM PE MA SA TO SA MA YA   MA NU PA LA YA   PE MA SA TO   TE NO PA TI TA DRI DO ME BA WA

སུ་ཏོ་ཁྱོ་མེ་བྷ་ཝ།   སུ་པོ་ཁྱོ་མེ་བྷ་ཝ།   ཨ་ནུ་རཀྟོ་མེ་བྷ་ཝ།   སརྦ་སིདྡྷི་མྲེ་ཏྲ་ཡ་ཙ

SU TO KOY YO ME BA WA   SU PO KOY YO ME BA WA   AH NU RAK TO ME BA WA   SAR VA SID DHI ME TRA YA TSA

སརྦ་ཀརྨ་སུ་ཙ་མེ་ཙི་ཏྟཾ་ཤྲི་ཡཿ   ཀུ་རུ་ཧཱུྃ་ཧ་ཧ་ཧ་ཧོཿ   ཧྲ་ག་ཝ་ན།

SAR VA KAR MA SU TSA ME TSI TANG SHI RI YA   KU RU HUNG HA HA HA HA HO   BAN GA WEN

སརྦ་ཏ་ཐཱ་ག་ཏ།   པདྨ་མེ་མུན་ཙ   པདྨ་བྷ་ཝ།   མ་ཧཱ་ས་མ་ཡ་ས་ཏོ་ཨཱཿ

SAR VA TA TA GA TA   PE MA ME MUN TSA   PE MA BA WA   MA HA SA MA YA SA TO AH

ཏེན་ཡོན་ན།   ཨོཾ།   །འདིར་ནི་རྟེན་དང་ལྷན་ཅིག་ཏུ། །འཁོར་བ་སྲིད་དུ་བཞུགས་ནས་ཀྱང་། །ན་མེད་ཚེ་དང་

HE YON NA   OM   DIR NI TEN DANG LHEN CHIG TU   K'OR WA SIE DU SH'UK NE KYANG   NE ME T'SE DANG

དབང་ཕྱུག་དང་། །མཆོག་རྣམས་ལེགས་པར་སྩལ་དུ་གསོལ། ཨོཾ་སུ་པྲ་ཏིཥྛ་བཛྲ་ཡེ་སྭ་ཧཱ།

WANG CH'UG DANG   CH'OG NAM LEK PAR TSAL DU SOL   OM SU TRA TIK TA BEN ZRA YE SO HA

With bodies as numerous as the particles in all the universes,
I bow before all those worthy of praise.
I pay homage with complete confidence
Entirely, with body, speech, and mind.

Repeat: OM MANI PEME HUNG

In the sky before me appears the Noble One of the Six Syllables.
He bathes me in the nectar that flows from his right hand;
The three veils of the mind vanish;
He is absorbed through the top of my head.

Please grant me your attention.
Under the power of agitation and stupor,
Our state of absorption lacks clarity,
And our recitation of mantras is imperfect.
Please look with benevolence upon this lack of clarity.

OM PE MA SA TO SA MA YA   MA NU PA LA YA
PE MA SA TO TE NO PA   TI TA DRI DO ME BA WA
SU TO KOY YO ME BA WA   SU PO KOY YO ME BA WA
AH NU RAK TO ME BA WA   SAR VA SID DHI ME TRA YA TSA
SAR VA KAR MA SU TSA ME   TSI TANG SHI RI YA
KU RU HUNG HA HA HA HA HO   BAN GA WEN
SAR VA TA TA GA TA   PE MA MA ME MUN TSA
PE MA BA WA MA HA SA MA YA SA TO AH

If we have a representation of the deity:

OM *By staying in this very place,*
United to this representation,
Spare us illness and grant us long life and power.
Grant us the sublime accomplishment
In the most excellent way.

OM SU TRA TIK TA BEN ZRA YE SO HA

།ཉེན་མེད་ན། ཨོཾ། །ཁྱེད་ཀྱི་སེམས་ཅན་དོན་ཀུན་མཛད། །རྗེས་སུ་མཐུན་པའི་དངོས་གྲུབ་སྩོལ།

OM   K'YE KYI SEM CHEN DON KUN DZE   JE SU T'UN PEI NGO DRUB TSOL

།སངས་རྒྱས་ཡུལ་དུ་གཤེགས་ནས་ཀྱང་། །སླར་ཡང་འབྱོན་པར་མཛད་དུ་གསོལ། བཛྲ་མུཿ

SANG GYE YUL DU SHEK NE KYANG   LAR YANG JON PAR DZE DU SOL   BEN ZRA MU

།མདུན་རྟེན་ཡོད་མེད་དང་བསྟན་པའི་གཤེགས་བརྟེན་གང་འགབ་ཏུ།

།བདག་ལྷ་ཐུགས་ཀའི་ཧྲཱིཿལས་ཐིམ། །དེ་ཡང་བློ་འདས་འོད་གསལ་དང་། །སླར་ཡང་ཞལ་གཅིག་ཕྱག་གཉིས་པའི།

DAG LHA T'UK KEI HRIH LA T'IM   DE YANG LO DE OE SAL DANG   LAR YANG SH'AL CHIG CH'AG NYI PEI

།ཐུགས་རྗེ་ཆེན་པོར་གསལ་བར་གྱུར། །དགེ་བ་འདི་ཡིས་མྱུར་དུ་བདག །སྤྱན་རས་གཟིགས་དབང་འགྲུབ་གྱུར་ནས།

T'UK JE CH'EN POR SAL WAR GYUR   GE WA DI YI NYUR DU DAG   CHEN RE ZIG WANG DRUB GYUR NE

།འགྲོ་བ་གཅིག་ཀྱང་མ་ལུས་པ། །དེ་ཡི་ས་ལ་འགོད་པར་ཤོག།། ॥

DRO WA CHIG KYANG MA LU PA   DE YI SA LA GOE PAR SHOK//

།།བཟང་སྤྱོད་སྨོན་ལམ་དང་བཀྲ་ཤིས་གང་བཏོང་བར་བྱའོ།། དེ་ལྟར་སྒྲུབ་པ་བཤགས་སྐུ་བྱ་བ་སོགས་རྒྱལ་བའི་དུས་ཆེན་བཞི་འཛ། དེ་མིན་སྐུ་བ་གང་ཡིན་གྱི་ཚ་བདུན་གསུམ་སྒྲོ་ཉིན་དངོས་བཞི་ཟིལ་བར་སྤྱོ་དངོས་གཞིས་ལ་ཚོག་གསུམ་ལྷུམ་རེ་དང་། རྗེས་གསོ་སྒྲོ་མ་གཏོགས་ཚ་ གཅིག་བྱེ་བའི་སྒྲུབ་གནས་རྣམ་དག་ལན་གཅིག་གིས་ནས་འགྲོའི་རྒྱུན་ལས་བཅད་པ་སོགས་མཐའ་ཡོན་བསྒྱགས་པ་མཐའ་ཡས་པའི་རྒྱུ་ཆེར་གནས་ལས་ ཚོགས་པར་བྱོས་ཤིག། འདི་ནི་ཁྱིམ་པ་ཕོ་མོ་སོགས་སྐྱག་ཆོག་རྒྱལ་བ་ལ་བཞིན་འཚམས་སུ་མི་ལོང་པར་ཐབ་ཕྱིར་ཚོ་གཅག་གཞུང་ཚང་ཐུབ་ལས་ཏུ་བུར་ བཅད་མཐུན་ཅུང་གསལ་ཆོལ་དུ་ཁྲིག་མི་ནུ་བའི་སྒྲུང་གནས་སྐབས་བཀག་གིས་ཐོང་ཟེར་ཏ་ཟན་ནས་སྒྲུང་བ་འབྲེལ་ཆད་འདི་གཏན་ཀུན་ཏུ་བཀྲ་ཤིས་པའི་རྒྱུ་ གྱུར་ཅིག།། ॥

If we have no representation of the deity:

OM You who realize the wishes of all beings,
Please grant us that same accomplishment.
Even though you have gone to the Buddha's country,
We implore you to return. BEN ZRA MU

(Recite only one of the two preceding prayers.)

I as the deity melt into light, which is absorbed into the HRIH in the heart.
This vanishes into the domain of clear light beyond all intellectualization.
Then I clearly appear as the Great Compassionate One, with one face and two arms.
Through this virtue, may I quickly achieve the realization of Mighty Chenrezig,
And may I bring every single being to that same state.

Thus one further concludes by saying the "Resolve to Practice Excellence" and then some good-omen prayers. The best time to practice is on the full moon of the fourth month of the lunar calendar, and on the four special anniversary days of the Buddha or on the eighth day of the lunar calendar, or on the full and new moon days. Make sure that the fasting day will be on an auspicious day.

Do the actual practice from beginning to end three times a day on both days. On the third day, except for the eight-precepts vow, do the entire practice once. In this way, one perfect Nyungne practice could shut the door to the three lower realms once and for all. In addition to that, many great benefits have been described. One should learn about those benefits from other sources.

This text is written for those ordinary beings who are not capable of practicing an extensive form of Nyungne practice and for this reason, from the main practice texts, I have included all the important aspects of the practice and have made this brief and clear text. At the time of Atir May Sho Ree Nyungne practice, I, Tashi Ozer, composed this text.

May it benefit all beings and bring auspiciousness to everyone.

Additional Prayers

ཁ་བསྔོ་བ་སྨོན་ལམ་ནི།

Dedication of Merit

བསོད་ནམས་འདི་ཡིས་ཐམས་ཅད་གཟིགས་པ་ཉིད།

SOE NAM DI YI T'AM CHE ZIG PA NYIE

By this merit may I attain omniscience.

སྐྱེ་རྒ་ན་འཆི་བ་རླབས་འཁྲུགས་པ་ཡི།

KYE GA NA CH'I BA LAB TR'UK PA YI

From the stormy waves of birth,
old age, illness, and death,

འཇམ་དཔལ་དཔའ་བོས་ཇི་ལྟར་མཁྱེན་པ་དང་།

JAM PAL PA WO JI TAR K'YEN PA DANG

Manjushri, the hero, knows how to
dedicate virtue,

དེ་དག་ཀུན་གྱི་རྗེས་སུ་བདག་སློབ་ཅིང་།

DE DAG KUN KYI JE SU DAG LOB CHING

Following the training of all
bodhisattvas,

དགེ་བ་འདི་ཡིས་སྐྱེ་བོ་ཀུན།

GE WA DI YI KYE WO KUN

By this virtue, may all beings

བསོད་ནམས་ཡེ་ཤེས་ལས་བྱུང་བ།

SOE NAM YE SHE LE JUNG WA

May they obtain the two sacred forms

ཐོབ་ནས་ཉེས་པའི་དགྲ་རྣམས་ཕམ་བྱས་ནས།

T'OB NE NYE PEI DRA NAM P'AM JE NE

May the enemy, wrong action, be overcome.

སྲིད་པའི་མཚོ་ལས་འགྲོ་བ་སྒྲོལ་བར་ཤོག

SIE PEI TS'O LE DRO WA DROL WAR SHOK

this ocean of existence, may all
beings be freed.

ཀུན་ཏུ་བཟང་པོ་དེ་ཡང་དེ་བཞིན་ཏེ།

KUN TU ZANG PO DE YANG DE SH'IN TE

as does Samantabhadra, too.

དགེ་བ་འདི་དག་ཐམས་ཅད་རབ་ཏུ་བསྔོ།

GE WA DI DAG T'AM CHE RAB TU NGO

I dedicate completely all this virtue.

བསོད་ནམས་ཡེ་ཤེས་ཚོགས་རྫོགས་ནས།

SOE NAM YE SHE TS'OK DZOK NE

complete the accumulation of merit
and wisdom.

དམ་པ་སྐུ་གཉིས་ཐོབ་པར་ཤོག

DAM PA KU NYI T'OB PAR SHOK

which arise from merit and wisdom.

།སངས་རྒྱས་སྐུ་གསུམ་བརྙེས་པའི་བྱིན་རླབས་དང་།

SANG GYE KU SUM NYE PEI JIN LAB DANG

By the blessings of having obtained the three bodies of Buddha,

།ཆོས་ཉིད་མི་འགྱུར་བདེན་པའི་བྱིན་རླབས་དང་།

CH'O NYIE MI GYUR DEN PEI JIN LAB DANG

by the blessings of the truth of unchanging dharmata,

།དགེ་འདུན་མི་ཕྱེད་འདུན་པའི་བྱིན་རླབས་ཀྱིས།

GE DUN MI CH'E DUN PEI JIN LAB KYI

By the blessings of the indestructible intentions of the sangha,

།ཇི་ལྟར་བསྔོ་བ་སྨོན་ལམ་འགྲུབ་པར་ཤོག།

JI TAR NGO WA MON LAM DRUB PAR SHOK//

may this dedication and aspiration be accomplished.

Offering Prayer (before a meal)

༄༅། སྟོན་པ་བླ་མེད་སངས་རྒྱས་རིན་པོ་ཆེ་

TON PA LA ME SANG GYE RIN PO CH'E

The Supreme Director is the precious Buddha.

སྐྱོབ་པ་བླ་མེད་དམ་ཆོས་རིན་པོ་ཆེ།

KYOB PA LA ME DAM CH'O RIN PO CH'E

The Supreme Protector is the precious Dharma.

འདྲེན་པ་བླ་མེད་དགེ་འདུན་རིན་པོ་ཆེ།

DEN PA LA ME GE DUN RIN PO CH'E

The Supreme Leader is the precious Sangha.

སྐྱབས་གནས་དཀོན་མཆོག་གསུམ་ལ་མཆོད་པ་འབུལ།

KYAB NE KON CH'OG SUM LA CH'OE PA BUL

To the Three Rare Precious Jewels, I make this offering.

ཇོ་བོ་སྐྱོན་གྱིས་མ་གོས་སྐུ་མདོག་དཀར།

JO WO KYON GYI MA GO KU DOG KAR

Lord with white body not veiled by fault,

རྫོགས་སངས་རྒྱས་ཀྱི་དབུ་ལ་རྒྱན།

DZOK SANG GYE KYI U LA GYEN

Whose head is adorned by a perfect buddha,

ཐུགས་རྗེ་ཅན་གྱི་འགྲོ་ལ་གཟིགས།

T'UK JE CHEN GYI DRO LA ZIG

Who looks upon all beings with the Eyes of Compassion,

སྤྱན་རས་གཟིགས་ལ་མཆོད་པ་འབུལ།

CHEN RE ZIG LA CH'OE PA BUL

To you, Chenrezig, I make this offering.

Printed in the United States
by Baker & Taylor Publisher Services